Group Care Practice
with Children
and Young People Revisited

Group Care Practice with Children and Young People Revisited has been co-published simultaneously as *Child & Youth Services*, Volume 27, Numbers 1/2 2005, and Volume 28, Numbers 1/2 2006.

Group Care Practice with Children and Young People Revisited

Leon C. Fulcher
Frank Ainsworth
Editors

Group Care Practice with Children and Young People Revisited has been co-published simultaneously as *Child & Youth Services*, Volume 27, Numbers 1/2 2005, and Volume 28, Numbers 1/2 2006.

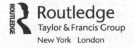

Routledge
Taylor & Francis Group
New York   London

First published by The Haworth Press, Inc.

10 Alice Street, Binghamton, N Y 13904-1580

This edition published 2012 by Routledge:

Routledge
Taylor & Francis Group
711 Third Avenue
New York, NY 10017

Routledge
Taylor & Francis Group
2 Park Square, Milton Park
Abingdon, Oxon OX14 4RN

Group Care Practice with Children and Young People Revisited has been co-published simultaneously as *Child & Youth Services,* Volume 27, Numbers 1/2 2005, and Volume 28, Numbers 1/2 2006.

The development, preparation, and publication of this work has been undertaken with great care. However, the publisher, employees, editors, and agents of The Haworth Press and all imprints of The Haworth Press, Inc., including The Haworth Medical Press® and Pharmaceutical Products Press®, are not responsible for any errors contained herein or for consequences that may ensue from use of materials or information contained in this work. With regard to case studies, identities and circumstances of individuals discussed herein have been changed to protect confidentiality. Any resemblance to actual persons, living or dead, is entirely coincidental.

The Haworth Press is committed to the dissemination of ideas and information according to the highest standards of intellectual freedom and the free exchange of ideas. Statements made and opinions expressed in this publication do not necessarily reflect the views of the Publisher, Directors, management, or staff of The Haworth Press, Inc., or an endorsement by them.

Cover design by Marylouise E. Doyle

Library of Congress Cataloging-in-Publication Data

Group care practice with children and young people revisited / Leon C. Fulcher, Frank Ainsworth, editors,
    p. cm.
    "Group Practice with Children and Young People Revisited has been co-published simultaneously as Child & Youth Services Volumes 27, Numbers 1/2 2005 and 28, Numbers 1/2 2006."
    Includes bibliographical references and index.
    ISBN-13: 978-0-7890-3279-9 (hard cover : alk. paper)
    ISBN-10: 0-7890-3279-1 (hard cover : alk. paper)
    ISBN-13: 978-0-7890-3280-5 (soft cover : alk. paper)
    ISBN-10: 0-7890-3280-5 (soft cover : alk. paper)
I. Social work with children. 2. Social work with youth. 3. Children-Institutional care.
4. Youth-Institutional care. I. Fulcher, Leon C. II. Ainsworth, Frank. III. Child & youth services.

HV713.G765 2006
362.7-dc22
                                         2005035636

Group Care Practice
with Children
and Young People Revisited

CONTENTS

ABOUT THE EDITORS

Leon C. Fulcher, PhD, is an international Child & Youth Care Consultant with experience in the USA, Canada, the United Kingdom and Ireland, New Zealand, Malaysia, China, and the United Arab Emirates. He is presently employed by the United Arab Emirates University as Assistant Provost and Dean of Students assisting with the task of making residential accommodation for 9,000 young people more student- and quality-oriented.

Frank Ainsworth, PhD, is a Senior Principal Research Fellow (Adjunct) in the School of Social Work and Community Welfare at James Cook University in Queensland, Australia. In addition he is also in private practice in Perth and Sydney as an Evaluation and Research Consultant. He has experience in the United Kingdom, USA, South Africa, and Australia.

About the Contributors

Gale E. Burford is Professor of Social Work and Director, Child Welfare Training Partnership at the University of Vermont and is an international consultant on the uses of Family Group Conferences to support family participation in decision-making about the health, well-being, and supervision of children and young people.

Stephen F. Casson has worked for nearly 40 years as a British practitioner, supervisor, manager, trainer, consultant and writer, in government, non-government and private sectors. His publications and consultancy work have focused particular attention on issues concerning teamwork and quality assurance in the delivery of child and youth care services.

Thom Garfat has been involved for 30 years in helping troubled children and their families, and the staff who work with them as a Canadian practitioner, supervisor, director, teacher, trainer, consultant and writer. He has distinguished himself as a Joint Editor of the *Journal of Relational Child and Youth Care Practice* as well as being one of the founding editors of the Child and Youth Care Network and CYC-Online, the international Internet magazine for child and youth care workers.

Martin Knapp is Professor of Social Policy, Director of the Personal Social Sciences Research Unit, and Chair of London School of Economics' Health and Social Care; and Professor of Health Economics and Director of the Centre for the Economics of Mental Health, Institute of Psychiatry, King's College London.

Mark Krueger is the Interim Dean of the School of Continuing Education at the University of Wisconsin, Milwaukee Campus. A long-established writer, scholar, practitioner, and leader in the field of child and youth care work in North America, Mark has been honoured by his profession for lifetime achievements and contributions to professional advancement of the field.

The late **Henry W. Maier** was acknowledged by many to be the leading authority in the field of his generation, and he devoted his life to mentoring, teaching, writing and encouraging the development of responsive child and youth care practices. As Emeritus Professor of Social Work at the University of Washington and a practice consultant of international renown, Henry was also the recipient of an Outstanding Achievement Award by his alma mater, the University of Minnesota, in 2000/2001.

Martha A. Mattingly is Emeritus Professor of Psychology in Education at the University of Pittsburgh; a highly respected teacher, researcher and writer of national standing in the child and youth care field; and recipient of the Distinguished Service Award for Outstanding Contribution to the Profession of Child and Youth Care Work by the Association for Child and Youth Care Practice in 2000.

Richard W. Small is the Executive Director of the Walker Home and School, a nationally accredited, non-profit organization based in Needham, Massachusetts, that provides a range of services to 3- to 22-year-old emotionally, behaviorally, and learning disabled students and their families. Through Walker's Campus Based Programs, the Walker Trieschman Center (a division of the Child Welfare League of America), Beacon High School, Walker Partnerships, and the Institute for Equity in Schools, Walker supports children, youth, families, and the professionals around the world who serve them.

Karen D. VanderVen is Professor of Psychology in the Faculty of Education at the University of Pittsburgh, with practice experience working with both normal and exceptional children, and families, in a variety of settings, including early childhood programs, psychiatric treatment facilities, and community mental health. She is a teacher, writer and consultant of international standing and is also a past recipient of the Albert E. Trieschman Memorial Award for distinguished service to the profession of child and youth care work.

Adrian Ward is a Senior Clinical Lecturer in Social Work at the Tavistock Clinic in London and an experienced practitioner, teacher, and writer in the field of Social Work, specialising in therapeutic work with children and young people. He is currently the editor of the *International Journal of Therapeutic Communities*.

Foreword

KEYWORDS. Residential care, residential treatment, child care, group living, care environments, group care, therapeutic communities

"Seven o'clock: Wake up kitchen boy." This stark command appeared at the head of a schedule for daily life at a residential centre in South London in the late 1970s, a centre to which I was being dispatched by the employers who had funded my professional training in social work. This place operated primarily as a "remand centre" for young men awaiting trial but also as an observation and assessment centre to which young people coming into care would be admitted whilst professional reports were written on them and decisions were made about suitable further placements. None of these young people had been convicted of any offence, and some were extremely vulnerable and would have been unlikely to commit an offence, but they were all submitted to the same brutalising process. They were "pushed through" the institution with all the efficiency of a sausage machine, which was how the Principal proudly described it.

Being of a sensitive disposition, and having studied the works of Charles Dickens and William Blake as part of my undergraduate degree, I immediately recognised the message behind the opening line of this schedule and decided that I needed to know no more. I explained to the Assistant Director of Social Services that this was not my idea of supportive group care for young people. Since there was no better option on offer, I decided there and then to break my contract (despite the promise from the boss that he would end my career in social work) and soon found employment with a far more enlightened employer. I never

---

Address correspondence to: Adrian Ward, Tavistock Clinic, 120 Belsize Lane, London, UK, NW3 5BA.

[Haworth co-indexing entry note]: "Foreword." Ward, Adrian. Co-published simultaneously in *Child & Youth Services* (The Haworth Press, Inc.) Vol. 27, No. 1/2, 2005, pp. xxi-xxxi; and: *Group Care Practice with Children and Young People Revisited* (ed: Leon C. Fulcher, and Frank Ainsworth) The Haworth Press, Inc., 2006, pp. xix-xxix. Single or multiple copies of this article are available for a fee from The Haworth Document Delivery Service [1-800-HAWORTH, 9:00 a.m. - 5:00 p.m. (EST). E-mail address: docdelivery@haworthpress.com].

forgot, however, the image of the kitchen boy as a kind of unpaid house servant (probably a position of some status, in fact), or the picture which it conjured up of the regimentalised and exploitative routine for these young men.

It is astonishing to realise that the above incident must have occurred at around the time that some of the chapters in *Group Care for Children: Concept and Issues* were being written, although it feels like a remnant from a different age entirely. As several of the authors acknowledge in the reflective introductions to their chapters in this updated collection, some things have changed beyond recognition in the intervening twenty years, while others have scarcely changed at all. I will not attempt to summarise all that has happened, as the authors themselves each offer their own perceptive account of these developments, but I will nevertheless make some comments on the literature, research, and evolving practice contexts of the intervening years from my location as a British practice educator. I will begin, however, by taking the opportunity to welcome the appearance of this volume, to reflect on the influence and range of the original books, and to comment on the new collection.

The two original volumes (Ainsworth & Fulcher, 1981; Fulcher & Ainsworth, 1985) were of enormous value to students, practitioners, managers, and policy makers alike, and especially to trainers and academics, because they brought together such a wealth of material from many of the leading researchers and thinkers of the day. Many of the papers that appear in this new edition were hugely influential in their time in terms of shaping our thinking about the range and potential of group care settings and practice. Several of the other papers from those volumes that have not found their way into today's collection were of equally great value. However, I would especially like to mention Henry Maier's (1981) paper on the "Essential Components in Care and Treatment Environments" and Karen VanderVen's (1985) chapter on "Activity Programming," each of which has enduring worth in attesting to the power and significance of the everyday in group care practice. This valuing of the everyday was a distinctive theme in the original volumes, appearing in many of the chapters, including Jim Whittaker's (1981) authoritative review of the major approaches to residential treatment, and it was summed up in Frank Ainsworth's (1981) eloquent argument that "group care practitioners take as the theatre for their work the actual living situations as shared with and experienced by the child" (p. 234). I think what made this such a significant phrase was the image, perhaps not fully developed in the text, of theatre with all its rich connotations of drama, role-performance, tragedy, comedy, and sometimes even absurdity; it also, incidentally, suggested a parallel with the "operating theatre" and associations with urgency, expertise, and the concerned care delivered by a professional team. If all the world's a stage, then certainly group care, in the Ainsworth and Fulcher formulation, represents one of the leading schools of theatre.

These volumes were not only true to the real life of everyday practice, however, they also provided the conceptual frameworks and professional contextualisation within which the whole phenomenon could be analysed, including such diverse matters as career development, research, and costing. Most of all, they established the very concept of "group care" as an inclusive term to cover both residential and day services as well as a range of related forms of provision. Until then, the concept of group care had appeared mainly in the work of Martin Wolins (1976) and one or two other writers, but these volumes proposed the case that there was enough in common between all of these activities for it to be useful and productive to consider them as aspects of the one phenomenon: "group care." As I argued some years later (Ward, 1993, 2006, in press), what the term sums up are the two central features of this practice: working in and with groups and "caring" as a professional activity. From then on, and not just in the child care sector, it became possible to think, plan, and teach much more inclusively about a whole spectrum of provisions, not only in terms of the focus of the workers in all parts of the service but also in terms of the experiences of the service users and their families.

Linking forward from those earlier volumes to the present re-visited collection, the most obvious connecting threads are in the editing and writings of Leon Fulcher and Frank Ainsworth, who have each remained both true to their original commitments and utterly authentic in their position as world scholars in this field. It has been enormously to the ultimate benefit of the young people (and their families and communities) who use group care services that such sharp but also sympathetic minds have applied themselves to this arena. It is good to discover in this new edition that the writing has lost none of its edge, and the editing is as clear and focused as ever. As one who grapples at times with both of these tasks, I salute them.

CHANGING CONTEXTS, EVOLVING PRACTICE

Times do change, though, and however valuable the original texts, they were bound to need updating for a new publication. This volume selects nearly a dozen of the earlier papers and re-presents them for to-day's audience, topped and tailed by new overviews from the editors. In each chapter the authors have provided helpful commentaries on their original work and discussion on the changes of the intervening years. The new collection thus remains just as sharp, as true, and as timely as the previous two, and the depth and breadth of coverage is certainly as comprehensive. I will not discuss each chapter in turn, since Chapter 1 includes just such a discussion, but I will add my thoughts on the overall picture. I must emphasize, however, that the following comments are written largely from a European (and UK-based) perspective rather from than a fully global one, although I do suspect they will find their echoes across the other continents.

In their new opening chapter Ainsworth and Fulcher helpfully identify some of the factors that have "reshaped the field of group care" (p. 8), principally in terms of six separate but linked social policy imperatives, including normalisation and de-institutionalisation. They argue convincingly that group care practice has been influenced by the interacting effect of these other factors such as the advent of the perma-nency planning, family preservation, and family reunification move-ments. To this list might be added a number of other factors which I will not have space to develop fully but which ought to be mentioned.

There is firstly the whole "marketisation of welfare" which has been intended to address supposed flaws in public welfare by exposing it to the full blast of commercial competition and private enterprise. Although implemented in differing ways throughout the Western world, this policy shift has had some unfortunate consequences. In the UK, for example, the child care field has experienced a huge expansion in the pri-vate sector, sometimes backed by investment from large venture capital funds, with all the predictable risks of the distortion of value-systems and the exploitation of the social needs of vulnerable groups for profit (Toynbee, 2005). More broadly, it is being increasingly recognised that there are considerable problems in using a market approach to welfare provision (Kendall, 2001; Le Grand, 1997), although the full impact of this approach in the child care sector has perhaps not yet been fully under-stood (Kirkpatrick, Kitchener, and Whipp, 2001).

Secondly, there has been the huge decline in the use of residential fa-cilities, not just in the UK but across the world, to the point that some administrations have tried to dispense with it altogether, although some-times just with the effect of shifting children from one category of resi-dential care to another (Cliffe & Berridge, 1991). This decline has been partly due to perceptions about costs (probably based on calculations simplistic, in contrast to Martin Knapp's comprehensive analysis) but also based on reaction against the perceived risks of residential care in the wake of an awful catalogue of abuse of children by care workers and others. This terrible history of abuse, to which Leon Fulcher makes powerful reference in the "Blues" section of Chapter 2, has in some cases almost destroyed the belief that residential care can ever be good for children (Corby, Doig, & Roberts, 2001), although there nevertheless remains firm evidence that residential care is viewed by many young people as a positive and even preferred alternative (Berridge, 2002).

Thirdly, and doubtless influenced by the anxieties generated by the history of abuse, there has been the growth of a culture of regulation and inspection that has sometimes felt oppressive and restrictive for practitioners. In the UK, at least, this development has led to a situation in which many young workers are guided far more by official regulation than they are by professional education or training, to which they have extremely limited access. While there can be no doubt that the increased regulatory framework was necessary or that it has improved some aspects of practice (Stuart & Baines, 2004), it can also be profoundly inhibiting of creativity and of the capacity for critically reflective engagement which is the hallmark of professional practice. Nevertheless good residential practice does continue to thrive and will be greatly supported by the present volume.

Fourthly and with greater optimism, I would mention the evolution of a growing spectrum of day-services for children, young people, and their families, including family centres, pre-school centres, drop-in, and other resources for young people on the street or misusing substances. While a few of these resources have emerged as direct replacements for residential units, most have evolved because of a recognition (sometimes implicit rather than explicit) of the "added value" offered by such typical group care elements as informal social interaction over shared mealtimes and peer support between those otherwise identified only as service-*users*. The enormous developing potential of what has been called "centre-based practice" has been recognised at a truly international level, with an emphasis on ecological practice (Warren-Adamson, 2001) that finds direct echoes in the present volume, and there would be much to be gained from further exchange of practice models between these various models.

I would also draw attention to the continuing growth in many countries of the "service-user movement" in which the voices of those using group care services have the opportunity not merely to make evaluative comment but in many cases also to contribute actively to the planning and redesign of both policy and practice. This is happening at both local and national levels and is often reflected in the programmes of national and international conferences in this field, for example, those hosted at the Scottish Institute for Residential Child Care (www.sircc.strath.ac. uk), which is itself worthy of mention as an international reference point for positive developments in group care for children. In parallel with the growth of the service-user movement has been the important development of the role of Children's Commissioners in several nations and the growing impact and implementation of the UN Convention on the Rights of the Child.

There is plenty more to be said on these and other developments in policy and practice over the last twenty years, and I do not mean to suggest that the present volume is lacking in this respect–rather that the wisdom of these collected papers remains vital for a proper analysis of these continually changing environments. In the next section I will suggest some further themes from the literature and offer the reader some signposts towards further information and discussion.

UNFOLDING KNOWLEDGE AND IDEAS

Just as practice and policy have evolved, so the group care literature has developed enormously over the last twenty years, both in terms of theory and of research. Again, it will not be appropriate here to attempt a full literature review, but it may be helpful to recognise some of the landmarks of these two decades, especially in the British and European context. Those wanting fuller reviews of the research, especially on residential care and treatment, would do well to consult the work of Bullock (1993) and colleagues and the overview of a series of studies in the UK funded by the Department of Health (1998). These reviews in turn are summarised and discussed by David Berridge (2002), who is one of the leading child care researchers in the UK and whose own contribution to research in various aspects of residential and foster care for children has been of great value (see, for example, Barter, Renold, Berridge, & Cawison, 2004).

Especially influential among the UK research studies have been the work of Sinclair and Gibbs (1998), who studied 48 children's homes and explored the influence on outcomes for children of a large number of factors, and of Whitaker, Archer, and Hicks (1998) who looked in depth at the work of group care practitioners in children's homes. The major development in research in this field over the last twenty years has been the growth of evidence-based practice and, in particular, the recognition of the need for outcomes studies, looking not only at short-term evaluations but also at longer-term outcomes of group care experience. This is a complex and challenging task, however, since it is very difficult to trace and prove causal connections between particular inputs and specific outcomes. One especially promising study in the field was by Brown, Bullock, Hobson, and Little (1998), who studied the structure and culture of homes and their impact on the experiences of young people.

One impact of the growth of evidence-based practice may be the closer collaboration between researchers and practice-theorists, since in order to find out "what works?" we firstly need to know "what happens?" In other words, we need more detailed description and analysis of the experience of group care from every viewpoint. A striking example of such a study may be found in the work of Jim Anglin (2002) whose study, *Pain, Normality, and the Struggle for Congruence*, draws explicit lessons for the delivery and organisation of practice from an in-depth analysis of everyday life and practice in a small number of children's homes. Overall, however, it can be argued that there remains a significant gap between the respective writings of the researchers and the practice-theorists, with insufficient cross-referencing between the two groups. Among the few who have bridged this gap are Malcolm Hill (Chakrabarti & Hill, 2000) and Frank Ainsworth in the present volume, both exploring the dynamics of family and kinship links.

Moving to the contributions to theory-for-practice in the English-language literature on residential care, I would draw attention to the contributions of John Burton (1993, 1998), who writes in a highly accessible style and with courage and conviction based on his own extensive practice experience. I would also mention the work of Roger Clough (2000), who co-edited a valuable analysis on the theme of "Groups and Groupings" in both residential and day centres (Brown & Clough, 1989). Each of these writers is strong in their discussion of the value-base for practice, a theme which has often been under-developed in the practice literature, although Stanley and Reed (1999) offer a broad analysis of "principled practice in health and social care institutions," and Leon Fulcher's own contribution in the present volume builds on his work in previous papers. Other useful volumes include Frost, Mills, and Stein's (1999) analysis of residential care in terms of empowerment, Jim Rose's (2002) account of working with young people in secure accommodation, and Crimmens and Pitts (2000) on "Positive Residential Practice." There have been a number of collections on aspects of residential treatment (e.g., Hardwick & Woodhead, 1999; Ward, Kasinski, Pooley & Worthington, 2003) and family centres (McMahon & Ward, 2001), and several European volumes (e.g., Colton, Hellicks, Ghesquiere & Williams, 1995; Eriksson & Tjelflaat, 2004), although generally there remains more work on residential care *per se* than on either day care services or on group care as a whole.

There has been a gradual growth in the influence of the European model of social pedagogy, which takes a truly integrated approach to the broad task of "bringing up children" (Petrie, 2002), and offers especially valuable models of integrated professional training for staff, although the whole question of professional training for group care personnel remains a matter of great concern (Residential Forum, 1998). It is interesting to observe that, as this volume appears, the UK government is attempting radical changes towards the integration of its provision for child health, welfare, and education with the aim of taking a more holistic approach to both preventative and interventive practices. It remains to be seen whether these changes will have the intended positive impact on children's lives.

Lastly, it seems important to recognise the increasing levels of international communication and understanding on themes of group care for children and youth. Compared to the mid-eighties, there is now far greater possibility for international exchange of ideas and concerns about practice, especially through e-mail and Internet communication. The possibilities of such methods are still only emerging, but it is particularly striking that on networks such as CYC-Net (www.cyc-net.com), there are daily and ongoing exchanges between practitioners, researchers, and teachers at all levels of experience and knowledge in a way that would have been inconceivable twenty years ago. Such discussions often serve to remind us that there remain huge areas of work to be done in terms of producing accessible theory for practice and in researching current policy and practice. We still know little about the connections between process and outcome in this field, and although the challenges are immense, even small progress proves invaluable. There are other networks that enable young people in the care system to talk with each other and compare notes about their experiences, and it is to be hoped that the influence of the service-user movement will lead to an increase in such resources.

RETURN TO THE FUTURE

Finally, I want to close by suggesting that there has been genuine progress in practice over these twenty years. I recently visited a small local children's residential facility that caters to young children who have been seriously traumatised by abusive experiences and helps them gradually towards regaining hope and faith in themselves and in the world, ultimately restoring them either to their birth family, if appropriate, or to foster care. In contrast to the harsh regime with which I opened this foreword, here I learned that the day opens with the children bringing their blankets and covers through into a shared quiet room, where they sit and chat together with their carers over a warm drink, gathering informal strength and support from each other before facing whatever the new day will bring. It is a picture of both peace and optimism, especially knowing the ghosts and anxieties with which such children grapple every day, and it confirms to me that the best quality group care is still alive, well, and thriving in the twenty-first century. I commend this volume, *Group Care Practice with Children and Young People Revisited*, to you as a splendid companion to practice and a genuine aid to the deeper understanding which needs to underpin our thinking about all the many dimensions of group care for children.

Adrian Ward

REFERENCES

Ainsworth, F. (1981). The training of personnel for group care with children. In F. Ainsworth, & L. C. Fulcher (Eds.), *Group care for children: Concept and issues.* London: Tavistock.

Ainsworth, F., & Fulcher, C. (Ed.). (1981). *Group care for children. Concept and issues.* London: Tavistock.

Anglin, J. (2002). *Pain, normality and the struggle for congruence: Reinterpreting residential care for children and youth.* New York: The Haworth Press, Inc.

Barter, C., Renold, E., Berridge, D., & Cawsion, P. (2004). *Peer violence in children's residential care.* Basingstoke, England: Palgrave Macmillan.

Berridge D. (2002). Residential care. In D. McNeish, T. Newman, & H. Roberts. (Eds.), *What works for children? Effective services for children and families.* Buckingham: Open University Press.

Brown, A., & Clough, R. (1989). *Groups and groupings: Life and work in day and residential centres.* London: Tavistock/Routledge.

Brown, E., Bullock, R., Hobson, C., & Little, M. (1998). *Making residential care work: Structure and culture in children's homes.* Aldershot: Ashgate.

Bullock, R., Little, M., & Millham, S. (1993). *Residential care for children: A review of the research.* London: HMSO.

Burton, J. (1993). *The handbook of residential care.* London: Routledge.

Burton, J. (1998). *Managing residential care.* London: Routledge.

Chakrabarti, M., & Hill, M. (Ed.). (2000). *Residential child care: International perspectives on links with families and peers.* London: Jessica Kingsley.

Cliffe, D., & Berridge, D. (1991). *Closing children's homes: An end to residential care?* London: National Children's Bureau.

Clough, R. (2000). *The practice of residential work.* Basingstoke, England: Macmillan.

Colton, M., Hellicks, W., Ghesquiere, P., & Williams, M. (Eds.). (1995). *The art and science of child care. Research, policy and practice in the European union.* Aldershot: Arena.

Corby, B., Doig, A., & Roberts, V. (2001). *Public inquiries into abuse of children in residential child care.* London: Jessica Kingsley Publishers.

Crimmens, D., & Pitts, J. (Eds.). (2000). *Positive residential practice. Learning the lessons of the '90s.* Lyme Regis, England: Russell House Publishing.

Department of Health, U.K. (1998). *Caring for children away from home.* Chichester, England: Wiley.

Eriksson H. G., & Tjelflaat, T. (Ed.). (2004). *Residential care. Horizons for the new century.* Aldershot, England: Ashgate.

Frost, N., Mills, S. A., & Stein, M. *Understanding residential child care.* Aldershot, England: Ashgate.

Fulcher, L. C., & Ainsworth, F. (Ed.). (1985). *Group care practice with children.* London: Tavistock.

Hardwick, A., & Woodhead, J. (Ed.). (1999). *Loving, hating and survival. A handbook for all who work with troubled children and young people.* Aldershot, England: Ashgate.

Hill, M. (2000). Inclusiveness in residential child care. In M. Chakrabarti, & M. Hill (Eds.), *Residential child care: International perspectives on links with families and peers* (pp. 31-66). London: Jessica Kingsley.

Kendall, J. (2001). Of knights, knaves, and merchants: The case of residential care for older people in England in the late 1990s. *Social Policy and Administration, 35*(4), 360-375.

Kirkpatrick, I., Kitchener, M., & Whipp, R. (2001). "Out of sight, out of mind:" Assessing the impact of markets for children's residential care. *Public Administration, 79*(1), 49-71.

Le Grand, J. (1997). Knights, knaves, or pawns? Human behaviour and social policy. *Journal of Social Policy, 26*(2), 149-169.

Little, M. (2000). Understanding the research. In A. Hardwick & J. Woodhead (Eds.), *Loving, hating and survival: A handbook for all who work with troubled children and young people* (pp. 95-107). Ashgate: Arena.

Maier, H. W. (1981). Essential components in care and treatment environments for children. In F. Ainsworth & L. C. Fulcher (Eds.), *Group care for children. Concept and issues.* London: Tavistock.

McMahon, L., & Ward, A. (2001). *Helping families in family centres: Towards therapeutic practice.* London: Jessica Kingsley Publishers.

Petrie, P. (2003). Coming to terms with pedagogy. Re-conceptualising work with children. In B. Littlechild & K. Lyons (Eds.), *Locating the occupational space for social work: International perspectives.* Birmingham: BASW/Venture Press.

Residential Forum. (1998). *A golden opportunity?* London: NISW.

Rose, J. (2002). *Working with young people in secure accommodation.* Hove, England: Brunner-Routledge.

Sinclair, I., & Gibbs, I. (1998). *Children's homes. A study in diversity.* Chichester, England: Wiley.

Stanley, D., & Reed, J. (1999). *Opening up care. Achieving principled practice in health and social care institutions.* London: Arnold.

Stuart, M., & Baines, C. (2004). *Progress on safeguards for children living away from home: A review of action since the people like us report.* London: Joseph Rowntree Foundation.

Toynbee, P. (2005, January 28th). Pity the little goldmines. *The Guardian.* Downloaded from *http://politics.guardian.co.uk/columnist/story/0,9321,1400463,00.html*

VanderVen, K. (1985). Activity programming: Its developmental and therapeutic role in group care. In L. C. Fulcher, & F. Ainsworth (Eds.), *Group care practice with children.* London: Tavistock.

Ward, A. (1993 & 2006, in press). *Working in group care. Social work in residential and day care settings.* Birmingham, England: Venture Press. New edition due 2006, Policy Press, Bristol.

Ward, A., Kasinski, K., Pooley, J., & Worthington, A. (Eds.). (2003). *Therapeutic communities for children and young people.* London: Jessica Kingsley.

Warren-Adamson, C. (Ed.). (2001). *Family centres and their international role in social action. Social work as informal education.* Aldershot, Education: Ashgate.

Whitaker, D., Archer, L., & Hicks, L. (1998). *Working in children's homes: Challenges and complexities.* Chichester, England: Wiley.

Whitaker, J. (1981). Major approaches to residential treatment. In F. Ainsworth & L. C. Fulcher (Eds.), *Group care for children: Concept and issues.* London: Tavistock.

Wolins, M. (Ed.). (1976). *Successful group care.* Chicago: Aldine.

Preface

KEYWORDS. Group care, residential care, residential treatment

For many of us *Group Care for Children* (1981) and *Group Care Practice with Children* (1985) were published at a time in our professional careers when we were shaping our views of the field. These volumes served as a primary source of reference for our writing and thinking. The editors, Leon Fulcher and Frank Ainsworth, along with their contributors, broadened our perspectives and gave us several new ways to think about our work. So when I heard they were at it again, I was excited. I wanted the new volume sooner rather than later so I could read the collection of chapters that I knew would play a major role in defining our field in the 21st century.

Since publication of the first two volumes, many changes have occurred. In the U.S., for example, we have moved through an era in which many of the trends and policies described in the first two volumes have taken hold such as normalization, deinstitutionalization, use of less restrictive environments, mainstreaming, permanency planning, and accountability. Many group care organizations have been restructured into multifaceted agencies with continuums of services ranging from less restrictive family support and case management services to the more restrictive patterns of group care. Members of organizations and communities are now trying to collaborate and place children, young people, and families with the proper services in the continuum of care at the proper time and to be flexible in moving back and forth from least to most restrictive programs as required, based on need.

Address correspondence to: Mark Krueger, Youthwork Learning Center, University of Wisconsin-Milwaukee, 161 West Wisconsin Avenue, Milwaukee, WI 53202.

[Haworth co-indexing entry note]: "Preface." Krueger, Mark. Co-published simultaneously in *Child & Youth Services* (The Haworth Press, Inc.) Vol. 27, No. 1/2, 2005, pp. xxxiii-xxxiv; and: *Group Care Practice with Children and Young People Revisited* (ed: Leon C. Fulcher, and Frank Ainsworth) The Haworth Press, Inc., 2006, pp. xxxi-xxxii. Single or multiple copies of this article are available for a fee from The Haworth Document Delivery Service [1-800-HAWORTH, 9:00 a.m. - 5:00 p.m. (EST). E-mail address: docdelivery@haworthpress.com].

Within the continuum of services, group care has been asked to do more with less. Funds have been reduced, lengths of stay have been shortened, and only the most difficult children and young people are referred to group care with the emphasis on getting them back home or into foster care as soon as possible. Group care has also been asked to help prepare a large number of young people who do not have families or permanent placements to "make it on their own" when they reach the age of eighteen and achieve legal emancipation.

While the system in general and lengths of stay have changed, many of the major challenges facing group care remain the same: to create opportunities for children, young people, families, kin groups, and foster parents to strengthen relationships and to make the connections and discoveries considered essential to help them succeed and live fulfilling lives. Experience and research have taught us a great deal about how to address these challenges through reinforcing the developmental strengths and needs of children and young people. New methods for engaging and working with families have also been discovered. As part of a global group care community, we have increasingly learned and been influenced by innovations in other countries. We have also learned how to speak across the spaces of our diverse cultures and design programs that take into consideration the unique stories that each child, young person and adult brings to group care.

Yet there is still a long way to go. We need new research, approaches and policies to ensure that children and young people living in out-of-home care receive the permanence and success we all wish for them. We also need innovative ways to support, educate and compensate the people who do group care work as well as strategies to convince our governments and communities that children and young people in group care are worthy of a larger investment of resources.

For all these reasons, this is a crucial time for a new contribution that revisits organizational issues, conceptual models and best practices aimed at helping countries, communities, programs, managers and practitioners learn from each other; to garner public and political support; to improve practice; to promote staff development, to mitigate problems of misunderstanding; and to move the field forward in a positive policy direction. Like the first two volumes, *Group Care Practice with Children and Young People Revisited* is much welcomed. It will often be in our hands, used in classrooms, and referenced during planning meetings, not simply left to sit on bookshelves gathering dust.

Mark Krueger

Chapter 1

Group Care Practice
with Children Revisited

Leon C. Fulcher
Frank Ainsworth

SUMMARY. Using a comparative analysis group care for children and young people is examined as an occupational focus, as a field of study and as a domain of practice in programs that range from residential institutions to group homes and kin group foster care. Structural issues that shape the interplay between organizational dynamics and interpersonal processes are considered, as well as the ways in which group care services have evolved historically and continue to feature prominently in the health, education, justice and welfare systems of both developed and developing countries. *[Article copies available for a fee from The Haworth Document Delivery Service: 1-800-HAWORTH. E-mail address: <docdelivery@haworthpress.com> Website: <http://www.HaworthPress.com> © 2005 by The Haworth Press, Inc. All rights reserved.]*

Address correspondence to: Leon C. Fulcher, 64 Cameron Street, Dunfermline, Scotland KY12 8DP, UK.

[Haworth co-indexing entry note]: "Group Care Practice with Children Revisited." Fulcher, Leon C., and Frank Ainsworth. Co-published simultaneously in *Child & Youth Services* (The Haworth Press, Inc.) Vol. 27, No. 1/2, 2005, pp. 1-26; and: *Group Care Practice with Children and Young People Revisited* (ed: Leon C. Fulcher, and Frank Ainsworth) The Haworth Press, Inc., 2005, pp. 1-26. Single or multiple copies of this article are available for a fee from The Haworth Document Delivery Service [1-800-HAWORTH, 9:00 a.m. - 5:00 p.m. (EST). E-mail address: docdelivery@haworthpress.com].

doi:10.1300/J024v27n01_01

KEYWORDS. Group care, residential care, residential treatment, group homes, youth work, youthwork, group work, at-risk youth, deinstitutionalisation, mainstreaming, least restrictive environment

After receiving many requests for a new edition of *Group Care for Children* (Ainsworth & Fulcher, 1981) and *Group Care Practice with Children* (Fulcher & Ainsworth, 1985), originally published in the United Kingdom, we decided to develop a single volume drawing on selected materials from these publications. Interestingly, over the past two decades the term "group care" has acquired a wider currency as evidenced by the number of subsequent publications that now use this terminology (Ainsworth, 1997; Anglin, 2003; Carman & Small, 1989; Davison, 1995; Epstein & Zimmerman, 2003; Gitelson & Emery, 1989; Levy, 1993; Powell, 2000; Rossenfeld & Wasserman, 1990; Zimmerman, Epstein, Leichtman, & Leichtman, 2003).

In this new volume the aim has been to once again draw together materials from both sides of the Atlantic and draw on knowledge from Australia and New Zealand–and South Pacific island nations influenced by trans-Tasman policy and practice perspectives–as well as Indonesia and Malaysia. These perspectives have become familiar to the authors since publication of the original volumes through experiences that have confirmed the continuing relevance of the concepts and issues identified in the 1980s. Added to this are views about various developments that have influenced the field since that time. Former contributors to the original volumes were invited to reflect on developments that have taken place in their substantive fields of enquiry since publication of the original materials and to re-visit those themes still considered central to "best practice" in the field of group care. In so doing our commitment to comparative international and historical methods of enquiry has been maintained while addressing the continuing development of services for children and young people.

GROUP CARE AS A FIELD OF STUDY

By way of introduction to this new volume, the notion of group care is again set out and examined as a unique field of study. A number of devices are used in order to achieve this. First, it is noted how group care facilities are found in each of society's major resource systems: health care, education, social welfare, and criminal justice. This is achieved by highlighting the presence of comparable large institutions in each of these systems: mental hospitals in health care, boarding schools in education, orphanages and community homes in social welfare, and prisons or reformatories in criminal justice. The extent to which institutions such as these reflect the historical development of the field of group care is also acknowledged, as is the manner in which client populations in each type of institution may overlap. The presence of different types of institution in each of society's major resource systems is highlighted in Table 1.

Attention is also directed towards the emergence in each of the four resource systems of a range of smaller group living situations; these are often developed in response to criticisms of the debilitating nature of life in large institutions. These smaller group living situations are identified as residential nurseries, family group homes, peer group residences, hostels, refuges, shelters, or semi-independent group living units. Finally, it is noted how there has been the apparently simultaneous growth across all four resource systems of various types of day service provisions, each with a designated centre of activity where services are delivered to individuals through the medium of group care, as illustrated in Table 2.

Thus it is possible to delineate a composite profile of the group care field as it incorporates institutional care, residential group living, and day care services operating across all four of society's major resource systems, as shown in Figure 1.

What is excluded are community-based services such as general practice health care, community nursing, classroom teaching, clinical social work, counselling, and probation. As a result of the foregoing analysis, it is possible to delineate the field of group care.

TABLE 1. Large Institutions Across the Major Resource Systems

Health Care	Education	Social Welfare	Criminal Justice
Asylums	Day & Boarding Schools for	Orphanages	Prisons
Mental Hospitals	Normal, Maladjusted, & Emo-	Lodging Houses	Reformatories
Hospitals for the	tionally Disturbed Children	Emergency Care	Remand/Detention
Mentally Retarded	Hotels	Centres	Centres
General Hospitals	Residential Colleges	Community Homes	Training Schools
	Halls of Residence		

(Ainsworth & Fulcher, 1981, p. 4)

Group care incorporates those areas of service such as institutional care, residential group living (including–but not necessarily re-quiring–twenty-four hour, seven day-per-week care), and other community-based day services covering lesser time periods that supply a range of developmentally enhancing services for groups of consumers. The location of a service in the group care field re-sults from identifying how each type of service places emphasis on shared living and learning arrangements in a specified centre of activity. (Ainsworth & Fulcher, 1981, p. 8)

TABLE 2. Range of Day Services Across the Major Resource Systems

Health Care	Education	Social Welfare	Criminal Justice
Day Hospitals	Youth & Community	Day Care	Community Service
Day Clinics	Centres	Child Care Centres	Centres
Health Centres	Recreation & Leisure	Play Groups	Day & Project Centres
Day Nurseries	Centres	Activity Programs	Intermediate Treatment
	Day Nurseries	Intermediate Treatment	Units
	Day Schools	Units	
	Intermediate Treatment		
	Units		
	Alternative Schools		

(Ainsworth & Fucher, 1981, p. 8)

FIGURE 1. The Field of Group Care Across the Major Resource Systems

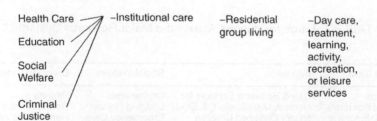

Health Care	–Institutional care	–Residential	–Day care,
Education		group living	treatment,
			learning,
Social			activity,
Welfare			recreation,
			or leisure
			services
Criminal			
Justice			

Excluded: Other community-based services such as general practice health care, community nursing, classroom teaching, clinical social work, counselling and probation.

(Ainsworth & Fulcher, 1981, p. 8)

In making such a statement, efforts were made to resist a superficial dichotomy that has prevailed in the human services where institutional care is located at one end of the continuum of care with day services located at the other extreme (Jones & Fowles, 1984). Such a dichotomy between institutional and community-based services is resisted since it is based primarily on a social policy perspective and fails to acknowledge the structural, organizational, and interpersonal processes that require stronger emphasis (Glaser & Strauss, 1967).

All forms of institutional care, residential group living, and day services operate with a group focus using the physical and social characteristics of a service centre to produce a shared life-space (Lewin, 1952; Redl, 1959) between those in receipt of care and those who provide it. By identifying the field of group care as it spans each of society's four major resource systems and by drawing attention to common characteristics of programs in this field, it is possible to identify group care as a discrete area of practice that needs to take its rightful place alongside other services offering benefits to children, young people, and their families.

THE PURPOSE OF GROUP CARE FOR CHILDREN AND YOUNG PEOPLE

Before examining the methodological basis of group care practice with children and young people, some comment is necessary about the purposes or functions of group care identified in *Group Care for Children: Concept and Issues* as "supplying a range of developmentally enhancing services for children and young people" (Ainsworth & Fulcher, 1981, p. 8). Health care, education, social welfare, and criminal justice are, of course, much broader in conception than the field of group care as defined above. In fact, each system has evolved over time in response to widely held notions of personal and societal need. It is thus worth clarifying the central notion or purpose that underpins each of the systems in question. The major purpose for health care is to treat, for education to teach, for social welfare to nurture, and for the criminal justice system to control.

Inevitably, each system embraces value preferences, organisational features, and occupational characteristics that reflect its own primary purpose or tasks. As far as group care services for children and young people are concerned, this creates a dilemma irrespective of the resource system that sponsors such services. In each instance, these functions must be woven firstly and importantly around what Maier (1979; 1981) described as the "core of care" as without such expression and care experience by the individual patient, student, client, or inmate, developmental change is unlikely to occur, and treatment, learning, development, or rehabilitation goals will not be achieved.

Yet experience has shown that such a care ethos is difficult to achieve. It is frequently compromised, since most group care centres are dominated by the single–yet simplistic–purpose that underpins the sponsor of its resource system. This results in an incomplete response to the personal and behavioural needs of children and young people who are searching for developmentally enhancing services.

Figure 2 enables one to explore some of these issues more clearly. First, it is possible to examine a largely static portrayal of the ways in which each of society's resource systems reflects a single purpose and how group care centres, sponsored by that system, are likely to emphasize a specific purpose or primary task. By including illustrations of group care services that combine more than one purpose or that seek to transcend the boundaries between systems, the intention has been to offer a more dynamic or interactive perspective, for example, residential

FIGURE 2. Resource System, Underlying Purpose, and Areas of Overlap in Group Care

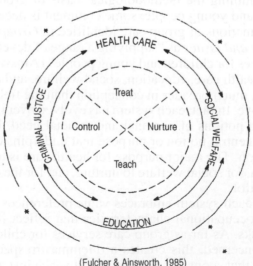

(Fulcher & Ainsworth, 1985)

treatment centres for emotionally disturbed children that provide both education and psychiatric services (i.e., social welfare, education, and health care), a children's hospital that provides schooling for long-stay patients (i.e., health care and education), or a detention centre for young offenders that offers in-house education and psychiatric services (i.e., criminal justice, education, and health care). It is worth noting, however, that centres seeking to transcend boundaries–and thereby address broader conceptions of children's developmental needs–are all too often faced with controversy.

Public debate frequently surrounds the operation of what might be called *hybrid* programs. This is the case even when a multiple focus or a blending of functions may be in the best interests of young people and their developmental progress. Having made this point, it is thus possible to proceed to a consideration of the methods or skills basis of group care practice.

GROUP CARE METHODS AND SKILLS

In Chapter 9 of *Group Care for Children*, about the training of group care personnel, Ainsworth (1981) divided practice into direct and indirect care as a way of starting to map out group care practice methods and skills. The intention of Figure 3 below is to highlight the ways in which both areas of skills have to interact in a dynamic yet ordered manner if responsive care is to be guaranteed.

Direct care involves working face-to-face with children and young people, while indirect care involves work carried out for and on behalf of children but not necessarily with them directly. Such a distinction helps to clarify the tasks carried out by different practitioners and the variety of activities that take place in any group care program. Of

FIGURE 3. Group Care Methods and Skills

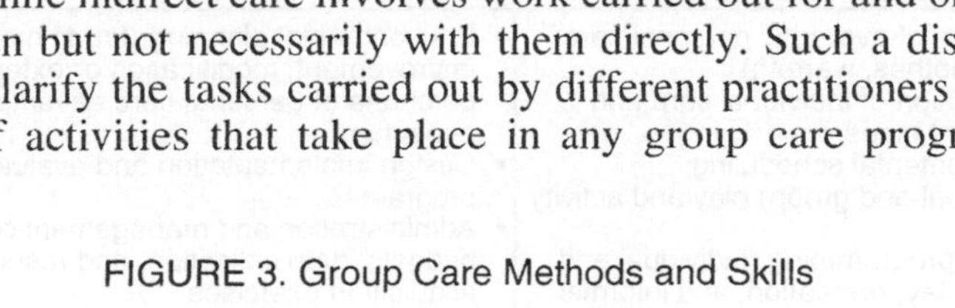

course, it is important to guard against the static picture that Figure 3 can convey, for there is no wish to reduce complex relationships to an unrealistic level of simplicity. Both direct and indirect methods and skills are important to the operational life of group care practice.

However, in order to understand these features and to converse about them in ways that might assist practitioners to use them, it is necessary to identify the component parts of each area to assist in understanding these skills and their accompanying processes as well as their relevance for work with children, young people, and their families. The material highlighted in Table 3 provides further clarification of these issues.

Now that the group care field has been delineated as it spans society's major resource systems, the underlying purpose of group care programs and the methods and skills base of good practice attention turns to an examination of factors that have reshaped the group care field since the late 1970s.

FACTORS THAT HAVE RE-SHAPED
THE FIELD OF GROUP CARE

Firstly, various social policy imperatives have impacted group care services in most Western countries. These imperatives are largely derived from six ideological tenets: normalisation, deinstitutionalisation,

TABLE 3. Group Care Methods and Skills in Direct and Indirect Care Work

Direct Care (work with children)	Indirect Care (work for/on behalf of children)
• Provision of everyday personal care (food, clothes, warmth) • Formulation of individual care and treatment plans • Developmental scheduling (individual and group) play and activity based • Activity programming (individual and group) play, recreation, and informal education • Group work (educational, activity, and therapeutic formats) • Life-space counselling (individual and group) • Program planning, unit level	• Environmental planning (fabric maintenance improvement, modification or extension and purchase of personal care essentials and equipment) • Design implementation and evaluation of unit program • Administration and management of program budgets, data collection, and resource acquisition exercises • External relations with media, local community, kindred systems, and significant others • Program leadership and team development • Selection, training, and assessment of performance of practitioners • Supervision and monitoring of practitioners' work and program achievements

(From Ainsworth, 1981, p. 240)

mainstreaming, minimal intervention, diversion, and use of the least restrictive environment. Each ideology, already impacting group care by the 1980s, was derived from work carried out primarily in the United States and Scandinavia between 1950 and 1980 in mental health, developmental disability, education, and criminal justice services (Ainsworth, 1999; Fulcher & Ainsworth, 1994). Table 4 lists these ideologies and notes their origin in particular service systems.

Each of these ideologies and related theoretical developments have had a major impact on group care services for children and young people across all of society's major resource systems during the past quarter century. Each of these ideologies is examined more closely in what follows.

Normalisation

This notion was imported into the United States through the promotional efforts of Wolfensberger (1972). From that point onwards, Wolfensberger gradually became the hero of professionals committed to services for the developmentally disabled across the Western world. The origins of his ideas about normalisation lay in attempts to reform services for developmentally disabled or mentally handicapped children (and adults) in Scandinavia during the 1960s. This policy initiative emerged in Denmark during the late 1950s (Banks-Mikkelsen, 1969) but came to impact directly on services in other Scandinavian countries (Nirje, 1969; Pedlar, 1990). Simply stated, normalisation promotes the use of

TABLE 4. Systems of Origin for Contemporary Policy and Practice Ideologies

Ideology	System
Normalisation	Developmental Disability
Deinstitutionalisation	Mental Health
	Developmental Disability
Mainstreaming	Education
Least Restrictive Environment	Education
Minimal Intervention	Criminal Justice, Especially Juvenile Justice
Diversion	Criminal Justice, Especially Juvenile Justice

(Adapted from: Ainsworth, 1999)

. . . means which are as culturally normative as possible to establish and/or maintain personal behaviours and characteristics which
are as culturally normative as possible. . . . Within this framework,
life satisfaction, self-esteem, and personal competence are viewed
as products of involvement with mainstream activities of society.
Also, participation in atypical, segregated, or specialised environments [compounded by] affiliations with other *socially devalued
persons* [have been] considered detrimental to an individual's development. (Landsman & Butterfield, 1987, p. 810)

It is difficult to disagree with the aims of normalisation when the arguments that promote it are so simple and their claims so important. It is
precisely *because* of these relatively simple truths that ardent believers
and followers were then attracted. Normalisation thus started being
used as justification for policy reforms offering rationales for reorganis-
ing health, education, social welfare, and criminal justice services in
virtually all Western economies. The normalisation *movement* was
aided by a "research instrument" that purported to measure coherence
of services for developmentally disabled people when compared against
a normalisation ideal (Wolfensberger & Glenn, 1975; Wolfensberger &
Thomas, 1983) along with a so-called *social role valorisation* theory
(Wolfensberger, 1983).

Deinstitutionalisation

From the 1930s onwards and prior to the idea of a welfare state, the
response of most Western economies to traditional social problems involved an *indoor relief* or institutional bias (Ainsworth & Fulcher,
1981; Jones & Fowles, 1984; Lerman, 1985). Such an historical preference expedited the construction of a range of traditional institutions in
most Western countries including lunatic asylums, mental hospitals,
alms houses, orphanages, children's homes, residential schools, training centres for the retarded, and institutions for wayward and delinquent
youths (Fulcher & Ainsworth, 1985).

By the late 1950s, there was growing disillusionment with institutional solutions to many of these social problems, with populations of
state mental hospitals and state schools for the mentally retarded reaching all-time highs (Hunter, Shannon, & Sambrook, 1986). Deinstitutionalisation was also promoted by studies of mental hospitals and
prisons in the U.S. and Britain undertaken in the 1950s, 1960s, and
1970s, including Barton's *Institutional Neurosis* (1959), Goffman's

Asylums (1961), Vaizey's *Scenes from Institutional Life* (1959), and Scull's (1977) *Decarceration*. All the studies generated powerful anti-institutional images and sentiments. Such sentiments–fueled through misinformed professional education–captured the hearts and minds of a generation of social welfare personnel who quickly absorbed such material and generalised the findings to all group care programs to which the word "institutional" was frequently–but wrongly–attached.

From that point onwards, all group care programs, irrespective of differences and contrary evidence (Ainsworth, 2001) have tended to be viewed as negative. And the ideals of deinstitutionalisation and developments of community-based services as the only viable alternative took on the trappings of a social movement. While aided by the introduction of psychotropic drugs (Gronfein, 1988), the more significant influence to promote deinstitutionalisation were claims that community-based services would cost less than institutional care (Scull, 1977), although this is now seen as highly debatable.

Other influences included the growth of the anti-psychiatry lobby, questions about the effectiveness of particular treatments, as well as issues relating to the guarantee of human rights for all patients and inmates (Brown, 1981). Instances of inhumane and abusive practices in a range of institutional settings helped fuel the deinstitutionalisation and community care agenda (Biklen, 1979a; Wooden, 1976). Within a remarkably short period, institutional care ceased to be the preferred intervention and became the *choice of last resort* for professional decision-makers working in health care, education, social welfare, and criminal justice services. It is interesting to note that traditional boarding schools remain the one clear exception to this pattern. These have retained a prominent place in the education of children and young people in all Western countries, providing almost exclusively for the offspring of each country's economic and political elite.

Mainstreaming

Through emphasis on culturally normative activities and the negative influence of segregated settings, the idea of normalisation also helped to promote the educational principle of mainstreaming, a policy ideal that claims all individuals are capable of learning, including those who are developmentally delayed, disabled or impaired. Mainstreaming argues that education for disabled or handicapped individuals should occur in regular community schools rather than in segregated special schools or classrooms (Connolly, 1990; Zigler & Muenchow, 1979). Community schools are expected to make special provision for such students, either within regular classrooms or, if absolutely necessary, in special education classrooms that are integrated with other regular school activities. Separation of disadvantaged students into special classes should only be used as a last resort.

Least Restrictive Environment

The idea of the "least restrictive environment" became a legal principle in the USA from the 1960s onwards (Biklen, 1979b), leading to claims that all segregated settings are too restrictive. The notion of least restrictive environment is different from mainstreaming in that it refers to the optimal environment that brings the child closest to their learning potential whilst still providing for their unique educational needs.

However, the ideal and the actuality are frequently miles apart. For example, the Education for All Handicapped Children Act of 1975 (POLE 94-142) guaranteed free, appropriate public education in the least restrictive environment for all American children. However, because of funding arrangements for local schools across the United States, massive variations continue to exist in the application of this laudable ideal. Litigation by parent and children's rights groups aimed at forcing the state to provide for excluded children became common. In Australia, mainstreaming and use of the least restrictive environment were embraced enthusiastically where segregated special education centres were reassessed as being too restrictive and handicapped children needed to be *mainstreamed* into regular classrooms. Those with behaviour problems and who could not cope with the regular classrooms were frequently excluded from the education system.

Similar developments occurred in New Zealand following introduction of the "Tomorrow's Schools" initiatives (Education Amendment Act, 1989) that placed charter obligations on all schools to make provision for children with special needs. Government argued that resources were included within the bulk funding arrangements that enabled each Board of Trustees to decide how they responded to all students enrolled at their school. So long as charter obligations were seen to be addressed, there was no government interference in the way services were provided, and intensive services for children with special needs largely disappeared. Many have argued that services for these children became more limited than at any time since the 1950s.

Minimal Intervention

Disillusionment with the American juvenile justice system became rampant in the 1950s and 1960s as many began questioning the capacity of this system to prevent delinquent children and young people from progressing to adult correctional facilities through the use of institutionally based services. High rates of recidivism, staff abuses of detained youths, and appalling conditions associated with solitary confinement (Wooden, 1976) generated serious questions about the extent to which the system had lost sight of its real mission. Institutions had become overcrowded, rigid, and custodial bureaucracies. The system as a whole was both expensive and stigmatising, and there were far too many young people being institutionalised as neglected, incorrigible, or delinquent. There were claims that delinquent behaviour was actually being reinforced in institutional settings, not reduced, so reform was inevitable and occurred dramatically in some places.

In Massachusetts, for example, all state institutions for delinquents were closed abruptly during the course of a few weeks (Scull, 1977). In New Zealand, significant policy reforms were implemented in the late 1980s in response to the Ministerial Review of a Maori Perspective for the Department of Social Welfare (1986; Department of Child, Youth and Families, 2003). In the United Kingdom, change was more gradual (Wagner, 1988) but the notion became prominent that state intervention in the lives of delinquent youths may serve only to compound the problem. Proponents of *radical non-intervention* claimed that if only adults will be patient, young people will cease being delinquent as they grew older (LeVine & Greer, 1984; Schur, 1965).

For many children and young people, such a response is appropriate. But for others, it is now known that rather than grow out of delinquent activity, some youth simply escalate their activities ensuring incarceration as in adult institutions. Unfortunately, minimal intervention became a panacea rather than a strategy to be applied selectively when appropriate.

Diversion

In a policy environment informed by normalisation, mainstreaming, and minimal intervention, it is easy to see why diversionary programs proliferated rapidly with the aim of keeping delinquent children and young people out of the system. Minimal intervention, diversion, and the use of alternatives to institutional care became required strategies

(Nelson, 1982) still popular more than two decades later. Linked as it was to the policy ideal of deinstitutionalisation, diversion can be traced to the 1967 U.S. Presidential Commission on Law Enforcement and Administration of Justice (Parbon, 1978) that urged correctional authorities to develop diversionary programs where "the prevailing assumption [was] that by placing delinquents in non-coercive organisations outside the legal area, the negative effects of labelling will be decreased" (Parbon, 1978, p. 492).

It was further argued that a consequence of such action would mean fewer juveniles would progress to adult correctional facilities. An extensive literature (e.g., Canagarayar, 1980; O'Brien, 1984; Pogrebin, Poole, & Regoli, 1984; Severy & Whitaker, 1984; Stewart & Ray, 1984) can be found that examines the variety of diversion programs introduced as the result of this 1967 policy.

In New Zealand, the Children, Young Persons, and Their Families Act (1989) gave statutory momentum to the diversion of children and young people away from institutions. While the statutory requirement of a family group conference became internationally recognised as a significant development in the delivery of child and youth services, the legislated ideal in New Zealand was dramatically eroded through fiscal limitations imposed by Treasury and a Government preoccupied with reducing public expenditure. Fiscal constraint limited the extent to which extended family members could participate in decision-making about the futures of their children. Diversion succeeded, however, in helping to reduce public expenditure on child and youth services with a

> . . . reduction in the number of residential care beds available for young people from around 1,000 beds in the late 1970s to around 100 beds by 1996 [through emphasis being placed] on family placements, kin-based care or family-like situations in the community. By the mid-1990s it became apparent that the pendulum had swung too far, and that residential capacity was no longer adequate to meet demand. . . . In April, 2002, reflecting its wish to minimise the number of young people held on remand in police cells because of inadequate residential options, Cabinet directed its Child, Youth, and Family Service to review its 1996 Residential Services Strategy. (New Zealand Child, Youth and Family Services, 1996, p. 4)

In summary, all six practice ideologies–normalisation, deinstitutionalisation, mainstreaming, use of the least restrictive environment, diversion, and minimal intervention–have featured prominently in the reform of group care services in Western communities across all of society's major resource systems. Each practice ideology has shaped the development of child and youth care services with such principles now enshrined in statutes. Normalisation and deinstitutionalization have been used to dramatically reduce the number of children and young people in institutions and, but for extreme circumstances, have limited the time that any young person can be held in an institutional placement.

Mainstreaming and use of the least restrictive environment are now key principles that shape the education of children and young people. At the same time, minimal intervention and diversion have become justifications used to support families caring for their own children without state interference. In spite of these developments, however, group care services persist and are still prominent in most Western countries, although to varying degrees, in delivering specialist services for society's most vulnerable children and young people.

It should be noted that efforts to apply these ideologies are less advanced in many non-Western countries on the African and Indian subcontinents and in the Asia-Pacific region as well as in Eastern and Central Europe. Where the physical survival of children and young people is the prime concern in countries that have experienced economic chaos, famine, and even civil war, large children's institutions often remain. Social stability and certain levels of economic growth are required before the above ideologies can flourish. Until then large children's institutions represent humanitarian responses by churches, non-government agencies, and international aid organizations to the plight of children and young people. Such initiatives reflect an approach that economic prosperity, greater understanding of child development, as noted below, and the growth of children's rights in Western countries have superseded.

OTHER INFLUENCES

In the same era that gave rise to the policy imperatives and their excesses, there were other influences that also impacted the field of group care. The theoretical writings of Bowlby (1951, 1978) and Winnicott (1965) were influential as were the remarkable Robertson films, *A Two Year Old Goes to Hospital* (1952) and *Going to Hospital with Mother* (1958), illustrating the importance of attachment theory. Both films were shot in a London children's hospital ward and day nursery that by our definition are part of the group care field. These images and writings led to a realisation that long-term placement in poor quality 24-hour group care programs could have devastating effects on young children and youth such that community-based care rather than group care often, but not always, was the appropriate placement, especially for young children. These also impacted services in health care, education, and criminal justice. In health care the pattern of parental visiting to children and youth in hospital was fundamentally altered.

Even more radically, parents were allowed to stay in hospital with their children while treatment took place. Similarly, boarding schools revised their attitudes towards parents and parental visiting. And educational services for emotionally disturbed children began to focus on day centre or clinic settings and less on residential schools. Criminal justice services began to factor in the effects of disrupted attachment relationships as potential causes for delinquent behaviour, with the result that visiting arrangements in juvenile justice centres were liberalized.

Other factors in the broader social welfare systems in Western countries that were influential in the 1980s and 1990s were the advent of the permanency planning, family preservation, and family reunification movements that fueled the decline of 24-hour living components of the group care field (Lahti, Green, Emlen, Clarkson, Quinton, & Kuehelo, 1982; Pine, Warsh, & Maluccio, 1993; Warsh, Pine, & Maluccio, 1994; Warsh, Pine, & Maluccio, 1996; Whittaker, Kinney, Tracy, & Booth, 1990) all of which are to some extent manifestations of ideologies mentioned above.

Lahti's research in Oregon (1982) rightly drew attention to children and young people who languished in group care programs through an agency's failure to search for families and kin who might provide these individuals with a permanent family placement. Similarly, the Homebuilders' model of family preservation that began in 1974 (Kinney, Haapala, Booth, & Leavitt, 1990) aimed to prevent unnecessary group care placements. This approach was buttressed through notions of the best interest of the child (Goldstein, Freud, & Solnit, 1973), drawing heavily on attachment theory (Bowlby, 1978; Howe, Brandon, Hinings, & Schofield, 1999).

Paradoxically, under the same best interest of the child banner, family reunification services (Goldstein, Freud, & Solnit, 1973; Maluccio, Pine, & Warsh, 1993; Pine, Warsh, & Maluccio, 1993) emphasised the importance of the birth family and a values perspective articulated as "the modern defense of birth family rights" (Fox-Harding, 1981). All of the above in turn led to attempts to reunify as swiftly as possible children placed in 24-hour group care programs with their families. These three movements, combined with the six social policy ideologies detailed earlier, proved to be powerful forces that reshaped the field of group care in dramatic ways.

Collectively, these ideologies, theoretical perspectives, and service developments emphasised a reduction of admissions to 24-hour group living programs, imposition of time limitations on the use of such programs, and early discharge whenever used. Not surprisingly, all these perspectives were gratefully embraced by Western economic rationalists throughout the 1980s and 1990s in searching for ways to reduce expenditure on all forms of government services, including those for children and young people (Fulcher & Ainsworth, 1994).

This alliance between ideology and economic rationalism combined to dramatically reshape health, education, social welfare, and criminal justice services, becoming powerful moral injunctions cast as social justice and human rights imperatives that impact directly on child and youth services. Not all of the above developments were entirely negative, and the application of these ideologies and theoretical perspectives on social welfare generally–and group care programs in particular–have borne much welcome fruit. For example, large children's institutions that were already in the process of decay during the 1970s no longer dot the landscape of Western towns and cities, even though they are still found in some Asia-Pacific countries and, as noted, in other developing regions.

Instead, family foster care and, increasingly, kinship care (Cuddeback, 2004; Geen, 2004; National Forum, 2004) are the dominant form of care when children cannot live with their family. There are also fewer children in 24-hour group care programs than ever before (Bath, 1994, 1997; Budde et al., 2004). Children and young people who are now placed in 24-hour group care programs are likely to be in less least restrictive settings, and many attend mainstream public schools as part of a local community.

This approach is a far cry from an earlier era when these children lived long-term on an institutional campus, ate and slept in congregate facilities, and attended an internal school with few opportunities for interaction with children not in care or with the surrounding community. For the children who require out-of-home care and whose principal needs are nurturing care, educational and other developmentally focused opportunities combined, where possible, with planned early family reunification have been positive changes.

In response, 24-hour group care programs across all systems, especially social welfare, have sought to offer more specialised services, e.g., programs for adolescent sex offenders, those that specialise in treating conduct disorders, and programs for children and young people with challenging behaviours.

Having delineated the field of group care and examined Western practice ideologies and theoretical perspectives that have impacted this field over the past half century, consideration turns to the distinct occupational focus of group care and what this means for those working in this field.

GROUP CARE AS AN OCCUPATIONAL FOCUS

It is worth noting how group care personnel in each of society's four major resource systems are assigned diverse occupational titles, and children or young people with whom they work are also labelled differently. In health care, for example, group care practitioners are usually called nurses, and the children or young people with whom they work are referred to as patients. In education, the workforce is identified as teachers and the young people with whom they work are students or pupils. Social welfare offers a greater diversity of occupational titles with group care practitioners being referred to as child and youth care workers (in North America or South Africa) or social workers (residential child care workers or social care workers in Britain and in Australia as youth workers), while children are identified as clients or residents.

Finally, occupational titles in the criminal justice system may vary widely from officer, warden, warder, guard, or correctional counsellor, while young people are referred to as detainees, prisoners, or inmates. Each occupational title assigned to workers or ascribed to the young people reflects the dominant service function found in each system be this, as noted, treatment, teaching, nurturing, or control. It is important also to note how the broad disciplinary titles like nurse, teacher, or social worker also apply to broader categories of personnel not identified as group care practitioners, since many such professionals can be found working in services outside the group care field.

A brief review of professional training orientations adopted for group care practitioners within the four resource systems also highlights how, in current training endeavours for nurses, teachers, social workers, and criminal justice personnel, scant attention is given to core issues associated with group care practice. Practice concerns associated with group composition and peer helping skills (Gibbs, Potter, & Goldstein, 1995; Vorrath & Brendtro, 1985), therapeutic crisis management (Bath, 1998), life-space counselling (Fescer & Long, 2000) and environmental characteristics of the service centre are rarely considered.

There has also been a failure to integrate training materials from the broad orientations of education, recreation, counselling, and social care. This is a matter of serious concern, since these diverse orientations underpin the methodological basis from which responsive group care practice develops. An emphasis on person-environment transactions, on the use of normal life events, and on the positive exploitation of environmental influences to support developmental processes is, of course, entirely compatible with formulations about the ecology of human development (Bronfenbrenner, 1979).

Interestingly, such an orientation also reinforces the *triggering function* that group care practitioners perform in their relations with young people. Practitioners perform this function by seeking to "set in motion or mobilize [a child's] coping capacities, natural life processes, and striving towards growth" (Maluccio, 1981, p. 22). In that respect group care practice embraces a contemporary strengths perspective (Saleebey, 1992).

GROUP CARE PRACTICE WITH CHILDREN REVISITED

This volume is divided into three main sections, each of which develops from the foregoing discussion. The first section, focusing on *Working Directly with Children, Young People and Their Families*, is introduced with a chapter by Leon Fulcher on responsive care for children and young people at home or away from home. The knowledge base that underpins child and youth care work is reexamined through the device of a musical metaphor introducing six voices that impact responsive practices with children, young people, and their families.

The *soul* of child and youth care is located in guarantees of physical safety and security and attending to bodily comforts, routines, and preferences. *Rhythms* of proactive caring build through the unique developmental patterns presented by each child or young person cared for at home or away from home. The *blues* of child and youth care are recorded in every social history and care order, presenting stark emotions about significant life events, personal pain, cultural safety, risk-taking, acting out, self-mutilation, and escape.

Richard Small and Leon Fulcher then explore relationships between group care practice and education, thinking of a child's environment as a curriculum for teaching competencies and learning outcomes important to daily living. Conscious effort is required to deal with a young person's functioning in the present so as to avoid diagnostic conclusions that emphasize difficulties in one area of their life as the cause of complex learning problems.

In Chapter 4, Frank Ainsworth explores how group care programs and their workforce can easily become hostile to families, blaming birth parents or adult care givers for the emotional pain and difficult behaviours of at-risk children and young people who populate these programs. If child and youth care workers are to successfully undertake family work, they must first move away from blaming parents and become family-centred, clarifying their roles as workers with families as essential partners in decision-making and shared care activities with their children and young people. This material extends the methods and skills repertoire of group care personnel as identified in Chapter 1.

The second section focuses on *Working Indirectly to Support Children, Young People, and Families*. In Chapter 5, Henry Maier examines the inherent strains that operate when primary care is provided in secondary settings. In this classic manuscript in the child and youth care literature, Maier explores the struggles associated with reconciling primary care requirements for children and young people living in group care programs with secondary organizational demands imposed by external agency expectations and administrative requirements, a struggle that finds its expression and potential balance in the daily work of staff.

In Chapter 6, Stephen Casson explores the importance of a shared language and practice in any group care centre. In addressing the issue of program planning at unit level, this chapter outlines an action planning approach to practice which should be of particular interest to managers and team leaders as well as group care teams working in the social welfare and social services sector.

In Chapter 7, the authors explore the culture of group care further, drawing attention to the developmental conditions provided by a centre, issues of organizational design, the physical environment, team functioning, and the importance of group development along with personal development for each young person in the centre. In Chapter 8, Gale Burford and Leon Fulcher explore the extent to which resident group composition influences the overall functioning of group care teams. Reporting on practice research carried out in the 1980s, this material is still unique for its research design and its confirmation of practice wisdom suggesting that different types of residents influence group care workers and teamwork in very significant ways.

The final section is concerned with *Organisational Influences on Practice*. In Chapter 9, Martha Mattingly reassesses the importance of managing occupational stresses in group care practice. While the personal and professional well-being of practitioners has long been addressed in the training and supervision of human service workers, serious efforts to identify problems confronting these workers and potential consequences for both staff and residents are comparatively recent. This classic contribution to the literature highlights ways in which child and youth care has provided leadership in the management of occupational stress in direct service activities with children and young people.

In Chapter 10, Karen VanderVen re-examines patterns of career development in the field of child and youth care, highlighting roles that involve working directly with children in specific settings as well as roles that involve working indirectly in support of children through working with other adults such as parents, other caregivers, or professionals. Other child and youth care career roles involve working in support of human service systems that impact the care of children and young people to influence family welfare or, working at the macro-level, to promote caring communities that support the health and well-being of children. Each career role presents important challenges and offers valuable opportunities for influencing the lives of children, young people, and their families.

Finally, in Chapter 11, Martin Knapp re-examines economic influences that have significantly impacted the provision of group care services for children, young people, and their families in communities around the world. The dynamic of cost has reshaped both the nature as well as the provision of group care services, transforming the nature of caring services offered in local communities. In a reappraisal of themes identified in his seminal contribution more than two decades ago, this leading authority looks back at key themes impacting on the economics of social care that shape group care services.

In conclusion, we return to the question of challenges facing the future of group care services for children, young people, and their families at the start of the 21st century. Attention is drawn to themes thought likely to influence the continuing development of group care in the decade ahead. Evidence-based practice and outcomes research are highlighted for their significant contributions that impact on the future provision of culturally appropriate, responsive, community and family-oriented services. As with our two earlier volumes, this volume is not intended to provide a total statement about group care practice with children and young people. Rather, it gathers together current thinking from both sides of the Atlantic, as well as from the Asia-Pacific region, and addresses a number of practice concerns that confront workers in this field.

In this respect, it is hoped that the volume will contribute to an expanding literature to enhance understanding of group care practice and promote interest in the positive contributions that services in this field can offer children and families in the decades ahead.

REFERENCES

Ainsworth, F. (1981). The training of personnel for group care with children. In F. Ainsworth & L. C. Fulcher (Eds.), *Group care for children: Concept and issues* (pp. 225-244). London: Tavistock.

Ainsworth, F. (1985). Residential programs for children and youth: An exercise in reframing. *British Journal of Social Work, 15*, 145-154.

Ainsworth, F. (1997). *Family centered group care: Model building.* Aldershot, Hampshire: Ashgate Publishing.

Ainsworth, F. (1999). Social injustice for "at risk" adolescents and their families. *Children Australia, 24, 1*, 14-18.

Ainsworth, F. (2001). After ideology: The effectiveness of residential programs for "at risk" adolescents. *Children Australia, 26*, 11-18.

Ainsworth, F., & Fulcher, L. C. (Eds.). (1981). *Group care for children: Concept and issues.* London: Tavistock.

Anglin, J. P. (2003). *Pain, normality, and the struggle for congruence: Reinterpreting residential care for children and youth.* New York: The Haworth Press, Inc.

Banks-Mikkelson, N. E. (1969). A metropolitan area of Denmark, Copenhagen. In R. Krugel & W. Wolfensberger (Eds.), *Changing patterns in residential services for the mentally retarded.* Washington, DC: National Committee on Mental Retardation.

Barton, R. (1959). *Institutional neurosis.* London: Wright.

Bath H. (1994). Out-of-home care of children in Australia: A state-by-state comparison. *Children Australia, 19, 4*, 4-10.

Bath H. (1997). Recent trends in out-of-home care of children in Australia. *Children Australia, 22, 2*, 4-8.

Bath, H. (1998). *Therapeutic crisis management: Training manual.* Canberra: Marymead Child and Family Centre.

Biklen, D. (1979a). The case of deinstitutionalization. *Social Policy, 10*(1), 48-54.

Biklen, D. (1979b). The least restrictive environment: Its application in education. *Child & Youth Services*, 5(1/2), 121-144.

Bowlby, J. (1951). *Child care and the growth of love*. London: Penguin.

Bowlby, J. (1951). *Attachment and loss* (Vol. 1). London: Penguin.

Bronfenbrenner, U. (1979). *The ecology of human development*. Cambridge, MA: Harvard University Press.

Brown, P. (1981). The mental patients' rights movement and mental health institutional change. *International Journal of Human Services*, 11(4), 523-540.

Budde, S., Mayer, S., Zinn, A., Lippoid, M., Avrushin, A., Bromberg, A., George, R., & Courtney, M. (2004). *Residential care in Illinois: Trends and alternatives*. Chicago, IL: Chapin Hall Centre for Children.

Canagarayar, J. K. (1980). Diversion: A new perspective in criminal justice. *Canadian Journal of Criminology*, 22(2), 168-175.

Carman, G. D., & Small, R. W. (1989). *Permanence and family support: Changing practice in group child care*. Washington, DC: Child Welfare League of America

Child Welfare League of America. *Family reunification: A sourcebook*. Washington, DC: Author.

Children, Young Persons, and their Families Act of New Zealand. (1989).

Connolly, R. E. (1990). Public law 94-142: The Education For All Handicapped Children Act. *New England Journal of Human Services*, 9(1), 21-27.

Cuddeback, G. S. (2004). Kinship family foster care: A methodological and substantive synthesis of research. *Children and Youth Services Review*, 26, 623-639.

Davison, A. J. (1995). *Residential care: The provision of quality care in residential and educational group care*. Aldershot, Hampshire: Aldgate Publishing.

Department of Child, Youth & Family Services. (2003). *Review of the residential services strategy 1996*. Wellington, New Zealand: Government Printing Office.

Department of Social Welfare. (1986). *Puao-te-Ata-tu (Daybreak): Report of the ministerial advisory committee on a Maori perspective for the Department of Social Welfare*. Wellington, New Zealand: Government Printing Office.

Epstein, R. A., & Zimmerman, D. P. (2003). *Transitions from group care: Homeward bound*. New York: The Haworth Press, Inc.

Fescer, A. F., & Long, N. J. (2000). *Life space crisis intervention*. Hagerstown, MD: Institute for Psycho-Educational Training.

Fox-Harding, L. (1991) *Perspectives in child care policy*. London: Longman.

Fulcher, L. C., & Ainsworth, F. (Eds.). (1985). *Group care practice with children*. London: Tavistock.

Fulcher, L. C., & Ainsworth, F. (1994). Child welfare abandoned? Ideology and the economics of contemporary service reform in New Zealand. *Social Work Review*, 6(5), 2-13.

Geen, R. (2004). The evolution of kinship care policy and practice. *The Future of Children*, 14(1), 31-150.

Gibbs, J. C., Potter, G. B., & Goldstein, A. P. (1995) *The EQUIP program. Teaching youth to think and act responsibly through a peer-helping approach*. Champaign, IL: Research Press.

Gittlson, P., & Emery, L. J. (1989). *Serving HIV-infected children, youth and their families: A guide for residential group care providers*. Washington, DC: Child Welfare League of America.

Glaser, B. G., & Strauss, A. L. (1967). *The discovery of grounded theory: Strategies for qualitative research.* New York: Aldine.

Goffman, E. (1961). *Asylums.* New York: Doubleday.

Goldstein, J., Freud, A., & Solnit, A. (1973) *Beyond the best interests of the child.* New York: Free Press.

Gronfein, W. (1985). Psychotropic drugs and the origins of deinstitutionalization, *Social Problems, 32*(5), 437-454.

Howe, D., Brandon, M., Hinnings, D., & Schofield, G. (Eds.). (1999). *Attachment theory, child maltreatment and family support.* London: Macmillan.

Hunter, J. M., Shannon, G. W., & Sambrook, S. L. (1986). Rings of madness: Service areas of 19th century asylums in North America. *Social Science and Medicine, 23*(10), 1033-1050.

Jones, K., & Fowles, A. J. (1984). *Ideas on institutions: Analysing the literature on long-term care and custody.* London: Routledge & Kegan Paul.

Kinney, J., Haapala, D., Booth, C., & Leavitt, S. (1990). The Homebuilders model. In J. K. Whittaker, J. Kinney, E. M. Tracy, & C. Booth (Eds.), *Reaching high risk families: Intensive family preservation services.* New York: Aldine de Gruyter.

Lahti, J., Green, K., Emlen, A., Clarkson, J., Quinton, D., & Kuehel, M. (1982). *A follow-up study of the Oregon project.* Portland, OR: Regional Research Human Services, Portland State University.

Landesman, S., & Butterfield, E. C. (1987). Normalization and deinstitutionalization of mentally retarded individuals: Controversy and fact. *American Psychologist, 42*(8), 809-816.

Lerman, P. (1985). Deinstitutionalization and welfare policies. *Annals of the American Academy of Political and Social Science, 5,* 132-155.

LeVine, E., & Greer, M. (1984). Long-term effectiveness of the adolescent learning center: A challenge to the concept of least restrictive environment. *Adolescence 19*(75), 521-526.

Levy, Z. (1993). *Negotiating positive identity in a group care community: Reclaiming uprooted youth.* New York: The Haworth Press, Inc.

Lewin, K. (1952). *Field theory in social sciences.* London: Tavistock.

Maier, H. W. (1979). The core of care: Essential ingredients for the development of children at home or away from home. *Child Care Quarterly, 8*(3), 161-173.

Maier, H. W. (1981). Essential components in care and treatment environments for children. In F. Ainsworth & L. C. Fulcher (Eds.), *Group care for children: Concept and issues* (pp. 19-70). London: Tavistock.

Maluccio, A. N. (Ed.). (1981). *Promoting competence in clients: A new/old approach to social work practice.* New York: Free Press.

McMaster, J. M. (Ed.). (1982a). *Methods in social and educational caring.* Aldershot, England: Gower Publishing.

McMaster, J. M. (1982b). *Skills in social and educational caring.* Aldershot, England: Gower Publishing.

National Forum. (2004).

Nelson, G. (1982). Services to status offenders and delinquents under Title XX. *Social Work, 27*(4), 348-353.

New Zealand Child, Youth, and Family Services. (1996). *Review of the Residential Services Strategy.*

Nirje, B. (1969). The normalization principle–Implications and comment. *Journal of Mental Subnormality, 16*(1), 62-70.

O'Brien, D. (1984). Juvenile diversion: An issues perspective from the Atlantic provinces. *Canadian Journal of Criminology, 26*(2), 217-230.

Parbon, E. (1978). Changes in juvenile justice: Evolution or reform, *Social Work, 23*(6), 494-497.

Pedlar, A. (1990). Normalization and integration: A look at the Swedish experience. *Mental Retardation, 28*(5), 275-282.

Pine, B. A., Warsh, R., & Maluccio, A. N. (1993). (Eds.). *Together again. Family reunification from foster care.* Washington, DC: Child Welfare League of America.

Pogrebin, M. R., Poole, E. D., & Regoli, R. M. (1984). Constructing and implementing a model juvenile diversion program. *Youth and Society, 15*(3), 305-324.

Powell, J. Y. (2000). *Family-centered services in residential treatment: New approaches for group care.* New York: The Haworth Press, Inc.

Redl, F. (1959). Strategy and technique of the life space interview. *American Journal of Orthopsychiatry, 29*(I), 1-18.

Rosenfeld, A., & Wasserman, S. (1990). *Healing the heart: A therapeutic approach to disturbed children in group care.* Washington, DC: Child Welfare League of America.

Saleebey, D. (Ed.). (1992). *The strengths perspective in social work.* New York: Longman.

Schur, E. M. (1965). *Radical non-intervention: Rethinking the delinquency problem.* Englewood Cliffs, NJ: Prentice Hall.

Scull, A. (1977). *Decarceration, community treatment, and the deviant: A radical view.* Lexington, MA: Prentice-Hall.

Severy, L., & Whitaker, J. (1984). Memphis-metro youth diversion program: Final report. *Child Welfare, 63*(3), 269-299.

Stewart, M., & Ray, R. (1984). Truants and the court: A diversionary program. *Social Work in Education, 6*(3), 179-192.

Vaizey, J. (1959). *Scenes from institutional life.* London: Faber & Faber.

Vorrath, H. H., & Brendtro, L. (1985). *Positive peer culture* (2nd edition). New York: Aldine de Gruyter.

Warsh, R., Pine, B. A., & Maluccio, A. N. (1996). *Reconnecting families: A guide to strengthening family reunification services.* Washington, DC: Child Welfare League of America.

Whittaker, J. K., Kinney, J., Tracy, E. M., & Booth, C. (Eds.). (1990). *Reaching high risk families: Intensive family preservation services.* New York: Aldine de Gruyter.

Winnicott, D. (1965). *The family and individual development.* London: Tavistock Publications.

Wolfensberger, W. (1972). *Normalization: The principle of normalization in human services.* Toronto: National Institute for Medical Research.

Wolfensberger, W. (1983). Social role valorization: A proposed new term for the principle of normalization. *Mental Retardation, 21*(6), 234-239.

Wolfensberger, W., & Glenn, L. (1975). *Pass 3: Program analysis of service system: A method and qualitative evaluation of human services–Field manual.* Toronto: National Institute for Medical Research.

Wolfensberger, W., & Thomas, S. (1983). *Passing (promoting service systems' implementation of normalization criteria and ratings manual* (2nd Edition). Toronto: National Institute on Mental Retardation.

Wooden, K. (1976). *Weeping in the playtime of others*. New York: McGraw-Hill.

Zigler, E., & Muenchow, S. (1979) Mainstreaming: The proof is in the implementation. *American Psychologist, 34*(10), 993-996.

Zimmerman, D. P., Epstein, R. A., Leichtman, M., & Leichtman, M. L. (2003). *Psychotherapy in group care: Making life good enough*. New York: The Haworth Press, Inc.

SECTION 1:
WORKING DIRECTLY WITH CHILDREN, YOUNG PEOPLE, AND THEIR FAMILIES

Chapter 2

The Soul, Rhythms and Blues of Responsive Child and Youth Care at Home or Away from Home

Leon C. Fulcher

SUMMARY. The knowledge base that underpins child and youth care work is re-examined through the device of musical metaphor, introducing six voices that impact on responsive practices with children, young people, and their families. The *Soul* of child and youth care is located in guarantees of physical safety and security and attending to bodily comforts, routines, and preferences. *Rhythms* of proactive caring build through the

Address correspondence to: Leon C. Fulcher, 64 Cameron Street, Dunfermline, Scotland KY12 8DP, UK.

[Haworth co-indexing entry note]: "The Soul, Rhythms and Blues of Responsive Child and Youth Care at Home or Away from Home." Fulcher, Leon C. Co-published simultaneously in *Child & Youth Services* (The Haworth Press, Inc.) Vol. 27, No. 1/2, 2005, pp. 27-50; and: *Group Care Practice with Children and Young People Revisited* (ed: Leon C. Fulcher, and Frank Ainsworth) The Haworth Press, Inc.. 2006, pp. 27-50. Single or multiple copies of this article are available for a fee from The Haworth Document Delivery Service [1-800-HAWORTH, 9:00 a.m. - 5:00 p.m. (EST). E-mail address: docdelivery@haworthpress.com].

unique developmental patterns presented by each child or young person cared for at home or away from home. The *Blues* of care are recorded in each social history and care order, highlighting stark emotions around significant life events, personal and cultural safety, risk-taking, and acting out, self-mutilation or escape. Six comparative policy themes are highlighted, voicing challenges for child and youth services over the next decade. *[Article copies available for a fee from The Haworth Document Delivery Service: 1-800-HAWORTH. E-mail address: <docdelivery@haworthpress.com> Website: <http://www.HaworthPress.com> © 2005 by The Haworth Press, Inc. All rights reserved.]*

KEYWORDS. Group care, residential care, residential treatment, group homes, youth work, youthwork, at-risk youth, family-centered care

Enter almost any family home with teenagers or group care centre, especially in Western countries, and one will almost certainly hear music. Whether blaring from MTV or an alternative television channel, from a bedroom stereo, or from a portable audio player through earphones directly into the ears of a young person moving to particular sounds, most child and youth care workers will agree that music is never far away from the lives of young people in care. And the music to which young people listen is also telling. Quite commonly, the music of youth is different from that listened to by adult carers or parents. There are also important cultural variations to the music one hears. It has been the author's experience that soul music is more commonly the sound of choice for young people of colour. Similarly, R&B (or Rhythms and Blues for the uninitiated) is more common amongst inner city youth than it is amongst suburban middle class kids. Generalisations such as these are always risky, however, since musical tastes vary from young person to young person and from one family to another. But it is the consistent awareness of music in the lives of young people that inspired the core ideas around which this chapter developed.

I use the literary device of metaphor and, in particular, a musical metaphor to review the knowledge base that underpins a responsive child and youth care service, what Garfat (1998) called effective child and youth care interventions at home or away from home. An essential requirement of responsive practice is the need to locate the perspectives of children and young people at the centre of service planning and policy formation. Such an approach challenges the traditional "expert" model that assumes an inability on the part of children, young people, and their families to participate fully in care and treatment processes. Six voices[1] are introduced that sing of different facets of child and youth care practice, each singing a different language with distinctive justifications for the care and treatment of children and young people.

The first voice belongs to the children and young people for whom children's services are developed. When listening carefully to this voice, one hears many soulful tales about life in and out of care or, indeed, in and out of schools. While lip service is given to locating the voices of children and young people at the centre of care service planning and policy formation, it is, sadly, too often the case that other voices sing louder, sometimes with unfortunate consequences.

The second voice sings through encounters with family and extended family members. This voice may articulate clear family preferences about the shared care of their children, regardless of whether family participation in the care and education of children is taken seriously.

A third voice sings the language of health, education, and welfare professionals who, frequently, introduce discordant sounds of formality and technical jargon when explaining complex diagnostic outcomes and treatment processes. Whenever the professionals come together to plan for the needs of children or young people requiring "extra" care beyond that which is readily available from families, then the voices of experts commonly sing loudest to the exclusion of others. It was precisely because of this tendency for experts to exclude families from participation in decision-making about the futures of their children that the contemporary Family Group Conference, with its legacy in Maori culture, was enshrined in New Zealand child welfare law in 1989. The policy objective was to ensure that all three voices–young persons, family members, and experts (as well as victims and community members)–are heard in formal decision-making about the care and supervision of children or young people (Fulcher, 1999).

Special interest groups, politicians, policy makers, and the media represent a fourth public voice that sings about children and young people in all parts of the world. This voice has enormous economic influence and "buying power" at local and national levels, shaping marketing strategies for children and young people nationally and internationally. This voice broadcasts via MTV images, advertising, and profiling of children and young people living in all parts of the world. The same voice is beamed daily to the world via BBC World, Deutsche Weld, or CNN. Such images contribute to the ways in which child and youth policy is frequently shaped by reactions to a death, to legal crises, national disasters, or public outrage.

A fifth voice sings through regulatory policies and procedures that shape contemporary practices in all human service organisations. This voice uses a technical language of behavioural competencies and evaluative transparency to regulate "duty of care" requirements and "minimum standards" under contract law, proscribing service mandates that license, fund, operate, and regulate child and youth care in voluntary child care organisations.

Finally, there is a voice of scholars, researchers, and theorists singing mostly from Europe and North America (Payne, 1997) but also from Africa (Bukenya, 1996), Asia, and other Southern Hemisphere countries (Yahya, 1994). For the past half-century this voice has authenticated or refuted claims to a knowledge base for responsive child and youth care practice.[2] Over the past three decades this voice of research and scholarship has, at times, argued that nothing works or that out-of-family care almost always produces negative consequences for children, young people, and their families. It is through this sixth voice that our musical metaphor develops, aimed at reframing the debate about proactive caring and responsiveness in the delivery of children's services. The reader is left to decide whether the results actually represent a radical reframing of contemporary debates or is merely the call for a conscientious return to basics.

THE SOUL OF CARE FOR CHILDREN AT HOME AND AWAY FROM HOME

Thirty years of child and youth care practice, parenting, teaching, and research experience has reaffirmed the teachings of long-time mentor and friend, Professor Henry Maier, that scholar-practitioner and professional role model for so many child and youth care workers during the past half-century. In the early 1960s, after postgraduate study at Pittsburgh and then later in London, Professor Maier (1963) set out important arguments about why child care should be considered "*a method of social work.*" Maier identified a knowledge base associated with child and adolescent development that informs a truly responsive child and youth care practice, highlighting issues central to any managed care and treatment approach. At the start of the 21st century, that knowledge base remains (Maier, 1987; Milligan, 1998), offering a legacy of child and youth care precepts that support responsive practices with children, young people and their families.

In "The Core of Care for Children at Home and Away From Home,"[3] Maier's (1979) developmental arguments showed how bodily comfort and the physical safety of each child are key performance outcomes in the delivery of responsive child and youth care services. Those arguments highlight the question, "Is this child safe now?" Proactive care provides bodily comfort and physical safety in daily practices with children and young people. This holds whether responding to an emergency or family crisis; formulating, implementing, and managing short or medium-term plans with children; or in developing care strategies that extend beyond age 18 and emancipation (Fulcher & Fulcher, 1998). Claims to responsiveness by child and youth care workers are most clearly authenticated at the *"meeting places of practice."* This is where the first three voices–those of children or young people, their family or extended family members and child welfare professionals–lay legitimate claims to being heard and to expecting their respective contributions will be taken seriously.

At the core of a responsive service sings a voice that resonates from the soul of each child or young person in care. That voice will always reflect a distinctive regional dialect and cultural history as it *raps* on through the stories, visions, joys, and fears that touch the child in all of us. The second voice sometimes sings quietly but frequently shouts from the souls of mothers, fathers, brothers, sisters, grandparents, aunts, uncles, cousins, and community members to express cultural and social preferences about the care of particular children and young people (Fox-Harding, 1991). The third voice of child welfare professionals–whether social workers, teachers or health care providers–commonly sings of expert opinions about health care status, educational performance, or other social indicators of well-being (Small & Fulcher, 1985), regardless of whether the words they sing are understood by young people and their families. Central to Professor Maier's arguments about *The Core of Care* for children at home and away from home was the recognition that *while each child may be expected to achieve developmental milestones in terms of physical, cognitive, emotional, and social development, each is still different in its own special way.* Such differences contribute to the soul of child and youth care practice whether at home or in foster homes, residential schools, care centres, or institutions. Whether adapting to an abusive home environment or living rough in the jungle using squeaks for language, children and young people still go to enormous lengths to get their physical and bodily comfort needs met.

Each young person follows his or her own personal rhythms with respect to hunger, toileting, personal space, dress, cold and warmth, sleep, susceptibility to illness, moods, and habits. It follows, as Maier argued (1981, 1992), that each child needs his or her own unique rhythms of caring to promote cultural safety, cognitive and emotional development, learning, social maturation, and enhanced personal well-being. Such rhythms connect with the soul of responsive child and youth care practices. It is through engaging proactively in rhythms of caring with particular children or young people–whether through nurturing care, teaching, therapeutic interventions, or behavioural supervision and controls–that child and youth care gains professional and public endorsement for responsiveness and for the service outcomes produced (Ainsworth & Fulcher, 1981; Fulcher & Ainsworth, 1985).

Summary

The Soul of child and youth care practice is directly linked to the daily management and oversight of basic bodily comforts and personal safety needs for children and young people living at home and away from home. Because of developmental needs for physical safety and security, some children or young people live temporarily in out-of-home placements while life plans are being reshaped and implemented. Second, the Soul of responsive child and youth care is touched through engaging with the unique character of each child or young person receiving care. No matter how many developmental milestones are evaluated, children are still different, one from another.

Finally, the Soul of child and youth care practice focuses on personal rhythms and opportunity events with children or young people, where sensitive engagement in caring relationships will promote personal development and social maturation through interactions that are in many ways auto-therapeutic. In this metaphor of *Soul*, it is easy to see how musical rhythms introduced between children or young people and their carers become fundamental to the successful delivery of quality service outcomes. To examine this further, attention turns to a consideration of five important rhythms with associated musical rhythms that frame child and youth care practices at home and away from home. Understanding (and heeding) the importance of these rhythms is fundamental to the delivery of responsive children's services.

THE RHYTHMS OF RESPONSIVE CHILD AND YOUTH CARE

The first rhythms needing to be identified and proactively engaged are those associated with family and extended family members and connecting to rhythms of interaction with kinship networks that exist for each child or young person received into care (Ainsworth, 1997; Burford & Casson, 1989; Pennell & Burford, 1995). Family rhythms are closely associated with particular circumstances in each child's or young person's home environment that may have resulted in their requiring child welfare services or being admitted to a foster home, residential school, or other centre (Fulcher & Ainsworth, 1985). Family rhythms contribute to the socialisation and behavioural training each young person has received before coming to the attention of child and youth care professionals.

For all these reasons, it is essential that planned care and treatment give priority to the active participation of family and extended family members. Active consideration needs also to be given to the kinship networks that help give children and young people their social and cultural identities. It is difficult to ignore research evidence showing that, despite what child welfare professionals may wish or think, children and young people still resume contact and continue some involvement with family and extended family members after leaving care (Fanshel, Finch, & Grundy, 1990). Family connections and *rhythms* are closely associated with each child's sense of identity (Bronfenbrenner, 1979), connecting with his or her soul to shape a unique personal and social character.

Next, it is important to identify each child's *education, recreation,* and *learning* rhythms. These include both formal and informal rhythms associated with a child's capacity for learning, their formal educational activities and achievements, and recreational pursuits that contribute to large muscle and cardiovascular development, eye-hand coordination, and time-structuring through leisure activities (Small & Fulcher, 1985). The educational, recreational, and learning rhythms will have been severely disrupted for many children and young people placed in foster homes or residential care such that these rhythms are underdeveloped, as noted in Kendrick's (1999) study of Scottish children. Paradoxically, these are the very rhythms that connect children and young people to a peer group, giving opportunities for behavioural, social, and cultural learning so important to long-term future development and achievement (Maier, 1975, 1987). These educational, recreational, and learning rhythms are clearly influenced through the purposeful use of activities such as homework or work experiences, participation in sport or cultural activities, or directed learning through hobbies or youth clubs at home as well as in group care schools and centres (VanderVen, 1985).

Play therapy, individual and small group leisure activities, and participation in community life offer children and young people opportunities for activating and nurturing rhythms in education, recreation, and learning. As Maier (1979) put it, when children and young people experience predictability in caring and learning rhythms with their carers, it is then that they learn to trust and emotionally depend on personal relationships. Through this way of managing relationships with young people, the emphasis can shift from institutional controls to personalised behaviour training tailored for each young person in residence at home, in a foster home, residential school, or institution (Garfat, 1998). Multiple learning opportunities are used in such ways to support personalised care plans that are sensitively planned around the developmental needs and performance of each child or young person (Eisikovits, Beker, & Guttmann, 1991; Maier, 1981), adding *Soul* to the *Rhythms* of responsive child and youth care.

A third important set of rhythms are those associated with *group living* whether at home, foster home, summer camp, residential school, group home, or institution (Beker & Eisikovitz, 1991). When looking closely at the daily and weekly activities of children and young people, one quickly finds that each day follows particular rhythms associated with food, sleep, work, and play–all requiring sensitive daily management (Fulcher, 1996). Rhythms of group living are concerned with differences that can be found between weekday routines and activities and events that happen on weeknights and weekends. Weekly and monthly rhythms in child and youth care can often be discerned through an examination of admission and discharge practices. These highlight whether a service provides short-term respite care, crisis management, long-term supportive care, education, or residential supervision. Monthly and seasonal rhythms of child and youth care are also commonly associated with school, work, and holiday periods.

Residential schools and care centres sponsored by religious organisations frequently employ weekly, monthly, and seasonal rituals in the delivery of child and youth care or, as in Malaysia or other parts of the Islamic world, religious practices require the offering of prayers five times a day. An examination of annual reports required of child and youth care centres quickly demonstrates how yearly rhythms of care are also important, most graphically seen when a child turns 18 and is re-classified an adult. At such times, support services that young people and families rely upon are withdrawn or they may be referred on, as in the case of young people with developmental conditions becoming the responsibility of health and disability services.

Child and youth care practices need also to engage with a fourth set of rhythms associated with *community and peer group activities*. Responsive practices require attention to the needs of each child or young person for purposeful engagement in social experiences that help connect them to normative peer group activities (Fahlberg, 1990, 1991; Halverson, 1995). Children and young people in care, wherever they live, have had their community and peer group rhythms frequently disrupted as placement decisions are made without careful consideration for the unintended consequences in decision-making. As young people are moved from one setting to another or change schools, it follows that their friends are also moved and important relationships severed.

Young people in care quite often become involved with other young people in care or engage in peer group activities that have a deleterious effect on health and well-being whether through alcohol and drug abuse, sexual abuse and neglect, or physical abuse. Unless new relationships are formed through the management of purposeful activities with alternative peers, then children and young people in care have little choice but a return to old friends and activities. These old relationships and patterns of behaviour have all too often resulted in the untimely deaths of young people in care or histories of struggle for survival in abusive relationships. Rhythms associated with peer groups and communities of interest reach deep into the soul of children and young people, wherever they live (Maier, 1990, 1992). Responsive practices need fundamentally to build from recognition of how these rhythms impact on children and young people and how proactive engagement in community and peer group rhythms can benefit children, young people, and their families (Maier, 1991).

Finally, one must not ignore the *cultural and spiritual rhythms of caring* that operate informally as well as formally in the delivery of responsive child and youth care. Elsewhere (Fulcher, 1998; Tait-Rolleston, Cairns, Fulcher, Kereopa, & Nia Nia, 1997; Cairns et al., 1996) it was shown how cultural rituals of encounter and exchange are commonly overlooked in the delivery of social work and child and youth care services (Stewart, 1997; Wilcox et al., 1991). Images, sounds, and smells of child and youth care practice spring instantly to mind that reflect cultural and spiritual rhythms of caring. These operate in any family or foster home as well as in residential schools, group care centres, or institutions (Ramsden, 1997; Te Whaiti, McCarthy, & Durie, 1997).

Look again at people engaging and interacting with each other in an active child or youth care service. Do people sit on tables, at tables, or on chairs? Are there smells of sweet grass or incense burning? Do young people eat with their right hand without utensils? Do they use chopsticks? Do people use a knife and fork in each hand or manoeuvre their way through dinner with a fork or spoon, except when cutting meat? Is pork served? Do young people drink alcohol? Do young people appear in public without arms and legs covered? Are rituals of fasting and prayer evident?

One quickly sees why some cross-cultural competencies are required if child and youth care workers are to avoid significant gaffes that leave some children and carers feeling culturally unsafe (Leigh, 1998; Rangihau, 1986, 1987; Shook, 1985). Rudolph Steiner centres have taught the world a great deal about spiritual rhythms of caring and learning, seeking ways in which these rhythms can be carefully balanced for each child or living and learning group. Successful outcomes for children and families have been achieved through thoughtfully matching the personal styles and learning attributes of different children to overcome performance deficits and achieve complementary outcomes. Practices elsewhere in the so-called developing world offer important illustrations of how cultural and spiritual rhythms of caring seek balance with behavioural representations of wellness (Cairns, 1991; Ibeabuchi, 1986; Sali, 1996) that touch the *soul* of each child or young person in care (Rose, 1992).

Summary

Five rhythms of child and youth care practice have been identified that touch the souls of children and young people in care, rhythms that need sensitive management and oversight whether at home or away from home. Children are enmeshed within rhythms that connect them with family and extended family members–including kinship networks–that help locate each child or young person with particular people, places, and a cultural identity. Education, recreation, and learning rhythms–both formal and informal–require sensitive management if children and young people in care are to be offered a minimum guarantee that their lives should not be placed at greater risk as a consequence of having lived in a foster home, residential school, group home, or institution.

Rhythms associated with family and residential group living can be monitored, recorded, and reported by hour, shift, weekday, weeknight, weekend, month, holiday period, sick leave, or year. Community and peer group rhythms enable children and young people to engage in purposeful activities and social learning opportunities. Finally, much is to be learned about the management of cultural and spiritual rhythms of caring that help give meaning to the lives of children and young people in care.

Cultural safety and personal well-being are recurring themes in the stories and the *Blues* of child and youth care practice. As this musical metaphor fades from *Soulful Rhythms* to the *Blues* of children and young people in care, it is important to pause and acknowledge the emotional and physical pain experienced by children and young people in care and the tears they and their carers have shed so many times over the years. Whether through frustration or relief, happiness or pain, such emotions were closely aligned to the challenge of providing *good enough* care and daily services that could make a difference to the well-being and futures of children and young people.

THE BLUES OF CHILD AND YOUTH CARE AT HOME AND AWAY FROM HOME

The *Blues* of care are being sung well before any child or young person leaves home and arrives at a foster home, a residential school, group home, or institution (Kahan, 1989; Wagner, 1988). The formal imposition of care, supervision, or custody by care and protection or place of safety order,[4] youth justice sentencing, or indefinite detention follows on from an important social history (Scarr & Eisenberg, 1993; Scull, 1977; Seed, 1973). Throughout that history, the voices of a young person, family and extended family members, neighbours, teachers, child welfare professionals and others may not have been heard clearly amidst the *noise* of emotional turmoil. Most of the children or young people for whom child welfare organisations provide services have not been diverted away from a formal reception into care. If diverted initially to boarding school or extended family care, a care or supervision order may still have been issued at a later stage.

As noted in chapter one, for the past three decades child and youth care policies have been reshaped by six ideologies of best practice: normalisation, deinstitutionalisation, mainstreaming, use of the least restrictive environment, minimal intervention and diversion (Fulcher & Ainsworth, 1994). All six practice ideologies have impacted directly on the planning and management of contemporary services provided for children, young people, and their families (O'Brien & Murray, 1997). These secondary influences associated with the social policy environment, service organisations, and the delivery of agency services prompt a whole new musical line of the *Blues* as highlighted in Henry Maier's chapter later in this volume. Confirmation that failures by "the system" have a direct impact on the well-being of both young people and staff can be readily found when listening to managers and workers talk about working in multiply restructured organisations delivering contemporary child and youth care services (Casson & George, 1995).

Foster parents and child and youth care workers are reminded that they operate at crisis points in the lives of children and families where the *Blues* sung by each child or young person confront a discordant beat of *The System* (Fulcher, 1988). Most child and youth care services operate in a policy environment that is overtly shaped by fiscal considerations. Agencies are expected to operate as business units that manage capital and human resources to produce quality outcomes for individual children or young people and their significant others (Knapp, 1984). One refrain of the Blues in all this has been the growing recognition of work-related stresses and how professional fatigue impacts on teamwork in the delivery of child and youth care services (Fulcher, 1991).

As Maier noted (1979), care for the caregivers is a core feature of any quality care guarantees made to children, young people, and their families, a claim reinforced through research carried out by Burford (1990) and Fulcher (1983). The musical beat of soul, rhythms and blues impacts directly on all involved in child and youth care practice through contributing to an emotional climate and a living milieu in any home or centre. The beat impacts directly on the professional identity and personal well-being of every worker or prospective worker, influencing the collective performance of child and youth care teams as a whole (Burford & Fulcher, 1985).

On arrival at a foster home, residential school, group home, or institution a child or young person is initially confronted with a second line of the Blues that sings of *personal and cultural safety* amongst strangers (Dominelli, 1988; Fulcher, 1998). Cultural safety, that state of being in which a child or young person experiences that her or his personal well-being—as well as social and cultural frames of reference—are acknowledged, even if not fully understood, is highlighted each time a young person starts engaging with others in their new care environment. Questions like *"Are there any people like me here?"* become recurring emotional themes, along with other *Rhythm* and *Soul* themes like *"Are there people who speak like I do?" "Do they eat the way I do?" "Do they eat the same food?"* and *"Why are these other people here?"*

Rituals of group membership begin immediately after one enters the door of a child and youth care service centre (Fulcher, 1996). Responsive carers establish and maintain positive rituals of encounter that promote group membership for new members, students, care staff, domestic or catering workers, and other visitors to the centre. In residential group living situations, a new child or young person may be assisted through the formal rituals of group membership. However, they must also establish their own personal place within the sub-group hierarchies and alliances that operate in any resident group while establishing purposeful relationships with carers as well. Respect for individuality connects with a young person's personal identity and that sense of who they were before admission to care. This extends further to "Who are/were their people?" "Who cared about them and for them?" "What was happening that resulted in their being placed in care?" and "What happens next?" Personal and cultural safety, managing group membership(s), and reinforcing identity are all interwoven into the *Soul, Rhythms and Blues* of caring, reinforcing the importance of responsiveness to this aspect of practice (Maier, 1991).

A third strain of the Blues is heard whenever a child or young person feels *shy, embarrassed, ridiculed, or unsafe* whether living at home, in a foster home, attending school camp, or staying at a residential school, group home, or institution. Shyness and embarrassment have their own special meanings in the native languages spoken by each child admitted into care. New Zealand Maori families experience *whakamaa* or embarrassment about a child being placed in care, while in Malaysia, the parallel response involves feeling *malu*. The voice and dialect of each new resident or staff member is pinpointed very quickly through a variety of "*getting to know you rituals*." Being made the brunt of a joke or feeling ridicule from resident group members are recurring themes of the Blues in child and youth care practice. One is always hopeful that no child or young person in care will ever be made the subject of ridicule or abuse by staff, and yet history sadly documents an abusive legacy in residential child and youth care practice. That history has been made prominent since World War II through media disclosures of abuse in all parts of the Western world (see, for example, Australian Human Rights and Equal Opportunities Commission, 1997; Canadian Royal Commission on Aboriginal Peoples, 1997; Rangihau, 1986). When a child feels unsafe culturally, spiritually, emotionally, or physically, then her or his voice sings a special refrain of the Blues. Unless that voice and its special rendition is heard by child and youth care workers and responded to with sensitivity, then children or young people such as these are placed at even greater risk than before. Responsive child and youth care practices need to guarantee that, from the moment of first contact, no child or young person in care will be made to feel unsafe or be left in unsafe situations.

A fourth rendition of the Blues sings out in *anger or fear*. Young people frequently bring a lifetime of anger into out-of-home placements, and they are usually angry for very good reasons (Durst, 1992). Many young people feel anger towards teachers, parents or step-parents, boyfriends or girlfriends, and others for "letting them down." Children and young people also experience fear or apprehension when joining a new living or learning group. It is important to hear and respond sensitively to voices singing the Blues out of anger and fear. It is all too easy for these powerful emotions of group living to place children or young people in abusive situations where they end up singing the *Blues* of victim, perpetrator, or voyeur with consequences that may last a lifetime. Legal obligations in the duty of care form the basis for minimum guarantees that no child or young person shall be harmed nor become the victim of abuse of any kind while in receipt of state-mandated care. Such expectations are also voiced by family and extended family members, by child welfare professionals, by special interest groups and the media, and by those purchasing and administering cost-effective services for children, young people, and their families.

Finally, when a child or young person becomes *isolated* from peers, from their carers, from family members, from friends, and from virtually everyone around them, it is important that child and youth care workers hear loudly and clearly the Blues of risk that require careful attention (Guttman, 1991). Isolation and feelings of personal alienation should not be confused with times when children or young people seek moments of solitude or time out. Isolation Blues are those associated with life and death. Burning preoccupations about life and death issues are sometimes tattooed in prominent places on a young person's hands, arms, chest, or face and become symbolic reminders of moments of pain etched as a *moko*[5] into their being for a lifetime. Cutting or bruising on a young person's wrists, limbs, breasts, or genitals must always be a concern, and body language such as this should provoke action on the part of all child and youth care workers.

When the principle of physical safety and security is threatened through accidental or self-inflicted injury or through the death of a child in care, then the professional integrity of child welfare services is called into question. It is important to remember that children or young people can sometimes reach the stage when the very thought of fronting up for what they have done or experiences to which they have been subjected becomes either too worrisome or burdensome to contemplate. At times like these, attempted suicide or death through risk-taking with drugs, alcohol, cars, motorbikes, or weapons becomes a stark alternative to the painful reality that engulfs their very existence. Much can be learned through hindsight about the deaths of children or young people in care. These remain salutary reminders to all child or youth care workers who continue to ask whether anything might have been done differently or whether anything might have saved them. The *Blues* sung by children or young people who died in care must never fall on deaf ears nor cease to weigh heavily on hearts seemingly out of tune with the emotional pain in children or young people's lives.

Summary

So long as child and youth care workers "tune in" and actively listen to what is going on, the Blues are being sung every day by children and young people for whom care, special education, treatment, supervision, or custody has been authorised (Garfat, 1998). Personal accounts of emotional suffering as well as the blues of survival in "the system" are commonly heard. Physical and cultural safety in the crowds of group living can be overlooked very easily during school camps, in foster homes, residential schools, group homes, and institutions. Rituals associated with group membership and individuality are distinctive features of group living, regardless of whether these rituals are planned or unplanned. Responsive child and youth care requires vigilance in situations where a child or young person might feel embarrassed, shy, ridiculed, or unsafe.

Other more direct interventions are required when working with children or young people feeling angry, scared, abusive, or abused. Finally, when a child or young person becomes withdrawn, isolated, or perhaps other-worldly, it is important to recognize how they profile someone who could do something seriously reckless or stupid, leading to death by suicide or risk-taking with alcohol, drugs, cars, motorbikes, or weapons. The Blues of child and youth care are musical themes heard daily, while the sounds of Soul and Rhythms of caring promote health and well-being.

TOWARD A RADICAL REFRAMING OF CHILD AND YOUTH CARE PRACTICES

To conclude, the six voices introduced at the start of this chapter are used to call for a radical reframing of child and youth care services aimed at achieving increased responsiveness in the decade ahead. Each voice of child and youth care sings through its own particular speech pattern and dialect, highlighting the importance of planning and policy formation being much more tightly focused around the developmental needs of children and young people. That there are at least six voices, all demanding to speak, gives evidence for the need to better understand organisational complexities associated with responsive multi-disciplinary practices in this field. Sadly, the combined musical output of all six voices creates discord, where the more powerful voices dominate at the expense of others.

The Voices of Children and Young People at Home or Away from Home: "Walk the Talk!"

Children and young people are far more sophisticated than they were in previous generations when social mores expected children to be seen and not heard and decisions were made for young people and not with them. Contemporary young people are now presented with a range of stimuli through the media, the Internet, and modern challenges of daily life like drugs, HIV-AIDS, and expectations that they ask "Why?" Those involved in child and youth care need to practice what they preach or teach far more actively than before, engaging in purposeful activity and direct care services to children and families in collaboration with other health, education, and social services professionals.

The five rhythms of proactive, responsive caring need to place children and young people at the centre of planning and policy formulation. Think about how children or young people might participate in staff reviews of their performance week-to-week! There needs to be a radical reframing of ideas about the way service outcomes are monitored and evaluated with each child or young person in care. If child and youth care workers and managers are to lead by example then young people need active encouragement to participate in decision-making about what is happening or is about to happen in their lives.

The Voices of Family and Extended Family Members: "Think Outside the Box!"

While lip service is frequently paid to family participation in decision-making around the care, education, and supervision of children and young people, the realities of family participation often fail to match up with the rhetoric. Those engaged in the delivery of child and youth care services need to think and act more strategically with individual children and families. This means exploring ideas about how to resource more responsive practice opportunities with particular children or young people and working in much greater partnership with family and extended family members to achieve better outcomes. It also means thinking practically about the futures of each child or young person in care and what those futures might hold when they reach age 18 or older.

There is ample research to show how family participation in decision-making about children or young people placed in care helps to produce enhanced service outcomes (Burford & Hudson, 2000). Whether relying on formal family group conferences or less formal protocols that encourage family participation, it is difficult to ignore the way increased family participation usually means improved service outcomes and longer term benefits for children, young people, and their families.

The Voices of Child Welfare Professionals: "Get Real!"

For all the advances in science, technology, and the arts gained over the past half-century, there is still a paradox in how little has changed in direct practice encounters with children and young people in primary care settings in most child welfare services. The language of child welfare professionals is still filled with jargon and big words used by different professional disciplines, drawing attention to knowledge maintained by experts regardless of whether these are communicated with children or young people and families or not. Staff turnover in child welfare services still remains critically high, and the research evidence is virtually non-existent on how work rosters and staff-to-client ratios contribute to responsiveness and continuity in young people's lives as they move through developmental life transitions.

Status hierarchies continue to place front-line care workers at the bottom of organisational charts, giving limited acknowledgment to the strategic benefit from their responsive practices employed with children or young people day-by-day. Peer supervision and formal supervision are all too frequently neglected or abandoned altogether whether through work pressures or because of service restructuring driven by consultants lacking knowledge of the field who confuse professional supervision with management. Far from being a waste of public sector spending, it is argued that time set aside for professional networking between child welfare professionals is critical to achieving enhanced responsiveness in the delivery of child, youth, and family services.

The Voices of Public Opinion: "Who's Carin'?"

The future of responsive child and youth care services is closely aligned to investment in any nation's young people. Those claiming that "nothing works" in child and youth care have seen this message snapped up by supporters of monetarist economics as justification for massive cuts in public investment in the futures of children and young people. Few have bothered to explore what works with which young people or under which circumstances. Then, as enquiry after enquiry documents the abuse of children in local authority care, public opinion becomes disparaging about there being anything that can make a difference. Social Darwinist views such as these end up blaming children or young people for a DNA code that puts them beyond redemption. Having *"failed the cure"* that caring community services offered them, many come to symbolise the call in places like the U.S. for capital punishment as young adults, this being a seemingly logical solution for heinous crimes and ill behaviour towards others.

Advocates of targeted expenditure also fail to acknowledge the way that children or young people must now be labeled as problems before any assistance is justified, ignoring the unintended consequences of labeling on identity formation and self-esteem. Thus, while those lobbying for the corporate interests of industry and government employ millions to shape public opinion, where are the lobbyists for children, young people, and their families? The rhetoric of commitment rarely finds implementation in the realities of practice for those struggling to provide responsive child welfare services.

The Voices of Regulating Authority and Fiscal Accountability: "Transparency of Costs and Accountability for Outcomes!"

The last decade of the 20th century saw child and youth care services operating increasingly through purchase of service contracting arrangements with governments and public agencies. Services are now commonly monitored as business units that deliver specific performance outcomes to targeted clientele. Public sector accounting practices now shape child and youth care outcomes. Ironically, government services are filled increasingly with contract administrators, not practitioners, who expect more from the voluntary sector in exchange for funding than was ever expected of government services in the past. One result has been that voluntary child care organisations now spend as much time on servicing the new client of ministerial and governmental expectations, distracting attention away from the top priority of service responsiveness to the "traditional clients" who are real children, young people, and their families. After all the contract jargon, technical language, and accountancy-speak, the most important aspect of transparency is that which still focuses on the needs of every child or young person in care. Accountability begins with family and extended family views about how a child and youth care service assists with the care of their child(ren), a key argument supporting the use of family group conferences at the beginning and end of each care order[6] to reaffirm family participation at every stage of the service planning process.

The Voices of Research and Scholarship: "If Ya Pay Peanuts, Ya Get Monkeys!"

If child welfare services are to gain formal recognition for the strategic role played in support of a nation's future, there needs to be political commitment directly commensurate with the nation's strategic investment in the futures of children and young people. It has been said that New Zealand kept better records of its sheep population in the late 19th century than it did of its children. In the late 20th century, zookeepers and horse racing attendants were often paid more than child and youth care workers, perhaps because of heavy investment in bloodstock!

Meanwhile, children and young people in care remain very much at risk of under-achievement, ill health, and court involvement because adults in many parts of the world lack the political will to invest in more responsive child and youth care practices. Scandinavian examples throughout the past half-century have reaffirmed the importance of sustained political commitment to the professional registration of child and youth care workers, and that includes salaries and conditions that are commensurate with the job. Poor pay and poor conditions reflect the status given to care work and the value given to enhancing the lives and well-being of children and young people in care.

Recent disclosures of sexual abuse in British residential homes only reinforce this point. It is not that more research is required to determine future directions for the development of child welfare services. The challenge lies in a radical reframing of policies and practices that implement what has already been documented through repeated research outcomes. This requires more than re-structuring child and youth care organisations that have already struggled through three decades of service restructuring while attempting to respond proactively to the contemporary needs of children, young people, and their families. Planning needs to extend beyond the current financial year to establish a strategic vision for the futures of children or young people in care, in education, recreation, leisure and sport with a three to five year time line, updated yearly. Otherwise structural features of child welfare bureaucracy continue to undermine the futures of any nation's children and young people by failing to strategically invest in their sustainable futures.

In conclusion, there is much to be gained from tuning in to all voices that sing the *Soul, Rhythms,* and *Blues* of child and youth care practice. All six voices introduced here require particular attention and active listening. The Heart and Soul of child and youth care are embedded in acts of caring that attend to bodily comforts and physical safety that acknowledges what makes each child unique. Children follow their own personal rhythms around physical, cognitive, emotional, behavioural and social development. Five distinctive rhythms of child and youth care were highlighted: Family rhythms; educational, recreational, and learning rhythms; rhythms of daily living; community and peer group rhythms; and cultural/spiritual rhythms of caring. The Blues of child and youth care are sung through each care order; through engagement in rituals of group membership; during times of emotional vulnerability, anger, and pain, and; during times of fear, withdrawal, and isolation. The Blues of child and youth care are heard daily in foster homes and group care centres but proactive attention given to the Soul and the Rhythms of caring helps to remedy the Blues by promoting health and well-being for young people and carers alike. It is hoped that these musical reflections will challenge child and youth care workers and managers–plus the organisations that employ them–towards achieving even greater responsiveness to the developmental needs of their nation's children and young people.

NOTES

1. In choosing this term, the writer relied on the Scottish Chambers Dictionary for an ancient definition of French origin, where *voice* means "to act as mouthpiece of: to give utterance or expression to: and to endow with voice."

2. The author wishes to acknowledge limitations associated with the way this review was restricted due to being "Other-Than-English Challenged," making it impossible to

decipher much written material voiced in languages other than English. This is a huge limitation.

3. The First Aberlour Child Care Trust Lecture given at Strathclyde University in Scotland.

4. The UK and many Commonwealth countries like New Zealand and Malaysia use a Place of Safety Order as the legal device that transfers a child into care for protection.

5. Maori ceremonial tattooing of the face and body.

6. A "care order" is the legal instrument through which a British child or young person, as also found in other Commonwealth countries, may be placed in state supervised care.

REFERENCES

Ainsworth, F. (1997). *Family centred group care: Model building.* Aldershot, Hunts: Ashgate Publishing.

Ainsworth, F., & Fulcher, L. C. (Eds.). (1981). *Group care for children: Concept and issues.* London: Tavistock Publications.

Australian Human Rights and Equal Opportunities Commission (1997). *Bringing them home: Report of the national inquiry into the separation of aboriginal and Torres Strait Islander children from their families.* Canberra: Australian Government Publishing Service.

Beker, J., & Eisikovits, Z. (Eds.). (1991). *Knowledge utilization in residential child and youth care work.* Washington, DC: Child Welfare League of America.

Bronfenbrenner, U. (1979). *The ecology of human development.* Cambridge: Harvard University Press.

Bukenya, S. S. (1996). *The Ugandan experience, realities and dreams: Plenary papers from the international conference on residential child care.* Glasgow: Strathclyde University, 57-62.

Burford, G. (1990). *Assessing teamwork: A comparative study of group home teams in Newfoundland and Labrador.* Stirling, Scotland: Unpublished PhD thesis.

Burford, G., & Casson, S. (1989). Including families in residential work: Educational and agency tasks. *British Journal of Social Work, 19*(1), 19-37.

Burford, G., & Fulcher, L. C. (1985). Resident group influences on team functioning. In L. C. Fulcher & F. Ainsworth (Eds.), *Group care practice with children* (pp. 187-214). London: Tavistock Publications.

Burford, G., & Hudson, J. (2000). *Family group conferencing: New directions in community-centered child and family practice.* New York: Aldine de Gruyter.

Cairns, T. (1991). Whangai–caring for a child. In G. Maxwell, I. Hassall, & J. Robertson (Eds.), *Toward a child and family policy for New Zealand.* Wellington: Office of the Commissioner for Children.

Cairns, T., Fulcher, L. C., & Tait-Rolleston, W., with Kereopa, H., Kereopa, T., Nia Nia, P., & Waiariki, W. (1996). Puao-te-Ata-tu (Daybreak) revisited. In D. J. McDonald & L. R. Cleave (Eds.), *Partnerships that work? Proceedings of the 1995 Asia-Pacific Regional Social Services Conference* (pp. 44-47). Christchurch: University of Canterbury.

Casson, S., & George, C. (1995). *Culture change for total quality: An action guide for managers in social and health services.* London: Pitman Publishing.

Dominelli, L. (1988). *Anti-racist social work.* London: Macmillan.

Durst, D. (1992). The road to poverty is paved with good intentions: Social interventions and indigenous peoples. *International Social Work, 35*(2), 191-202.

Eisikovits, Z., Beker, J., & Guttmann, E. (1991). The known and the used in residential child and youth care work. In J. Beker & Z. Eisikovits (Eds.), *Knowledge utilization in residential child and youth care work* (pp. 3-23). Washington, DC: Child Welfare League of America.

Fahlberg, V. (Ed.). (1990). *Residential treatment: A tapestry of many therapies.* Indianapolis, IN: Perspective Press.

Fahlberg, V. (1991). *A child's journey through placement.* Indianapolis, IN: Perspective Press.

Fanshel, D., Finch, S. J., & Grundy, J. F. (1990). *Foster children in life course perspective.* New York: Columbia University Press.

Fox-Harding, L. (1991). *Perspectives on child care policy.* London: Longman.

Fulcher, L. C. (1988). *The worker, the work group and the organisational task: Corporate re-structuring and the social services in New Zealand.* Wellington: Victoria University Press.

Fulcher, L. C. (1991). Teamwork in residential care. In J. Beker & Z. Eisikovits (Eds.), *Knowledge utilization in residential child and youth care practice* (pp. 215-235). Washington, DC: Child Welfare League of America.

Fulcher, L. C. (1994). When you're up to your neck in alligators, its hard to remember that the original aim was to drain the swamp: Some lessons from New Zealand health sector reform. *Australian Social Work, 47*(2), 47-53.

Fulcher, L. C. (1996). Changing care in a changing world: The old and new worlds. *Social Work Review, VII*(1/2), 20-26.

Fulcher, L. C. (1998). Acknowledging culture in child and youth care practice. *Social Work Education, 17*(3), 321-338.

Fulcher, L. C. (1999). Cultural origins of the contemporary family group conference. *Child Care in Practice, 5*(4), 328-339.

Fulcher, L. C., & Ainsworth, F. (Eds.). (1985). *Group care practice with children.* London: Tavistock Publications.

Fulcher, L. C., & Ainsworth, F. (1994). Child welfare abandoned? The ideology and economics of contemporary service reform in New Zealand. *Social Work Review, VI*(5/6), 2-13.

Fulcher, L. C., & Fulcher, J. (1998). To intervene or not?–That is the question: Managing risk-taking behaviour in student halls of residence, *Journal of the Australian and New Zealand Student Services Association, 11*, 14-31.

Garfat, T. (1998). The effective child and youth care intervention: A phenomenological inquiry. *Journal of Child & Youth Care, 12*(1/2).

Guttmann, E. (1991). Immediacy in residential child and youth care: The fusion of experience, self-consciousness, and action. In J. Beker & Z. Eisikovits, (Eds.), *Knowledge utilization in residential child and youth care practice* (pp. 65-82). Washington, DC: Child Welfare League of America.

Halverson, A. (1995). The importance of caring and attachment in direct practice with adolescents. *Child and Youth Care Forum, 24*(3), 169.

Hudson, W. W., & Nurius, P. S. (1994). *Controversial issues in social work research.* Sydney: Allyn and Bacon.

Ibeabuchi, G. B. E. (1986). *Developing child and youth care services in Nigeria: An analysis of contemporary problems and needs.* University of Stirling, Scotland: Unpublished PhD Thesis.

Kahan, B. (1989). *Child care research, policy, and practice.* London: Hodder & Stoughton.

Kendrick, A. J. (1999). Residential child care in Scotland: A positive choice? In G. Barlow (Ed.), *Child care policies and structures: An international perspective* (pp. 3-8). Realities & Dreams International Conference on Residential Child Care, 3-6 September 1996, Glasgow: Centre for Residential Child Care.

Knapp, M. (1984). *The economics of social care.* London: Macmillan.

Leigh, J. W. (1998). *Communication for cultural competence.* Sydney: Allyn and Bacon.

Maier, H. (1963). Child care as a method of social work. In *Training manual for child care staff* (pp. 62-81). New York: Child Welfare League of America Publications.

Maier, H. W. (1975). Learning to learn and living to live in residential treatment. *Child Welfare, 54*(6), 406-420.

Maier, H. W. (1979). The core of care: Essential ingredients for the development of children at home and away from home. *Child Care Quarterly, 8*(3), 161-173.

Maier, H. W. (1981). Essential components in care and treatment environments for children. In F. Ainsworth & L. C. Fulcher (Eds.), *Group care for children: Concept and issues* (pp. 19-70). London: Tavistock.

Maier, H. W. (1985). Primary care in secondary settings: Inherent strains. In L. C. Fulcher & F. Ainsworth (Eds.), *Group care practice with children* (pp. 21-47). London: Tavistock Publications.

Maier, H. W. (1987). *Developmental group care of children and youth: Concepts and practice.* New York: The Haworth Press, Inc.

Maier, H. W. (1990). A developmental perspective for child and youth care. In J. Anglin, C. Denholm, R. Ferguson, & A. Pence (Eds.), *Perspectives in professional child and youth care* (pp. 7-24). Binghamton, NY: The Haworth Press, Inc.

Maier, H. W. (1991). An exploration of the substance of child and youth care practice. *Child and Youth Care Forum, 20*(6), 393-411.

Maier, H. W. (1992). Rhythmicity–a powerful force for experiencing unity and personal connections. *Journal of Child & Youth Care Work, 5*, 7-13.

Milligan, I. (1998). Residential child care is not social work! *Social Work Education, 17*(3), 275-285.

O'Brien, P., & Murray, R. (1997). *Human services: Towards partnership and support.* Palmerston North, NZ: Dunmore Press.

Payne, M. (1997). *Modern social work theory* (2nd edition). London: Macmillan.

Pennell, J., & Burford, G. (1995). *Family group decision making project implementation report* (volume 1). St. John's, Newfoundland: Memorial University of Newfoundland, School of Social Work.

Ramsden, I. (1997). Cultural safety: Implementing THE CONCEPT. In P. Te Whaiti, M. McCarthy, & A. Durie (Eds.), *Mai I Rangiatea: Maori wellbeing and development* (pp. 113-125). Auckland: Auckland University Press.

Rangihau, J. (1986). *Puao-te-Ata-tu (Daybreak): Report of the ministerial advisory committee on a Maori perspective for the Department of Social Welfare.* Wellington: Department of Social Welfare, Government Printing Office.

Rangihau, J. (1987). *Beyond crisis.* Keynote Address to the First New Zealand Conference on Social Work Education, Christchurch: Rehua Marae, University of Canterbury, Department of Social Work.

Rose, L. (1992). On being a child and youth care worker. *Journal of Child & Youth Care, 5*(1), 21-26.

Sali, G. W. (1996). *Law and order in contemporary Papua New Guinea: An examination of causes and policy options.* Victoria University of Wellington: Unpublished PhD Thesis.

Scarr, S., & Eisenberg, M. (1993). Child research: Issues, perspectives, and results. *Annual Research Psychology, 44*, 613-644.

Scull, A. (1977). *Decarceration.* Englewood Cliffs, NJ: Prentice-Hall.

Seed, P. (1973). Should any child be placed in care? The forgotten great debate 1841-1874. *British Journal of Social Work, 3*(3), 321-30.

Shook, E. F. (1985). *Ho'oponopono: Contemporary uses of a Hawaiian problem-solving process.* Honolulu: University of Hawaii Press.

Small, R., & Fulcher, L. C. (1985). Teaching competence in group care practice. In L. C. Fulcher & F. Ainsworth (Eds.), *Group care practice with children* (pp. 135-154). London: Tavistock Publications.

Stewart, T. (1997). Historical interfaces between Maori and psychology. In P. Te Whaiti, M. McCarthy, & A. Durie (Eds.), *Mai I Rangiatea: Maori wellbeing and development* (pp. 75-95). Auckland: Auckland University Press.

Tait-Rolleston, W., Cairns, T., Fulcher, L. C., Kereopa, H., & Nia Nia, P. (1997). He koha kii-na kui ma, na koro ma: A gift of words from our ancestors. *Social Work Review, IX*(4), 30-36.

Te Whaiti, P., McCarthy, M., & Durie, A. (Eds.). (1997). *Mai i rangiatea: Maori wellbeing and development.* Auckland: Auckland University Press.

VanderVen, K. D. (1985). Activity programming: Its developmental and therapeutic role in group care. In L. C. Fulcher & F. Ainsworth (Eds.), *Group care practice with children* (pp. 155-183). London: Tavistock Publications.

Wagner, G. (1988). *Residential care: The research reviewed.* London: Her Majesty's Stationery Office.

Wilcox, R., Smith, D., Moore, J., Hewitt, A., Allan, G., Walker, H., Ropata, M., Monu, L., & Featherstone, T. (1991). *Family decision making, family group conferences–Practitioner's views.* Lower Hutt, NZ: Practitioners Publishing.

Yahya, Z. (1994). *Resisting colonialist discourse.* Bangi, Malaysia: Penerbit, Universiti Kebangsaan Malaysia.

Chapter 3

Developing Social Competencies
in Group Care Practice

Richard W. Small
Leon C. Fulcher

SUMMARY. Any discussions about specialized helping environments for children or young people would be incomplete without reference to the relationships found between practices in group care centers and schools. This involves thinking of a child's total environment as a curriculum for teaching competencies and learning outcomes important to daily living. The task involves making a conscious effort to deal with a child's functioning in the present, thereby avoiding diagnostic conclusions that emphasize difficulties in one area of their life as the cause of learning problems. *[Article copies available for a fee from The Haworth Document Delivery Service: 1-800-HAWORTH. E-mail address: <docdelivery@ haworthpress.com> Website: <http://www.HaworthPress.com> © 2005 by The Haworth Press, Inc. All rights reserved.]*

KEYWORDS. Group care, residential care, residential treatment, group homes, youth work, youthwork, group work, at-risk youth, therapeutic milieu, cognitive-behavioural intervention, social competency

Address correspondence to: Richard W. Small, Executive Director, Walker Home and School, 1968 Central Ave., Needham, MA 02492.

[Haworth co-indexing entry note]: "Developing Social Competencies in Group Care Practice." Small, Richard W., and Leon C. Fulcher. Co-published simultaneously in *Child & Youth Services* (The Haworth Press, Inc.) Vol. 27, No. 1/2, 2005, pp. 51-73; and: *Group Care Practice with Children and Young People Revisited* (ed: Leon C. Fulcher, and Frank Ainsworth) The Haworth Press, Inc., 2006, pp. 51-73. Single or multiple copies of this article are available for a fee from The Haworth Document Delivery Service [1-800-HAWORTH, 9:00 a.m. - 5:00 p.m. (EST). E-mail address: docdelivery@haworthpress.com].

REFLECTIONS ON TWO DECADES OF DEVELOPMENT

It is interesting, and a little scary, to have the opportunity to review one's theories about practice from the perspective of more than twenty-five years real-life experience. When Robin Clark Cookson and Richard Small first developed the ideas on which this present chapter is based (Clark & Small, 1979), they were attempting to push the boundaries of a practice paradigm that had inspired both of them: Trieschman's (1969) "competence not care" conceptualization of therapeutic environments for troubled children.

These authors were interested in curing mental illness, in meeting children's needs, and undoing the crippling effects of the past. But they were equally–perhaps more–interested in challenging children with the adventure of life, in promoting improved capacity to deal with the struggles of human existence, and in anticipating the opportunities of the future. The adults in a milieu are not just suppliers of psychological medicine to empty, sick children; they are also the acknowledged companions of children in an adventure full of challenges, obstacles, and opportunities. By combining giving something to and expecting something of children, those working directly with children teach the lessons that promote love and competence.

Such a powerful vision of the therapeutic milieu felt (and still feels) right to us, but it also was incomplete. With a little bit of hindsight, it seems clear that Robin and Rick were trying to deconstruct Trieschman's original formulation by making three basic points:

- The notion of "therapeutic milieu" as a powerful helping intervention is best operationalized as "total learning environment," fully integrating life space and school.
- The troubled and troubling behaviors of the children in our care are best understood not as symptoms of psychopathology but as rooted in brain-based social learning disabilities.
- If we really are interested in "teaching competence," we need to be clear about the targeted, measurable skills that make up developmental competence *and* the strengths and weaknesses of each children's individual learning style as these mediate developmental learning.

A quarter century later, these ideas about practice still ring true to us at Walker School, though it is humbling to acknowledge how much we still struggle. Walker now serves a wide range of children and young people from 3 to 22 years of age, across a range of helping programs. Though diagnostic fashions have been everchanging over the past three decades, we come to see it most useful to understand the complicated behaviors of our youngsters in terms of a cluster of developmental difficulties:

- Learned expectations of failure, victimization, and helplessness that significantly distort experiential learning.
- Significant attachment problems, including poor self-regulation, anxiety, anger, and basic mistrust resulting from insecure connections to parental figures. More recently, we are working with children who also suffer from much more serious distortions of reciprocal human relationships resulting from organic impairment and/or severely disturbed, traumatic, or absent connections to parental figures.
- Language-based learning disabilities, non-verbal learning disabilities, and other "soft" neurological impairments that inhibit social learning, distort feedback from the environment, distort communication with significant others, and magnify cognitive distortions associated with depression and low self-esteem.
- Limited repertoire of learned social behaviors, especially prosocial assertiveness and social problem-solving skills.

In the face of such challenges we try to focus our whole array of helping interventions as parts of a curriculum of corrective learning experiences for each child and family. The blueprint for this approach to the therapeutic milieu is simple to articulate:

- Come to the best understanding possible of each child's individual learning style.
- Use this understanding to teach new, more successful and measurable cognitions and behaviors.
- Give each child autonomous opportunities to practice new behaviors in school, at home, and in the community.
- Make sure each child leaves our care with an expanded behavioral tool kit for building the rest of their lives.

Of course, day in and day out workers often fall short of our aspirations, but every day brings new teaching opportunities. This is the hopeful power of a focus on competence. The 1985 revision of this chapter sought to make it more accessible to child and youth care workers, managers, and educators in Great Britain and Ireland as well as Australia and New Zealand. The chapter has been revised further in this edition to make its focus on social competencies more consistent with contemporary notions about developmental assets and, hopefully, even more usable for those wishing to adopt social learning strategies in their work with children, young people, and their families. The authors hope this material will continue to stimulate discussion and promote further explorations into the survival skills that children and young people bring with them into care and those they leave care having incorporated into their personal styles of being in their worlds.

INTRODUCTION

Any discussion of specialized helping environments for children and young people would be incomplete without reference to relationships between group care practice centers and in what happens in schools. After all, a large proportion of each young person's day is normally spent in some type of formal classroom experience. Moreover, many of the advances in the education of children and young people with special needs (Mann & Sabatino, 1974) pose important implications for group care practice with children and young people. Piaget (1970) and Montessori (1964, 1973), amongst others, have influenced the development of teaching methods based on children's interactions with their physical environment in all learning situations. Some of the approaches derived from their work help to inform activity programming outside the classroom (Silberman, 1973; Weihs, 1971). Other educators have contributed directly to the knowledge base about practice with children and young people with learning disabilities (Bangs, 1968; Cruickshank, 1971; Cruickshank & Johnson, 1975; Frostig & Maslow, 1973; Frostig, 1976; Kirk, 1966). The development of social learning techniques in the special education classroom paralleled advances in the wider field of child and youth care, especially in the United States. The literature provides a rich source of practical advice for those working with children in the group care field (cf. Bijou, 1971; Bradfield, 1971; Brown & Christie, 1981; Hewett, 1969; Homme, 1969; Meisels, 1974; Pizzat, 1973). Special education has given considerable attention to the management of surface behavior in the classroom. Swift and Spivak (1974) highlighted the contributions made by teachers in this area of practice.

However, in spite of the potential for common ground between teachers and group care workers, such common ground frequently remains unrecognized in practice. Some have attempted to illuminate the common themes between special education and group care practice, most notably Apter (1982); Brendtro & Ness (1983); Brown & Christie (1981); Hobbs (1966); Kashti (1979); and Nash (1976) amongst others. From an ecological perspective, the school classroom plays a significant part in the lives of children, young people, and their families. More importantly, school classrooms need to be considered an integral part of group care practice with children and young people. Both the school and the group care center offer a sophisticated technology and legitimate goals that can be used for teaching social competencies to children and young people with special learning needs.

INDIVIDUAL LEARNING STYLES AND THE DEVELOPMENT OF SOCIAL COMPETENCIES

When attempting to think of a young person's total environment as a curriculum for teaching and learning social competencies, one is faced with the problem of connecting the practice goals and techniques used by group care workers with those used by classroom teachers and others. In many respects, shared practice involves finding a language that all staff can share, as suggested by Casson elsewhere in this volume. In other respects the task involves making a conscious effort to deal with a young person's functioning in the present, thereby avoiding the temptation to make diagnostic conclusions which over-emphasize difficulties in one area as the cause of overall learning problems. The initial strategy for effective competency development should be to set aside–at least temporarily–the labels and stereotypes children bring with them so that observable behaviors can be assessed and provisional conclusions reached about what is likely to work best with each child or young person. In this way, it is possible to build a common vocabulary for the development of competencies by looking at a child's *personal learning style*.

Learning style is something far more comprehensive than the rate at which a child or young person acquires learning or his/her overall temperament. Here, learning style refers to the level of competencies that each child or young person brings to the tasks of learning. Competence is shaped by a particular balance of developmental assets, strengths, and weaknesses that can be observed, recorded, and supplemented by specific developmental strategies (Lerner & Benson, 2002). Implicit in this notion is a view of the learning process that considers each child or young person as a *whole person*: as a unique being who receives, associates, and expresses him/herself through perception, cognitive functioning, affect, language, and motor functioning. Assessment of competencies in each mode of functioning helps to assist workers in responding more directly to the special needs of children and young people in group care practice.

Perception

The manner by which the brain interprets stimuli received by the sense organs–or perception–depends on the integration of previous sensory experiences and individual neurological patterns. Perception skills are critical for learning and can vary greatly from one young person to another. Children or young people who are referred to group care services frequently have difficulties with perceiving or working out what is expected from them both in relation to interactions with others and perception of basic visual and auditory cues. Competence in the area of visual perception influences the extent to which a young person is able to "tune in" to learning situations. Some children and young people are especially oriented to visual experiences and apparently learn most effectively through this channel.

However, a young person who is seriously lacking in developmental competencies or assets may consistently lose their place when reading, be unable to find things when they are right in front of them, or become disoriented in familiar surroundings. If a young person is unable to judge distances and spatial relationships with some level of confidence, then she or he may exaggerate footsteps when moving up or down stairs or move awkwardly across open ground. Many of the social behaviors associated with the condition known as dyslexia are related to such visual-perceptual confusion.

A developmental learning environment that reinforces structure, repetition, and consistency can help a child or young person to organize the day around specific tasks and is therefore strongly indicated for children and young people with visual-perceptual difficulties. Some of the elements that are likely to influence practice relationships include:

- *Laterality:* Social competence is affected by a young person's ability to see him or herself as the central figure in a space, distinguish right side from left side, top from bottom, and front from back. Development of social competencies with laterality are necessary for such tasks as moving through crowded spaces (a busy train, a shopping center, rugged terrain) or distinguishing right and left body parts (getting dressed, personal hygiene).

- *Directional Tendency:* A young person's social competence is influenced by the ability to orient his or her body towards a space outside him or herself. Development of social competencies of this type are necessary for such tasks as map reading, following directions to school or the shops, or helping with the laundry.
- *Figure-Ground Relations:* Social competencies are limited by a young person's ability to perceive objects in the foreground while at the same time blocking out background distractions. Developmental competencies in this area are necessary for such tasks as focusing attention on one word on a page while reading or finding a cooking utensil in a drawer while helping to prepare a meal.
- *Discrimination:* Social competencies in this area involve the ability to identify and respond to fine visual detail when required to distinguish between one form or object and another. Developmental competencies in this area are necessary in order to discriminate between the letters *f* and *t* and in order distinguish between a smile and a frown.
- *Closure:* A young person's social competencies frequently require being able to fill in the missing parts of an object when only some parts are shown. Such developmental competencies are necessary for tasks such as spelling in written form, reading road signs while riding on a bus, or playing video games.
- *Position in Space:* Children and young people are frequently required to discriminate between objects which have the same general form but vary in their spatial position. Developmental competencies such as these are necessary for such tasks as recognizing that the letters *b*, *d*, and *p* are different while reading, drawing pictures or geometric patterns on sheets of paper, or locating a room in a high-rise office block when invited to attend for an interview.

While some children and young people are "all eyes" as they make sense out of their environment though visual means, others are "all ears," learning most efficiently through the auditory channel. A young person with weak auditory perception is likely to say, "Huh?" as a first response to questions or instructions even when having little difficulty hearing what was said. Such a young person may forget instructions or follow them in the wrong sequence. During a lesson when the teacher is speaking, such a young person may pay more attention to workers and birds or motor sounds outside the classroom window. When asked to bring something to class the next day, she or he may forget or bring the wrong object. As with children who have problems of visual perception, young people with limited social competencies with audio perception may encounter as well as create a great deal of frustration in their social relations. Such young people may become withdrawn or stubbornly "deaf" in situations where they feel uncertain or frightened.

Auditory perception is the interpretation of stimuli sent from the ear to the brain. When working with young people who lack competencies with audio perception, practitioners need to resist making quick interpretations of emotional conflict or resistance (even though these may be apparent symptoms). Until simple accommodations are made by young people to their immediate environment, they will be unable to engage in learning. Practice tasks may include providing a quiet place for the child or young person to work or play, presenting tasks one at a time, using pictures of words for items and activities in the environment, emphasizing hand movements, and insisting on eye contact so that a child can "hear" what is said through watching the speaker's lips. Some of the elements group care workers can expect to encounter in their practice relationships include:

- *Foreground-Background:* Social competence in this area involves a young person's ability to focus on foreground sounds and block out background sounds. Social competencies in this area are necessary for such tasks as hearing a parent, teacher, or care worker give instructions in a noisy dining room or paying attention to the directions given by an adult in a busy shopping mall during a shopping trip.
- *Discrimination:* Social competencies are limited for a young person if she or he is unable to discriminate between different sounds or auditory stimuli. Social competencies are required in this area in order to hear the difference between *sat* and *sad* during a spelling test or the difference between *no* and *now* when an adult is giving instructions.
- *Sequencing:* A young person's social competencies are dependent upon the ability to interpret what is heard in the correct order of presentation. Such competencies are necessary in order to perform such tasks as hearing the difference between *bets* and *best* or discerning which is done first when making breakfast: put the egg

into a pan of boiling water or put the egg into a pan of water and bring it to the boil.

• *Closure:* Social competencies are affected by a young person's ability to fill in missing parts of a whole word or meaningful sequence of sounds. Such developmental competencies are important in order to learn new words, discern accents, or speak with proficiency to someone over the telephone.

Cognitive Functioning

It is tempting for teachers and some group care workers to dwell on cognitive functioning as the most important determinant of personal learning style. Cognitive ability certainly plays an important part in all areas of physical and social development but, in practice, it is not always easy to identify the precise nature of a child's social competencies in this area as distinct from others. An arbitrary distinction is made in what follows between language competencies and specific, measurable skills associated with cognitive functioning. It is hoped that such a distinction might assist practitioners to distinguish more clearly between several aspects of a young person's social competencies in the cognitive area.

The ability to think clearly, to move beyond concrete events to abstract reasoning, to develop complex ideas, and to assign objects or ideas to categories are but a few of the cognitive skills necessary in learning social competencies. As with language, the precise manner in which the brain develops and carries out these operations is not entirely understood. On the evidence available, it would seem that cognitive skills are partly constitutional and partly based on the relative variety and intensity of sensory experiences during early childhood (Piaget, 1963; Piaget & Inhelder, 1969). Actual opportunities to manipulate, touch, smell, or otherwise experience concrete objects and social encounters can be said to aid concept formation throughout life. Some of the essential cognitive operations associated with learning social competencies include:

• *Abstraction:* Social competencies of this type are required if a young person is to discern between numerous concrete events, elements, characteristics, and relationships. Such developmental competencies are necessary, for example, if a child or young person is to find his or her home in a row of similar-looking terraced houses. This requires dealing with the idea of home as different from the other houses that look the same as the one in which the child or young person lives.

* *Categorization:* A young person's social competencies in this area involve the ability to group experiences and objects into classes or categories based on similarity of type or function. Developmental competencies of this type are necessary in order for a young person to understand basic geometry, handle tools, or simply separate the laundry.

* *Generalization:* Social competence will be restricted in this area if a young person lacks the ability to infer causal relationships between specific events and particular consequences. Competencies in this area are necessary in order for a young person to use the Highway Code while riding a bicycle across town as compared with simply knowing how to ride a bicycle. Understanding the rules associated with advanced arithmetic or figuring out that hitting the baby will always make mother angry are other cognitive skills that require generalization from one situation to another.

* *Time Sense:* Social competencies in this area involve the ability to remain oriented to time and changes measured in time. Developmental competencies in this area are necessary in order to plan ahead or for matching available energies to the duration of a given task. Transfer of learning from home or classrooms to specific employment situations also requires such competencies.

* *Number Concepts:* In this area, a young person's social competencies are influenced by the ability to count and use simple numbers to represent quantity. Developmental competencies are required in relation to number concepts if a young person is to engage actively in the variety of social encounters required in a technological age.

* *Arithmetic Reasoning:* Social competencies in this area involve the ability to manage such concepts as equality, inequality, computation, and distribution in daily life. Developmental competencies in this area are necessary in order to complete tasks such as shopping, managing pocket money, and estimating costs.

A young person with noticeable confusion in patterns of cognitive functioning may seem far more of a puzzle than other youngsters in a group. Such a young person might have persistent trouble with "simple" tasks such as grouping, counting, or sorting objects by category. She or he may become confused when asked to list everything that is used in a workshop or may be unable to predict adult responses following repeated episodes of interaction. Young people like these may count on their fingers and be unable to give change or tell time. In many ways, a group care placement is ideally suited to the task of managing cognitive difficulty given the potential for restructuring and reinterpreting the social environment for each young person. The primary tasks for parents, teachers, and group care workers in these contexts can be seen as promoting a young person's inner organization by shaping learning environments which make sense for each child. Classroom or group homes can provide the venue in which young people can rehearse social competencies for use in future social environments.

Affect

Social competencies relating to affect or emotional functioning can be said to involve a broad category of skills that influence a child or young person's overall pattern of functioning. Mastery in this area includes the skills required to manage emotional turmoil, personal thoughts, and feelings. Competencies in this area also involve a range of skills associated with presentation of self in interpersonal relations. Affect competencies are highlighted with respect to the following areas:

- *Self-Image:* These developmental competencies involve a young person having accurate and positive thoughts and feelings about oneself. Such competencies are necessary for meaningful social interactions and for such tasks as tolerating one's own mistakes or learning to be more assertive in social relationships.
- *Impulse Control:* A young person's social competencies in this area involve the ability to monitor and control personal thoughts and actions. These competencies are necessary in order for a child to sustain attention in a given task or to learn to wait their turn.
- *Social Perception:* Social competencies in this area involve a young person's ability to "read" the emotional communications of others and to "hear" what is expected in given social situations. These developmental competencies are necessary for learning to make friends, for becoming part of a group, or avoiding expulsion from formal settings such as a library.
- *Social Judgment:* A young person's social competencies are influenced by the ability to weigh alternatives, probabilities, and potential consequences of actions in different social situations. Developmental competencies in this area are necessary for weighing up situations such as when to be assertive, when to walk away from a

fight, and working out how to save face in socially demanding circumstances.

- *Delayed Reward:* Social competencies are restricted for one who is unable to postpone gratification for future gain. Developmental competencies in this area are necessary for such tasks as saving one's pocket money to buy an expensive item of clothing or budgeting for personal care items between one pay packet and another.
- *Foresight:* These social competencies involve the ability to contemplate future events in the midst of current activities and circumstances. Developmental competencies in this area are necessary for planning ahead, developing action plans, and for maintaining conscious self-control of behaviors.
- *Motivation:* A young person's social competencies in this area involve the ability to take pleasure in and derive satisfaction from semi-autonomous achievement. Such developmental competencies are necessary if a young person is to learn how to read for pleasure, pursue hobbies, ride a bicycle, or engage in any other type of self-learning activity.
- *Adaptability:* Social competencies in this area involve a young person's ability to remain calm, focused, and persevering in the face of change. Developmental competencies in this area are necessary for mastering anxieties involved with change and transitions such as moving to another town, changing schools, starting work, ending a relationship, and so forth.
- *Body Image:* Social competencies for a young person in this area involve an internal awareness of bodily feelings as well as a conscious awareness of body feelings in space and time. Such developmental competencies are necessary to help a young person prepare for a first date, to modify impulses to behave dangerously, or to maintain purposeful involvement with selected peers.

Learning is clearly inhibited when a young person is handicapped by anxieties, rage, or a distorted self-image. Learning is also impaired when a child is unable to give and receive affection. In more subtle ways, learning is hampered in young people who cannot deal with sadness, joy, excitement, or who repeatedly stumbles in social situations because of misreading the emotional responses of others and her or his impact on others. A young person lacking in emotional competencies may be incapable of heeding danger in the face of risk-taking behavior or helplessly paralysed by anxiety. She or he may be unable to think and plan ahead, to know when the teacher or foster parents are angry, or to understand why other children in the playground avoid playing with her or him. Finally, she or he may be unable to take risks in relationships for fear of making mistakes, even though risk-taking is an important part of social learning.

Language

Most children and young people learn to manipulate language from a very early age. Word games and the nuances of meaning are often a source of continuing delight to them. For some young people, however, language may be slow or problematic. For these children, words and the use of words may be less a tool of social interaction than a perplexing barrier to full participation in social life. Several processes involved in language functioning and developmental competencies with language are outlined below:

- *Simple Vowel and Consonant Sounds:* Social competencies in this area include the ability to discriminate among language sounds and to produce particular sounds correctly. Such developmental competencies are necessary for pronouncing words correctly or for learning a foreign language.
- *Vocabulary:* The social competencies involve a young person's ability to understand the meaning of words including the comprehension of different meanings in different contexts. These developmental competencies are necessary for the correct interpretation of written and spoken communication and for fluency of speech.
- *Grammar:* A young person requires basic social competencies in this area in order to understand both surface and depth structures of sentences. Such developmental competencies are necessary for determining when a collection of words is a sentence, when sentences have meaning, when sentences with different word order can mean the same thing, and how the arrangement of words in a sentence indicates their relationship to each other. These social competencies may be critically important when a young person goes for a job interview or when explaining one's actions when interviewed by the police.
- *Auditory and Visual Reception:*[1] Social competencies in this area involve a young person's ability to derive meaning from oral communication or from information presented visually via rulebooks, guides, posters, or signboards. Developmental competencies of this kind are necessary for grasping the complex differences in-

volved in the question, "Did you hit Jimmy or did he hit you?" following a fight in the dining room. Such developmental competencies are also necessary in order to understand the action in a comic strip or to read non-verbal expressions on the face of an adult.

- *Auditory and Visual Association:* In this area, social competencies involve a young person's ability to understand relationships between words or concepts presented orally and visually. These developmental competencies are necessary for tasks such as filling the salt cellar and sugar bowl with a white, granular substance, selecting categories of picture on a video screen, or for anticipating danger when seeing a young child run into the street.

- *Verbal and Manual Expression:* Social competencies in this area involve the ability to express simple and complex meanings through both verbal and non-verbal means. Developmental competencies of this kind are necessary for a young person to tell a friend or adult about a school outing or when a child needs to explain which hand tool is needed if its name has been forgotten. In short, developmental competencies in this area are necessary for complete communication in almost all social situations.

Emotionally closed-up youngsters who also have distinct language difficulties may refuse to speak or may use mostly single words and simple sentences in their speech. Sentences they do use may seem confusing. In dealing with such young people, both teachers and group care workers need to be aware of a young person's difficulties with language and what this means for that child. The meaning of words in communications with others can become easily distorted by young people because of this difficulty. In order to be certain that a meaningful exchange is taking place, adults need to determine whether the young person cannot understand what is expected or whether she or he understands but is unable give a response. If the child cannot understand what is heard, she or he can be helped to attain enhance competencies by allowing more time to respond, by simplifying sentences, or by using pictures and gestures to facilitate meaning-making. If the young person has trouble with expression, assistance can be provided by adults asking questions that elicit more precise responses. For example, if an open-ended question such as "What would you like to do this afternoon?" elicits no response, then a closed question like "Would you like to go shopping?" may yield a more successful outcome.

Motor Functioning

An accurate evaluation of a young person's motor abilities is critically important for teachers as well as group care workers if responsive learning activities are to be implemented. Many children function best when they are actively involved physically in learning tasks. Movement and activity are likely to be distinctive features of their learning style in most situations. For the young person who is reasonably competent in terms of motor functioning, workers need to provide positive means for such skills to be exercised as well as maintaining a focus on the control of excess energy.

Young people with weak motor skills may be able to read or watch television but be unable to write legibly. For such children, classroom teachers may need to provide a tape recorder in order to avoid struggles related more to a child's physical difficulties with shaping words on paper than with emotional blocks to expression. Similarly, group care workers may need to arrange personal practice sessions before exposing a young person with under-developed motor skills to competitive play situations where she or he may experience failure and humiliation.

The general area of motor functioning may be examined as the development of social competencies that integrate large and small muscle activity. Developmental competencies with motor skills area are likely to include the following elements of performance:

- *Gross Motor Skills:* These social competencies involve the ability to use and coordinate the large muscles of the body including legs, arms, and back. Such developmental competencies are necessary for activities like running, jumping, or climbing.
- *Fine Motor Skills:* In this area, social competencies involve the ability to use and coordinate the small muscles of the body including fingers and wrist, ankles and toes, and so on. These developmental competencies are necessary for such activities as drawing, writing or cutting with scissors, ice skating, and dancing.
- *Eye-Hand Coordination:* Social competencies in this area involve the ability to control both eyes and hands at the same time to perform a task. Such developmental competencies are necessary for gross motor activities such as catching or kicking a ball. Such competencies are also necessary for such fine motor activities as drawing a picture, sewing, or operating a self-powered wheelchair.
- *Balance:* Social competencies in this area involve the ability to coordinate large and small muscles to maintain balance equilibrium.

These developmental competencies are necessary for a young person to engage in activities such as riding a bicycle, climbing a ladder, or hopping on one foot.

• *Posture:* In this area, social competencies involve a young person's ability to hold the body erect. Such developmental competencies are necessary for sustained activities such as sitting, standing, walking, or bicycle riding.

Motor skills are important for adaptation to every part of a young person's social environment. Motor functioning is a particular area where practice goals in the life-space of group care and curriculum goals in the classroom overlap. With opportunities for motor skill training such as football or dance practice during recreation periods, a young person can increase physical proficiency as well as develop social skills for interacting more responsively and competently with a peer group. Furthermore, motor skill training also helps improve body awareness, enhance self-confidence, and even extend specific skills such as keyboard skills in a classroom or computer lab. There is great deal of potential in this area for positive collaboration between teachers and group care workers, collaboration that will enhance their practice responsiveness with children and young people.

To summarize, consideration has been given to five developmental modes of functioning that shape individual learning styles and social competencies amongst children and young people. These five developmental modes are *perception, cognitive functioning, affect, language,* and *motor functioning.* It must be emphasized again, however, that learning is very much a dynamic process in which interaction takes place between all five developmental modes. In short, some level of integration is achieved across all five modes of functioning, integration that is likely to shape learning styles and social competencies for children and young people. Other abilities, such as attention and memory, are also influenced by each child or young person's integration of developmental skills. A young person's ability to pay attention when involved in a particular task is the most delicate of all developmental competencies. Memory is also a highly variable capacity for each person. Some young people have difficulties with specific recall of words and names while others can recite the alphabet backwards. Some children may have the uncanny ability to remember details in physical space while others keep asking directions to the bus station. Social competencies for children and young people in receipt of group care services require the support and encouragement of teachers and group care workers whose practices are complementary.

LEARNING STYLE AND THE LEARNING ENVIRONMENT

The value of looking at the whole person and emphasizing developmental competencies with observable skills is that workers can be eclectic in their approach to learning tasks with children and young people. More to the point, the emphasis on individual differences in learning style rather than individual pathology may assist workers to make more practical sense out of assessments and to formulate practical goals in learning environments committed to developing social competencies. Since the focus of attention is the child or young person as a whole person with a consistent learning style, then the *methodological emphasis* of any program changes as interventions are redefined and take on a strengths-based perspective.

As attention shifts to helping each child or young person to develop social competencies in any or all areas of functioning, workers can thus reinforce personal strengths and shift attention away from individual weaknesses. This represents an important technical and clinical shift in thinking for those engaged in group care practice. Although a young person's weak or problem areas are acknowledged, primary attention is given to existing competencies and developmental assets that can be nurtured (and which a child can learn to use on his/her own) in new learning situations. The whole group care program thus becomes a comprehensive learning environment responsive to different learning styles as well as special learning needs. Several program features require consideration if workers are to use their group care center as a learning environment for children and young people, where social competencies become the focus of primary attention.

Assessment of Competencies

In setting up responsive learning environments, group care workers need to record details about the personal learning style of each child or young person. Such a record may be informally held amongst a team of workers or, more helpfully, written in summary form in a quickly referenced file, as in Kardex or Problem-Oriented Record systems. Compiling a record of information about a young person's functioning must be understood as involving a process of continuous assessment rather than a diagnosis of the child's "problem." All too frequently workers are tempted to use assessment typologies to diagnose a child's problems and, just as frequently, approaches such as these have resulted in constant struggles around a young person's incompetence in social situations. With the focus on deficiency, everyone working with a child or young person and, more importantly, the young person him/herself, may be blind to areas of strength in the overall pattern of functioning. Even the most seriously handicapped or developmentally delayed young person has some capacity to learn, and she or he approaches learning with a special combination of strengths and aspirations as well as weaknesses.

The Daily Curriculum

In daily programming terms, an emphasis on social competencies requires that the learning opportunities available for children and young people should possess at least three basic attributes. First, the daily curriculum and expectations for every participant in the program needs to be easily comprehended by each young person. A young person should be able to understand where she or he is headed with particular learning tasks, what skills she or he is using or struggling to master in a given task, and how she or he can use existing skills to engage in problem solving.

Second, the daily curriculum needs to be directed at specific formal academic goals as well as goals associated with daily living. Non-specific or esoteric objectives may result in basic survival skills–reading, writing, and arithmetic–being unlearned, thus undermining social competencies that a child or young person requires when reaching school-leaving age. Basic cooking, laundry, and self-care skills are examples of concrete goals that might be established in any group care center for adolescents.

Finally, the daily curriculum needs to be seamless in that formal academic learning parallels learning in other areas of a young person's life. Ideally, a young person should experience learning to read as part of the process of growing up and changing that also includes learning how to make friends, purchase an item of clothing at a shopping center, or deal with angry feelings after an argument.

Selection of Curriculum Materials

The books, games, papers, puzzles, and other objects a teacher brings into a classroom as aids to learning are important factors in defining the physical impact of the classroom as a learning environment. In similar ways, group care centers make use of curriculum materials that can be used in the development of social competencies where a variety of materials are adapted to the learning styles of different children or young people. Two things are implied by such an approach. To begin with, curriculum materials need to include variety to take into account different learning styles, different learning content, and changes in the weather. Both indoor and outdoor curriculum materials are required so that children and young people can attain social competencies which can be used in a wide range of situations. The second point implied by this approach is that curriculum materials need to be chosen with maximum flexibility in mind. Here, the idea is that materials need to be used with more than one child or young person in different situations and in different combinations with other materials. In group care centers this applies to recreation and leisure-time materials including games, equipment, or craft supplies.

Use of Physical Space

Teachers can use their classroom environment as a physical instrument that enables implementation of curriculum objectives. In similar ways, group care workers can use their center as a learning environment for teaching social competencies. To begin with, teachers and group care workers need to consider how responsive the physical environment (classroom or center) is to individual learning styles and the competing demands that are made by children or young people and staff. As Maier (1982) suggested, "The Space We Create Controls Us" in many subtle and not so subtle ways. A second consideration involves the question of whether the physical environment is instructive, communicating the message that this is a learning environment where social skills are used and where developmental competencies can be learned. The physical environment can invite or intimidate those who inhabit that environment. To use a theatrical metaphor, the physical environment does not provide the script used in the learning drama which unfolds. The script is provided by the actors and actresses, each with a personal learning style. The physical environment provides the staging and props which give context to the drama and thereby influences the intensity of a given sequence of activities.

Social Climate in the Learning Environment

At least five important features require consideration if the climate of a group care and treatment center is to facilitate learning of social com-

petencies. One of the most obvious features involves a climate of respect for individual differences. Since few behavior management
techniques are both effective and meaningful for every child in a group,
it follows that workers should be willing and able to adjust certain rules
or regulations accordingly. A second feature which influences the climate of a center involves clarity of expectations in all areas. There
should be no unnecessary mysteries or surprises in a classroom or group
care center. Each part of the developmental living and learning curriculum should be as clear and unambiguous as possible. A third feature is
the attitude of support that is present within the climate of a center. Low
staff morale, disinterest, boredom, or preoccupations with priorities
elsewhere can have a significant impact on the learning potential available in a center.

This climatic feature is frequently influenced by a fourth feature involving the presence of sufficient back-up support that can be instantly
available to help manage disruptive behavior. No one person can be expected to engage extremely disruptive behavior on his or her own. Management of disruptive behavior needs to arouse as little attention as
possible to avoid either active or covert positive reinforcement until
both young person and worker(s) can agree to resume their shared
learning tasks. Such an approach requires high levels of staff teamwork
and acceptance of back-up assistance as another of the learning resources available, not a sign of staff weakness. Finally, careful attention
to group composition helps to minimize extreme variability in the behavior patterns of a group of children or young people, a feature considered further by Burford and Fulcher elsewhere in this volume.

Collaboration with and Support from Others

When seeking to establish learning environments that teach developmental competencies, it is necessary to consider all those in direct contact with children and young people as being teachers in the broadest
sense. The classroom teacher orients his or her learning objectives towards one set of goals, while group care workers are oriented to another
set of goals. To the extent that learning goals are complementary in both
school classrooms and group care centers, then the learning of social
competencies can be facilitated. The same argument holds for the service goals pursued by an attached social worker, a detached social
worker, or social service managers. Each staff member working with individual children or young persons or a group of young people will benefit from knowing which learning approaches work best for the other

workers. It may be helpful if time can be scheduled for different workers to spend some time working in the others' domains, such as a teacher being involved in after-school activities, a group care worker helping in the classroom, or a social worker helping with recreation activities. Such overlaps help to generate a fuller appreciation of the importance of coordinating all aspects of the learning environment. Administrative supports available at any group care center need to include arrangements for bringing workers together to share their daily experiences with children and young people. Rigid scheduling patterns and territorial boundary disputes can, and frequently do, undermine collaborative efforts in group care practice. In this way, important sources of support can be removed from workers and young people in their shared task of developing social competencies.

CONCLUSIONS

An overall commitment to promoting competencies rather than curing illness is perhaps one of the most important goals of practice in the group care field. Such a goal is more readily achieved if all those working with a young person take account of his or her overall pattern of functioning and personal learning style. Functioning in the areas of perception, cognitive functioning, affect, language, and motor skills are all important considerations in teaching children and young people skills that will enhance their social competencies in different situations. Assessment of competencies, as compared with diagnosing the problem, will help to inform the daily curriculum of practice and the curriculum materials needed to promote learning.

Planned uses of the physical environment can help to facilitate a social climate in the center that encourages learning. Finally, collaboration with others involved in a young person's life can offer valuable support to both children and caregivers alike. In short, the whole center program is a learning environment in which the goals of formal education in the classroom and goals in the life space of group care are closely intertwined.

NOTE

1. The Reception, Association, and Expressive categories used in this section on language functioning are based on the comprehensive work by Kirk (1966).

REFERENCES

Apter, S. J. (1982). *Troubled children/troubled systems*. Oxford: Pergamon Press.

Bangs, T. (1968). *Language and learning disorders of the pre-academic child*. New York: Appleton-Century-Crofts.

Bijou, S. (1971). *The exceptional child: Conditional learning and teaching ideas*. New York: M. S. S. Information Corporation.

Bradfield, R. (1971). *Behavior modification of learning disabilities*. San Rafael, CA: Academic Therapy Press.

Brendtro, L. K., & Ness, A. E. (1983). *Re-educating troubled youth: Environments for teaching and treatments*. New York: Aldine.

Brown, B. J., & Christie, M. (1981). *Social learning practice in residential child care*. Oxford: Pergamon Press.

Clarke, R. B., & Small, R. W. (1979). Schools as partners in helping. In J. K. Whitaker (Ed.), *Caring for troubled children*. San Francisco: Jossey-Bass.

Cruickshank, W. M. (1971). *Learning disabilities in home, school, and community*. Syracuse, NY: Syracuse University Press.

Cruickshank, W. M., & Johnson, G. (1975). *Education of exceptional children and youth*. Englewood Cliffs, NJ: Prentice-Hall.

Frostig, M. (1976). *Education for dignity*. New York: Grune & Stratton.

Frostig, M., & Maslow, P. (1973). *Learning problems in the classroom*. New York: Grune & Stratton.

Hewett, F. (1969). *The emotionally disturbed child in the classroom*. Boston: Allyn & Bacon.

Hobbs, N. (1966). Helping disturbed children: Psychological and ecological strategies. *American Psychologist, 21*(12), 1105-1151.

Homme, L. (1969). *How to use contingency contracting in the classroom*. Champaign, IL: Research Press.

Kashti, Y. (1979). *The socializing community: Disadvantaged adolescents in Israeli youth villages* (Monograph No. 1). Tel Aviv: University of Tel Aviv, Studies in Educational Evaluation.

Kirk, S. A. (1966). *The diagnosis and remediation of psycholinguistic abilities*. Urbana, IL: University of Illinois Press.

Lerner, R. M., & Benson, P. L. (Eds.). (2002). *Developmental assets and asset building communities: Implications for research, policy and practice*. New York: Kluwer Academic/Plenum Publishers.

Maier, H. W. (1982). The space we create controls us. *Residential Group Care and Treatment, 1*(1), 51-59.

Mann, L., & Sabatino, D. (1974). *The second review of special education*. New York: Grune & Stratton.

Meisels, L. (1974). The student's social contract: Learning social competence in the classroom. *Teaching Exceptional Children, 7*(1), 34-36.

Montessori, M. (1964). *The Montessori method* [1912]. New York: Schocken Books.

Montessori, M. (1973). *From child to adolescence* [1939]. New York: Schocken Books.

Nash, C. (1976). *The learning environment: A practical approach to the education of the three-, four-, and five-year-old*. Toronto: Methuen.

Piaget, J. (1963). *The language and thought of the child*. New York: Basic Books.

Piaget, J. (1970). *Science of education and the psychology of the child.* New York: Grossman, Orion Press.

Piaget, J., & Inhelder, B. (1969). *The psychology of the child.* New York: Basic Books.

Pizzat, F. (1973). *Behavior modification in residential treatment for children: Model of a program.* New York: Behavioral Publications.

Silberman, C. (1973). *The open classroom reader.* New York: Random House.

Swift, M., & Spivak, G. (1974). Therapeutic teaching: A review of teaching methods for behaviorally troubled children. *Journal of Special Education, 8*(3), 259-289.

Trieschman, A. E. (1969). Understanding the nature of a therapeutic milieu. In A. E. Trieschman, J. K. Whittaker, & L. K. Brentro (Eds.), *The other 23 hours: Child care work with emotionally disturbed children in a therapeutic milieu* (pp. 1-50). NY: Aldine de Gruyter.

Weihs, T. J. (1971). *Children in need of special care.* London: Souvenir Press.

Chapter 4

Group Care Practitioners as Family Workers

Frank Ainsworth

SUMMARY. This article sets out a rationale and provides a model for family work by group care practitioners. In doing so it points out that practitioners will need to avoid parent blaming attitudes and become family-centered rather than simply child-focused. Thus the critical issues to be addressed are how to ensure that a group care program is from an organization, policy, and practice perspective congruent with a family-centered model.

If it is not, then a program is unlikely to be able to work successfully with birth parents and family members. Birth parents and family members will instead feel alienated and, as a result, are unlikely to cooperate with the group care program and the practitioner workforce. In fact, the program will have failed to incorporate family members into the care and treatment plan and to work with them as partners in this process even when it is in the best interest of a child or youth. *[Article copies available for a fee from The Haworth Document Delivery Service: 1-800-HAWORTH. E-mail address: <docdelivery@ haworthpress.com> Website: <http://www.HaworthPress.com> © 2005 by The Haworth Press, Inc. All rights reserved.]*

Address correspondence to: Frank Ainsworth, School of Social Work and Community Welfare, James Cook University, Townsville 4811, Queensland, Australia.

[Haworth co-indexing entry note]: "Group Care Practitioners as Family Workers." Ainsworth, Frank. Co-published simultaneously in *Child & Youth Services* (The Haworth Press, Inc.) Vol. 27, No. 1/2, 2005, pp. 75-86; and: *Group Care Practice with Children and Young People Revisited* (ed: Leon C. Fulcher, and Frank Ainsworth) The Haworth Press, Inc., 2006, pp. 75-86. Single or multiple copies of this article are available for a fee from The Haworth Document Delivery Service [1-800-HAWORTH, 9:00 a.m. - 5:00 p.m. (EST). E-mail address: docdelivery@haworthpress.com].

doi:10.1300/J024v27n01_04

KEYWORDS. Group care, residential care, residential treatment, group homes, youth work, youthwork, group work, at-risk youth, family work, therapeutic milieu

INTRODUCTION

A decade has passed since Whittaker and Pfeiffer wrote that "there continues to be deep and enduring scepticism about the reformability of . . . group care settings" (1994, p. 584). Since then little has changed. Voices that advocate discontinuing the use of group care facilities for children and youth are still to be heard (Barth, 2002) while others attempt to diminish the value of group care (Chamberlain, 2003). For example, an alternative social intervention for antisocial youth, specifically, Multidimensional Treatment Foster Care (MTFC), is promoted by using group care programs as an example of failure (Chamberlain, 2003).

This approach is taken regardless of the fact that the research results about MTFC can stand alone and show that MTFC is effective and deserves to be one service option, just like group care, in a range of child and family welfare services. For Chamberlain (2003) this is not enough, and she makes a comparison between the outcomes of MTFC and group care to try to prove a point. To this end she uses aggregated data from 11 community-based group homes that do not conform to any identifiable group care program model as a comparison against which to measure MTFC. This is neither necessary nor appropriate, since group homes are at best an accommodation and support option and are not designed or resourced as treatment programs. The comparison is worthless. In the decade since Whittaker and Pfeiffer's (1994) analysis there has been a push to make group care programs child-focused and family-centered (Ainsworth, 1991, 1997; Ainsworth & Small, 1995; Ainsworth, Maluccio, & Small 1996; Landsman, Groza, Tyler, & Malone, 2001; Powell, 2000; Garfat, 2003). There has also been an attempt to map what is known about the effectiveness of group care programs (Ainsworth, 2001) rather than their ineffectiveness.

These efforts auger well for child and youth care workers as they give direction to the field. Child and youth care practice will have to increasingly be evidence-based if it is to gain continuing professional recognition and meet new demands for accountability (Ainsworth & Hansen, 2002). Of course, it can be argued that many group care programs and their practitioner work force are hostile to families and are keen to blame parents or adult caretakers for the mental health problems and difficult behaviors of those "at-risk" children and youth who populate these programs (Ainsworth, 1991; Ainsworth & Hansen, 2000; Reder, Duncan, & Gray 1993; Scott & O'Neil, 1996). If child and youth care workers are to successfully undertake family work there must be change from this position, and this is not an easy task.

A first step in the process of moving away from a position of blaming parents and becoming family-centered is an examination of the organizational and policy environment of a group care program. This has to be followed by clarification of the role of child and youth care workers in regard to work with families. This clarification then leads to the identification of the current areas of group care practice that offer opportunities for working with parents and family members. In addition, if their role is to be extended to include work with families, any new knowledge and skill child and youth care workers need has to be identified.

A DEFINITION

Before child and youth care workers can successfully engage in family work an essential prerequisite is an organizational and policy environment that supports practices that are compatible with a child-focused and family-centered approach. The following definition highlights these issues.

> Family centered group-care practice is characterized by institutional structures, services, and professional practices designed to preserve and, wherever possible, to strengthen connections between child(ren) in placement and their birth parents and family members. Whether the function of group care is to provide short-term shelter, long-term care or residential treatment, education or training, a primary goal is always to work towards the child's optimum involvement in family life, even in situations where total reunification is not possible. (Small, Ainsworth, & Hansen 1994)

Recognition of the importance of birth parents and extended family is well supported by research evidence from several sources about the search by adoptees for their family of origin (Depp, 1982; Triseliotis, 1973) and of the lifelong anguish of relinquishing mothers in regard to the child they bore yet gave away (Howe, 1991; Standing Committee on Social Issues, 2000; Wells, 1993). Further support is drawn from studies of children leaving group care without access to family networks which they then decide to reconstruct (Festinger, 1983; Jones & Moses, 1984; Stein & Carey, 1986). Other studies about children sent from Britain by child welfare organisations to Canada, South Africa, and Australia (Bean & Melville, 1989) who later engaged in searches for their relatives in distant lands also confirm this position.

They indicate the importance of incorporating birth parents and family members into group care programs as partners in the care and treatment process. This of course does not mean that parents and family members will always be able to be equal partners in this process. But it does mean that their contribution, no matter how small, will be respected and greatly appreciated.

Alongside this the empirical evidence from model-building research shows that group care programs that are family-centered score well on scales of services available to birth parents and families, parental involvement in decision making, and positive worker attitudes towards parents and family members (Ainsworth, 1997). A validated measurement instrument (Trieschman Family Centred Group Care Instrument [TFCGCI], 1997) that a group care program can use is also available to for those programs that want to measure the extent to which their policy and practice is compatible with a family-centered approach. The use of this instrument then allows group care programs to identify areas that require change if the program is to be truly family centered (Ainsworth, 2001).

Group care programs that embrace a family-centered approach have a very different structure compared to other facilities. Movement to a family-centered position requires attention to organisational change processes. Child and youth care workers also have to fully endorse this definition. This can be difficult, especially for inexperienced workers, when they are faced with demanding, aggressive and, at times, uncooperative behaviours from both birth parents, family members, and children and youth. Under these circumstances the temptation is to focus on rescuing the child or youth (VanderVen, 1981) and blaming the birth parent and family members for their child or youth's difficulties. This is self-defeating activity that only diminishes the impact of the group care program.

THE CHANGE PROCESS

The first step in the change process that moves a program from a traditional child-centered perspective toward a family-centered approach is the adoption of a values perspective that is consistent with what Fox-Harding (1991) has described as "the modern defence of birth family and parental rights." This perspective sees parents not solely as perpetrators of harm but as partners in the care and treatment process. It underlies the "no blame" approach to work with families (Ainsworth, 1991; Reder, Duncan, & Gray, 1993; Scott & O'Neil, 1996) who are often as vulnerable as the children and youth who are placed in a group care program.

This approach adopts the view that birth parents and families themselves are stressed psychologically and environmentally and have, as a consequence, restricted coping and adaptation capacity (McCubbin, Thompson, & McCubbin, 1996). The task is for a group care program and child and youth care workers to position themselves in such a way as to gain the confidence of the birth parents and family members so that they can work with both the child or youth and the parents as partners in any change effort. This has to be done in such a way as to ameliorate these stresses and any behaviours, from any party, that may negatively impact children or youth.

DIRECT WORK WITH PARENTS AND FAMILY MEMBERS

So what can child and youth care workers reasonably expect to be able to do with birth parents and other family members, given the inevitable role and time constraints? Should they be a child advocate, family counsellor, family mediator, family therapist, family support worker, parent educator or, as VanderVen (2003) suggests, an activity promoter or coordinator?

A starting point for consideration of this issue is Ainsworth's (1981) seven areas of child and youth worker activity and skill (Ainsworth, 1981; 1996; Ainsworth & Fulcher, 1985; Central Council for Training and Education in Social Work, 1983): organization of the care environment, team functioning, activity programming, working with groups, on the spot counselling, use of everyday life events, and developmental scheduling. Child and youth care workers have to have these areas of knowledge and skill to be effective practitioners. The four examples given below of what constitutes each skill area are not exhaustive, they are simply illustrative.

Organisation of the Care Environment

- Understanding how a group care program fits into the surrounding community environment and identification of any areas of discord, noting the consequences of this for participants in the program.

- Recognition of the advantages/disadvantages imposed by the programs' physical space.
- Assessment of the space and equipment usage in the program and how these positively or negatively affect privacy, confidentiality, and choice for program participants.
- Management of community relations, the program space, and equipment to maximize the physical and emotional comfort of program participants as a foundation for a healthy learning environment.

Team Functioning

- Capacity to maintain a positive involvement in team meetings and in contributing to team morale.
- Awareness of the impact on program participant of differing approaches by team members to a common issue or problem and a willingness to modify one's own approach where necessary.
- Ability to carry shared responsibility with another team member for a particular portfolio or area of activity.
- Capacity to work on behalf of the group care program with another external agency while keeping the team up to date with any developments.

Activity Programming

- Ability to plan, implement, and evaluate a successful recreational activity for program participants.
- Accept responsibility for marking an important life event for a program participant, for example, a birthday.
- Capacity to deliberately use a personal life interest as a means of providing program participants with new creative experiences and satisfaction.
- Ability to use an activity to teach program participants a range of basic life skills.

Working with Groups

- Capacity to monitor group processes and intervene if these processes take on a negative tone.

- Ability to plan, implement, and evaluate an agreed group work intervention on behalf of the team.
- Work with another team member to devise a recreational, educational, or therapeutic event for a group of program participants.
- Take a lead role, as necessary, in managing a key worker/participants program meeting.

On-the-Spot Counselling

- Provide immediate counselling support for program participants who are distressed or whose behaviour is unusual, difficult, or disruptive to the program.
- Recognise and respond to casually expressed concerns by program participants that indicate a recent or forthcoming event is causing an unusual level of stress or anxiety.
- Use the opportunity provided by shared living tasks to review difficulties that have arisen during the day and encourage new ways of dealing with such events.
- Intervene in areas of tension or conflict between program participants and resolve matters through mediation and negotiation, not through the use of power.

Use of Everyday Life Events

- Assist program participants to develop high level skills in ordinary everyday life tasks.
- Accept responsibility for involving program participants in important areas of daily living, for example, cleaning services.
- Discuss with program participants issues of personal presentation and hygiene and encourage a change in behaviour when necessary.
- Ensure that personal property and private space of program participants is respected.

Developmental Scheduling

- Assess the needs of a program participant and schedule activity that will enhance the participants' skill level, for example, interpersonal relating.
- Educate a program participant about the consequences of a particular condition that may limit future opportunities in such a way

that becomes less stressful and threatening, for example, asthma and diabetes.

- Teach a program participant a new skill that allows them to advance to the next life stage more confidently, for example, anger management.
- Encourage the growth of a neglected talent, for example, the playing of a musical instrument.

Finally, these skill areas need to interact with each other in order to make for a dynamic and effective group care teaching and learning environment (Ainsworth & Fulcher, 1985).

LEARNING, ROLE, KNOWLEDGE, AND SKILL

This list of skills and responsibilities helps one identify any additional knowledge and skills child and youth care workers may need. One area of knowledge that is required is in regard to the different ways children and youth and birth parents and family members learn. Ainsworth (1996a) describes Bronfenbrenner's three types of learning dyads:

> The first is the *observational dyad*, as when a parent sees a child and youth care worker managing a child's difficult behavior. The second type of dyad is a *joint activity dyad*, that allows for learning through shared experience, as when a birth parent or family member learns important household and management of the environment skills from a child and youth care worker through sharing a common task. This shared joint activity dyad consolidates the care process between child, birth parent, and child and youth care worker. Finally, we have the child and youth care worker and birth parents' *primary dyad*, which incorporates learning from both the observational dyad and the joint activity dyad. The importance of this primary dyad is that, in Bronfenbrenner's (1979) words, it "continues to exist phenomenologically for both participants even when they are not together" (p. 58). In this instance the child and youth care worker who has the potential to influence a birth parent's behavior even when he or she is no longer physically present. (p. 21)

Bearing these dyads in mind, child and youth care workers can use each of the seven areas of skill outlined in this model of family-centered group care practice (Ainsworth 1981, 1996b, 1997) to begin to undertake family work. Birth parents and family members can be incorporated at various times into each area of activity (Ainsworth & Hansen, 1986). In doing so child and youth care workers will be able to begin to do family work.

This is not through some exploration of a birth parent's internal psychological process or a family member's life-long grievances. It is through the use of real life situations and events as a way to engage hard to reach parents and family members and to teach child-rearing and nurturing skills. Child and youth care workers role in family work is not that of counsellor or therapist. Their roles are as a parent educator, trainer, and supporter. This is in line with recent empirical research that confirms that it is disruption to the parenting process as a product of macro-economic and environmental stress that leads to anti-social behavior in children and youth (Weatherburn & Lind, 2001). Child and youth care workers need to heed this new knowledge when making a family assessment or when designing a family-focused intervention. For example, teaching parents and family members new child-rearing and monitoring skills is likely to be helpful in reducing stress and anxiety and that in itself will be immensely therapeutic.

Added to the above are newer modes of practice that have the potential to enrich at least two of the Ainsworth (1981, 1996, 1997; Ainsworth & Fulcher, 1985) skills areas. Life Space Crisis Intervention (LSCI), a well developed modality for use in group situations in schools and group care programs, clearly enhances the skills required for on-the-spot counselling (Fecser & Long, 2000). Also of value is the Therapeutic Crisis Intervention (TCI) package that teaches deescalation and conflict resolution techniques (Bath, 1998). In addition, the EQUIP program (Gibbs, Potter, & Goldstein, 1995) that uses a group format to teach anger management and for promoting moral development through a peer helping approach, gives child and youth care workers a further avenue through which to advance their skills in working with groups. These new formats have yet to be fully integrated into child and youth care practice even though they seem to have much to offer practitioners as they struggle to make a difference to the lives of children and families.

CONCLUSION

The critical issues for child and youth care workers in relation to family work are how to ensure that the group care program is, from an organization, policy, practice, and worker attitudes perspective, congruent with a family-centered model of practice. If it is not, then the program is unlikely to be able to work successfully with birth parents and family members. Birth parents and family members will then feel alienated and are unlikely to cooperate with the group care program. In fact, the program will have failed to incorporate them into any care or treatment plan and to work with them as partners in the care and treatment process even when it is in the best interest of a child or youth.

REFERENCES

Ainsworth, F. (1981). The training of personnel for group care with children. In F. Ainsworth & L. C. Fulcher (Eds.), *Group care for children: Concept and issues* (pp. 225-244). London: Tavistock.

Ainsworth, F. (1991). A "no blame" approach to work with families of children and adolescents in residential care. *Child and Youth Care Forum, 20*(5), 301-311.

Ainsworth, F. (1996a). Group care workers as parent educators. *Child and Youth Care Forum, 25*(1), 17-28.

Ainsworth, F. (1996b). Parent education and training or family therapy: Does it matter which comes first? *Child and Youth Care Forum, 25*(2), 101-110.

Ainsworth, F. (1997). *Family centered group care: Model building.* Aldershot: Ashgate.

Ainsworth, F. (2001). After ideology: The effectiveness of residential programs for "at risk" adolescents. *Children Australia, 26*(2), 11-18.

Ainsworth, F., & Fulcher, L. C. (Eds.). (1985). Group care practice with children. In L. C. Fulcher & F. Ainsworth (Eds.), *Group care practice with children* (pp. 1-18). London: Tavistock.

Ainsworth, F., & Hansen, P. (1986). Incorporating natural family members into residential programs for children and youth. *Australian Child and Family Welfare 11*(1), 12-15.

Ainsworth, F., & Hansen, P. (2000). Social workers' view of parents of emotionally disturbed children: Replication of a U.S. study. *Australian Social Work, 53*(3), 37-43.

Ainsworth, F., & Hansen, P. (2002). Evidence-based social work practice: A reachable goal. *Social Work and Social Sciences Review, 10*(2), 36-49.

Ainsworth, F., & Small, R. W. (1995). Family-centered group care practice: Concept and implementation. *Journal of Child & Youth Care Work, 10*, 9-14.

Ainsworth, F., Maluccio, A. N., & Small, R. W. (1996). A framework for family centered group care practice: Guiding principles and practice implications. In D. Braziel (Ed.), *Family focused practice in out-of-home care: A handbook and resource directory* (pp. 35-55). Washington, DC: Child Welfare League of America.

Barth, R. (2002). *Institutions vs. foster homes. The empirical base for a century of action.* Report for the Annie E. Casey Foundation. Chapel Hill, NC: University of North Carolina, School of Social Work, Jordan Institute for Families.

Bath, H. (1998). *Therapeutic crisis management: Training manual.* Canberra: Marymead Child and Family Centre.

Bean, P., & Melville, J. (1989). *The lost children of the empire*. London: Unwin Hyman.
Bronfenbrenner, U. (1979). *The ecology of human development*. Cambridge: Harvard University Press.
Central Council for Education and Training in Social Work (1983). *A practice curriculum in group care*. London: CCETSW Paper 14.2.
Chamberlain, P. (2003). *Treating chronic juvenile offenders. Advances made through the Oregon multidimensional treatment foster care model*. Washington, DC: American Psychological Association.
Depp, D. C. (1982). After reunion: Perceptions of adoptees, adoptive parents, and birth parents. *Child Welfare, 61*(2), 115-119.
Fecser, A. F., & Long, N. J. (2000). *Life space crisis intervention*. Hagerstown, MD: Institute for Psychoeducational Training (available at www.air.org/cecp).
Festinger, T. (1983). *No one ever told us . . . postscript to foster care*. Washington, DC: Child Welfare League of America.
Fox Harding, L. (1991). *Perspectives in child care policy*. London: Longman.
Garfat, T. (Ed.). (2003). *A child and youth care approach to working with families*. New York: The Haworth Press, Inc.
Gibbs, J., Potter, G., & Goldstein, A. P. (1995). *The EQUIP program. Teaching youth to think and act responsibly through a peer helping approach*. Champaign, IL: Research Press.
Howe, D. (1991). *Half a million women*. London: Penguin Books.
Landsman, M., Groza, V., Tyler, M., & Malone, K. (2001). Outcomes of family-centered residential treatment. *Child Welfare, 80*(3), 351-379.
Jones, M. A., & Moses, B. (1984). *West Virginia's former foster children, their experience and lives as young adults*. Washington, DC: Child Welfare League of America.
McCubbin, H. I., Thompson, A. I., & McCubbin, M. A. (1996). *Family assessment: Resiliency, coping and adaptation*. Madison, WI: University of Wisconsin Publishers.
Powell, J. Y. (2000). *Family-centered services in residential treatment. New approaches for group care*. New York: The Haworth Press, Inc.
Reder, P., Duncan, S., & Gray, M. (1993). *Beyond blame: Child abuse tragedies revisited*. London: Routledge.
Scott, D., & O'Neil, D. (1996). *Beyond child rescue. Developing family centered practice at St Luke's*. Sydney, Australia: Allen and Unwin.
Small, R. W., Ainsworth, F., & Hansen, P. (1994). *The Carolina's project—Working paper No. 1*. Needham, MA: Albert E. Trieschman Center.
Standing Committee on Social Issues (2000). *Adoption in New South Wales*. Legislative Council. Sydney, Australia.
Stein, M., & Carey, K. (1986). *Leaving care*. Oxford: Basil Blackwell.
Trieschman Family Centred Group Care Instrument (TFCGCA). (1997). In F. Ainsworth (Ed.), *Family centered group care: Model building*. Aldershot: Ashgate.
Triseliotis, J. (1973). *In search of origins: The experience of adopted people*. London: Routledge Kegan Paul.
VanderVen, K. (1981). Patterns of career development in group care. In F. Ainsworth, & L. C. Fulcher (Eds.), *Group care for children: Concept and issues* (pp. 201-224). London: Tavistock.
VanderVen, K. (2003). Activity oriented family focused child and youth work in group care: Integrating streams of thought into a river of progress. In T. Garfat (Ed.),

Working with families: A child and youth care approach. New York: The Haworth Press, Inc.

Weatherburn, D., & Lind, B. (2001). *Delinquent-prone communities.* Cambridge: Cambridge University Press.

Wells, S. (1993). What do birth mothers want? *Adoption and Fostering, 17*(4), 22-26.

Whittaker, J. K., & Pfeiffer, S. I. (1994). Research priorities in residential group child care. *Child Welfare, 73*(5), 583-601.

SECTION 2:
WORKING INDIRECTLY
TO SUPPORT CHILDREN,
YOUNG PEOPLE, AND FAMILIES

Chapter 5

Primary Care in Secondary Settings:
Inherent Strains

Henry W. Maier

Introduction by Thom Garfat

SUMMARY. There is an ever present struggle associated with reconciling *primary* care requirements for children and young people living in group care programs with *secondary* organizational demands imposed by external agency expectations and administrative requirements. That struggle finds its expression and potential balance in the daily work of staff. This

[Haworth co-indexing entry note]: "Primary Care in Secondary Settings: Inherent Strains." Maier, Henry W., and Thom Garfat. Co-published simultaneously in *Child & Youth Services* (The Haworth Press, Inc.) Vol. 27, No. 1/2, 2005, pp. 87-116; and: *Group Care Practice with Children and Young People Revisited* (ed: Leon C. Fulcher, and Frank Ainsworth) The Haworth Press, Inc., 2006, pp. 87-116. Single or multiple copies of this article are available for a fee from The Haworth Document Delivery Service [1-800-HAWORTH, 9:00 a.m. - 5:00 p.m. (EST). E-mail address: docdelivery@haworthpress.com].

doi:10.1300/J024v27n01_05

classic manuscript in the literature of child and youth care offers an enduring analysis of the interplay between primary and secondary care issues that
shape responsive group care services. *[Article copies available for a fee from
The Haworth Document Delivery Service: 1-800-HAWORTH. E-mail address:
<docdelivery@haworthpress.com> Website: <http://www.HaworthPress.com>*

KEYWORDS. Group care, residential care, residential treatment, group
homes, youth work, youthwork, group work, at-risk youth, care workers,
ecology of care, direct care

IN BED AT NOON:
AN UPDATE TO HENRY MAIER'S ORIGINAL CHAPTER

To call a piece of writing a classic suggests that there is something
about it that endures through time and a changing field of service. In this
sense Henry Maier's chapter, written some 30 years ago, has become a
classic in group care practice with young people, because it has influenced the evolution of the field since its first writing. Suggesting that a
work is a classic also suggests that there is some enduring truth contained in the writing that has not altered with time. In this sense too,
Henry's chapter rests as a classic in the field. The material that Maier
has distilled for us here is based on the most soundly accepted systemic
and ecological principles which have, themselves, shown an enduring
strength. While it might be possible, therefore, in an "update" such as
this to draw new examples or call on new references, they would only
serve to highlight the original points, not expand on them. As Maier said
in this chapter, "In general, the tendency is for organizational requirements to modify special individual care requirements." This basic
theme, which permeates everything in the chapter, requires no updating: It is as true today as it was when first written.

Henry (he did prefer to be called Henry) made a distinction between
the primary and secondary demands or requirements placed on the caregiver working in the group care environment. He highlights the potentially restricting impact of the ecological organizational context on the
focus of staff and shows how the demands of the organization tend to
take precedence over the primary responsibility of the staff: the care and
treatment of the young people. This detailed concentration on the context of the child care workers' primary responsibility introduced clearly

to the field, as had some of Maier's earlier writings, the need to attend to how the organizational reality influences the work of the staff (Maier, 1979a, 1979b).

Subsequent years have seen an increased interest in this area. Durrant (1993), Fewster (1990), Garfat (1998), Krueger (1991), Osler (1993), Ricks (1989), VanderVen (1993), and even Henry (1994) have continued the call to attend to context, especially as it impacts on the interventions of the care worker. Yet while the impact of context on intervention has become to some extent another maxim of the field, little attention has been devoted within the field to the implications of the specific organizational context except to acknowledge its presence. While one occasionally finds acknowledgement that "certain characteristics of the agency, service system, and broader society impinge on the work situation such as agency policy, administration, and supervisory structure, the relative connectedness or isolation of the setting with regard to the larger community and the respect and esteem that the group care field is accorded" (Peters & Mandle, 1991, p. 297), little seems to have changed.

One is left to wonder why this is so and, perhaps, the only answer lies in the tendency of organizational management to perceive the organization as benevolent and supportive, allowing little room for a consideration of how this context impacts harmfully on the primary responsibilities of the care staff and what might be done to bring a greater balance between these two important demands. For it is surely as true today, as it was then when Henry originally presented this chapter, that "primary, individualized care concerns tend to give way to those of secondary, organizational power."

Interestingly, perhaps, is that the main concern to be taken from this chapter by the field as a whole is Henry's emphasis on "care for the caregiver." For buried here among observations on organizational context, the clinical work of caregiving, recognition of the importance of professional status, and the acknowledgment that, for example, team meetings are often overwhelmed by administrative demands, is a clear recognition that the caregiver is in need of care. To quote from this chapter again, "The quality of care and training of children is directly related to the sense of well-being experienced by their care-givers." Or, as Henry said later, "Caregivers are enriched or limited as agents of care according to the care they receive" (Maier, 1987, p. 19).

This call by Henry for care for the caregiver, echoing as it did the earlier work of Bronfenbrenner (1979) and Fulcher (1983), has found a permanent place in the literature of group care (see, for example,

Kerins, 1995; Ricks, 1992; Smith, 2002). Almost everything one reads about the quality of care offered to children and their families notes the need for support and nurture for the caregivers themselves. Yet it is a cry usually ignored by the organizations offering such services. While occasionally one hears of an agency within which caregivers do genuinely feel cared for, it would appear that such is the exception rather than the rule.

While we may have expanded our awareness of the needs of caregivers with regard to skills and knowledge (see, for example, *North American Consortium of Child and Youth Care Education Programs*), and self, including that of the caregiver, has become central to the effective intervention process (see, for example, Fewster, 1990; Garfat, McElwee, & Charles, in press), we have failed dismally as a field to heed Henry's call for a change in how we attend to the needs of the workers. Indeed, many would argue that with increased administrative demands, reducing budgets, and other additional strains, if anything, we have slipped backwards.

And, thus, this chapter remains a classic: filled with truths as yet unrealized, replete with significant recommendations as yet unfilled, and echoing still the cry for a different approach to acting on the context of caregiving. That it is republished here offers hope for a new generation of caregivers. Thanks, Henry.

Thom Garfat
Rosemere, Quebec

INTRODUCTION

The ever present struggle of reconciling primary care requirements of children and young people living in group care facilities with the program's secondary organizational demands finds its expression and potential balance in the daily work of the child and youth care staff. Actually, workers seem to be serving two masters. The following account of a staff meeting at a prestigious child care agency serving forty severely disturbed elementary and high-school age youngsters has all the symptoms of the aforementioned strain. I submit that the underlying themes[1] are inherent in staff deliberations almost anywhere.

Let us look in on a typical one-and-a-half-hour staff meeting. Forty minutes have been taken up with general announcements, enquiries, administrative admonitions, and "success proclamations." Finally, the main topic of the particular staff session was raised: In which way can we strengthen the group care components of the residential program? This topic was introduced and interpreted by the group life supervisor expressing the need for more precisely tailored individual approaches to the residents' therapeutic requirements. One worker immediately elaborated on her idea that she could do more for the children if she were to work solely on weekdays. It seemed that the children with whom she was the most involved tended to be away on weekends. Additionally, she pointed out, on Mondays and Tuesdays these children were apt to have their difficult days, coinciding with the time she was off-duty. Numerous other valid suggestions were brought up, each one involving potential alterations in each worker's investment in time or personal energy.

Workers also volunteered specific program suggestions for selected children and recommended different care practices for a particular sub-unit. These latter suggestions created both excitement and frustrations. A member of the administrative staff, in the midst of this lively discussion, wondered with serious concern whether or not these valid suggestions may not lead to a kaleidoscope of practices and potentially a separate group care program for each resident! Another worker quickly added that the administrator was right: The suggestions would result in a unit with extremely poor organization. Someone else added ironically: "These kids could then get up at any hour of the day. Maybe then the evening shift can see how it is to get the youngsters to straighten out their rooms rather than always creating a mess."

At this point, other workers voiced in turn their readiness for more personal involvement with the children. Several questioned with sincerity whether they could muster the energy for added personal care engagement, particularly with the difficult children under discussion. Somehow the perennial request surfaced about keeping the children's play areas free of office staff cars so that the children and care workers could play unhampered. This concern was pushed aside with embarrassed laughter and the meeting continued as before, by more or less acknowledging all input but dealing with none.

Towards the end of the allotted meeting time, a residential worker recommended a trade-off in more time with the kids in exchange for less paperwork. This suggestion, which received an affirmative sigh from many workers, reminded the agency director (who chaired the session) that he was about to take up the issue of recording with the care staff. He wanted their assistance in finding ways the agency could more effectively manage their recordings and to verify the residents' progress. He regretted that time had run out too quickly for this "lively and productive" staff meeting. The issue of alternative ways of recording was recommended as the major topic for next month's staff meeting.

What happened in this staff session seems to be merely an echo of what happens on the front lines of group care practice. In the treatment planning for each child, in the daily care activities, in the cooperation and stress of group care work, in programme planning, and in the scheduling of staff, an inherent struggle exists between provisions of personalized care and institutionalized demands for organizational accountability. We also noted that the primary care issues, though central to service delivery and the agenda of this particular staff meeting, still remained sandwiched between organizational concerns. The scenario offered above articulates the major thesis of this chapter, which is that provision of primary (personal) care within a secondary (organizational) care context always presents a difficult course but it can also offer challenging opportunities.

PRIMARY CARE WITHIN A SECONDARY CARE CONTEXT

Care in Everyday Life

The care received by children growing up in their own families is directly impacted by the quality of care rendered to their immediate caregivers. Infants have their parent(s) "at their command, families to protect the mothers or alternate caregivers, societies to support the structure of families, and traditions to give a cultural continuity to systems of tending and training" (Erikson, cited in Maier, 1973, pp. 89-90). It is common knowledge that the quality of care and training of children is directly related to the sense of well-being experienced by their caregivers. Emien's reminder, "If you care for children, then care for parents" (cited in Gabarino, 1982, p. 234), can be broadened and applied to all types of primary care-givers: grandparents, babysitters, foster parents, day care and, of course, residential care workers. In fact, a decisive factor in group care work is whether there is or is not "ample care for the caring" (Maier, 1979, p. 172). Bronfenbrenner pointedly asked, "Who cares for those who care?" (cited in Gabarino & Stocking, 1980, p. 3).

An Ecological Perspective About Care

Validation of the above notion was elaborated by Bronfenbrenner in his empirically grounded ecological formulations (Bronfenbrenner,

1979). An ecological systems perspective applies not only to interpersonal interactions but also to the mutually reinforcing processes and events between larger and smaller systems. Interconnectedness is part of the nature and pattern of life (Bronfenbrenner, 1979). In particular, we note that events in larger systems impact as much, if not more so, the nature of events in the relevant subordinate systems. In everyday life, for example, to cite Bronfenbrenner,

> A person's development is profoundly affected by events occurring in settings in which the person is not even present. . . . Among the most powerful influences affecting the development of young children in modern industrialized societies are the conditions of parental employment. (Bronfenbrenner, 1979, pp. 3-4)

The degree of work satisfaction, working hours, and take-home pay more strongly affect the degree of each parent's active and psychological availability and the nature of parent-child interactions than his or her personal qualifications for parenthood.

We note that much of a child's life is determined by secondary life systems that involve neither the developing persons as active participants nor the young persons' caregivers in their role as the children's nurturers. Significant events occur that affect what happens in the setting that contains the developing person (Bronfenbrenner, 1979, p. 25). It is important to note that members of the subordinate settings have little power to influence the very events that tend to influence strongly their own as well as the lives of care-receivers (Bronfenbrenner, 1979, pp. 255-56).

As illustrated, working hours, salaries or wages and, to an extent, work satisfaction, are beyond the control of the recipients. The labour market, policy makers, and other settings of power "control the allocation of resources and make decisions affecting what happens in other settings in the community or in the society at large" (Bronfenbrenner, 1979, p. 255). These decisions also reach into the lives of almost all individuals within their spheres and subsequently impact the course of each family.

Applied to our immediate concerns, the nature of primary care in any children's centre is strongly coloured by the employment policy and the institution's pronouncements on the workers' roles within the total scheme. Such factors operate quite independently of the workers' personal and professional qualifications or the staff members' personal commitments to daily work tasks.

The ecological impact of secondary systems upon primary relationships is applicable to group care situations, regardless of whether the children are in care for part of, most of, or continuous 24-hour services. We noted in the staff meeting described above that a worker's personal readiness to adapt her or his working periods to the requirements of a particular group of children hinged on the program's readiness to adapt to particular working arrangements. One can assume with relative certainty that the decision would ultimately be made on the basis of how feasible it was for scheduling changes to be instituted within administrative considerations, in other words, "making the fewest waves." It is unlikely that such a decision would be made on the basis of children's and workers' urgent need for each other.

At another point in the foregoing meeting, a clinical recommendation for greater individualization was immediately counteracted with the fear that increased attention to individual children's differential requirements would lead to a lack of clarity in oversight and would result in organizational "shambles." It is true that individualism in its extremes becomes the antithesis to organizational order, yet the reverse is also the case: Organizational rigidity negates individuality, which is apt to receive less emphasis on organizational deliberations.

Finally, we noted that a staff meeting, with an agenda focused upon the children's welfare, started and ended with organizational concerns. Service factors, such as whether recording for communication between staff would allow more intense therapeutic involvement, were easily overridden by administrative concerns. The professional dilemma of increased direct versus indirect service time became reframed into an organizational dilemma: the urgency of translating service gains into measurable standards of reporting. There is an ever-present pressure to account for the program's efficacy to the next larger systems, namely the sponsoring and controlling systems. Altogether the issue before us is that primary, individualized care concerns tend to give way to those of secondary, organizational power.

The dominance of administrative over immediate child and youth care concerns is not necessarily a peculiarity of the foregoing staff meeting. Rather it is inherent in the exchanges between two systems where the super-system or the organizational system substantially influences the norms, pace, limits, and flow of communication of its sub-systems. The sub-systems are those of the client, staff, group care, and physical domain systems. Each of the sub-systems, in turn, from time to time influences the organization. Only when persons associated with any one of the sub-systems are able to marshal sufficient thrust to counteract organizational "necessities" do such sub-system efforts prevail.

For instance, care workers might have collectively and in a determined manner insisted on a more flexible wakeup time for children travelling to a school some distance away. These children might have had their breakfast ahead of children attending the local school. The latter could proceed more leisurely, as they were also typically children who required more flexible time demands. It is possible that the straightening up of rooms could occur at varying points of the day. For some youngsters it is more important to start the day and get off to school with as little hassle as possible, whether their room is sufficiently tidied up or not.

Such a thrust from the care staff might have led to an organizational change where workers were employed and supported for their flexibility and adaptability to situational demands rather than for allegiance and conformity to institutional practices. Moreover, such a thrust from a sub-unit could bolster administrative adaptability and readiness to justify to its own workers and the outside that children's centres are for adaptive living rather than providing a showpiece in housekeeping. Unmade beds at noon can represent sure signs that certain children and staff are working actively on other issues vital in the developmental lives of these particular children. (No apologies or regrets are necessary, if such conditions are part of acceptable agency standards.)

In general, the tendency is for organizational requirements to modify special individual care requirements. Such a dilemma can be witnessed when plans for children who are ready to engage in a wider range of activities are throttled when an agency does not perceive itself as being ready to branch out. Many activities beyond the perimeter of a group care centre are prematurely curtailed for fear of unfavourable public relations. Other activities within the walls such as appropriate exceptions for some children, variations in procedures, and programmes for separate living units are discouraged or, worse, not even considered due to fear of destabilizing the programme's overall efficiency. The submergence of exceptions, special considerations, or a thrust towards greater diversity all have a slight ring of truthful imperative. Where would the children, the staff, and the service be if the stability of the agency or programme were endangered? But is it really such an either/or dichotomy?

The very struggle between individual freedom for personal initiative and adherence to organizational norms, the desire to serve individual children while remaining mindful of what others would say and, above all, the strain to become fully involved in child and youth care activities while remaining a faithful peer to one's fellow workers represent mind-boggling organizational nightmares. It is not unlike the everyday struggle of being a "good" parent as well as a full marriage partner or a "good" sales person who fully meets a customer's interests as well as her or his own, as a business person. All these activities elicit conflicting requirements, a notion considered more fully below.

In group care practice it is common that an intense involvement with one child readily creates a demand by other children for equal time. The result may be a rivalrous frown by coworkers with a possible warning against overinvolvement or at least a curt reminder that not every staff member can afford such a heavy investment. Similarly, the impulse to deal with children according to the situation, viewing rules as being flexible or not applicable at a particular time, can easily be interpreted as a worker operating without standards or denying support to fellow workers.

It is also true that a search for common guidelines in the care of children may be continuously disrupted by the awareness that such common rules cannot apply logically to a number of children or will not be carried out by some "notorious" care worker. In another instance, the hope that a token economy can provide a reliable and objective approach, rendering personal involvement unnecessary, is somewhat marred by empirical data revealing that private, interpersonal negotiations over the allotment of a token may be more important than the token system per se (Maier, 1981, pp. 49-50).

The complexities just described spell out the interactional conflict between the individual's worker role and the larger system–the work group. Actually, this inter-system strain exists between all individual and organizationally oriented processes and systems. Individual and peer group needs, situational and organizational procedures, and clinical and bureaucratic considerations are in continuous interaction, meaning that one cannot deny the other. All are part and partners within the same larger whole. While this is so, in this struggle it is a fact of life that the supra-system largely determines the eventual outcome (Resnick, 1980). The credence which is ultimately given to work with each child, to staff coordination, and to the creation of specific care procedures is not so much decided by the children's and staff's ongoing requirements as by the organization's capability and status to deal with these vexing issues. Child and youth care issues, clinical considerations, and staff investments decline or flourish in the arms of the bureaucratic organization.

BUREAUCRATIC AND CLINICAL ISSUES

It is taken for granted that much or most of an administrator's (director, superintendent, principal, chief, or others) time is necessarily absorbed with organizational concerns and the representation of the organization to the outside world (its supra-system). It is not surprising that much time is consequently spent separated from the day-to-day concerns of the service. When she or he does devote time to any particular feature of the programme, the impact of that agency administrator will be keenly felt, and how a particular programme segment is assessed will also influence the direction and quality of care delivery of the centre's staff.

In a visit to one centre, for instance, is the administrator concerned about the number of children in service, likely to focus on whether things are "going smoothly," whether the hot water supply is sufficient, or the reasons why two window panes are broken again? In another example, the administrator's interests might focus upon the residents' progress and, in particular, upon the difficulties and problems encountered by the staff, especially in the most recently emerging trouble spots. The former scenario of administrative emphasis is more common. That is understandable because this dimension relates to an administrator's working spheres. The latter foci of enquiry dip into the domain of care systems, also appropriate but more removed from the group care manager's view. It is little wonder then that care workers sense administrators' preoccupation with overall management; consequently administrators' preoccupations readily become part of the operational norms of a staff team.

The Clinical Aspect of Group Care Work

Practice in group care entails clinical work, that is, care provided on the basis of actual observation of individuals' requirements in contrast to a provision of group care on the basis of generalized expectations for members of a circumscribed group–a class of people.[2] Clinical means selected care for a specific individual in terms of his or her idiosyncratic situation on the basis of the group care worker's best professional understanding and skills.

The Bureaucratic Aspects of Group Care Work

Practice in group care also entails bureaucratic performance. This inherently requires that a worker fulfills and enhances the service obligations of a particular organization, simultaneously delivering such service efficiently, regularly, and impartially. Child and youth care, when it is bureaucratically couched, means providing care of equal quality to all residents without regard to personal discriminatory differences or personal whims. Bureaucratic service means performance by established norms, applicable as decreed or agreed, regardless of individual reservations or inconveniences. Both clinical and bureaucratic perspectives, considered here as primary and secondary care, have their legitimate claims for existence. While both systems may seem to be diametrically opposing forces, both exist within the same interactive field in group care practice with children. A closer look at this interlocking of primary and secondary care (or clinical and bureaucratic) systems may be helpful.

A CONCEPTUAL LOOK AT PRIMARY (CLINICAL) AND SECONDARY (BUREAUCRATIC) CARE SYSTEMS

The individual and organizational strains and dilemmas mentioned above may be understood and explained through reference to system analysis (Parsons, 1964) and, in particular, Herman Resnick's (1980) explication.

Historical Vestiges

Group care centres, in many ways, possess some stark vestiges of pre-industrial economic society where kinship controlled the occupational system. Members of the kinship system virtually owed their lives to their place of work with its intense face-to-face encounters, strong authority structure, and close kinship alliances. By contrast, modern society assures economic success through mobility, loyalty to the task rather than persons, and entails depersonalization of face-to-face contacts (Litwak & Szelenyi, 1969).[3]

The interpersonal linking functions of the former kinship system are, in general, maintained by the family but also by other modern primary systems: friendships, clubs, community groups, and group care centres. The ecological, economic, and political functions of kinship systems are now distributed over many modem structures such as government, worlds of business, the trades, and professions. This professional realm also includes the service delivery aspects of group care. The two contemporary spheres of everyday social functioning–the *interpersonal* and the *economic/political* spheres of group care practice–can be likened to a kinship economy.

Sociological Manifestations

Parsons (1964) and Resnick (1980) established that in contemporary society we are confronted with two distinctly separate *group* systems and system patterns of interactions. *Primary systems* comprise face-to-face small groups in close association like teams, cliques, and gangs as well as socially engineered primary systems. Such socially engineered systems might include communes, educational classes, military platoons, therapy and encounter groups, as well as day care or around-the-clock care groups.

Secondary systems, on the other hand, are organizational, usually large impersonal systems, for example, business, religious, professional, military, industrial, recreational, and other societal organizations, including group care service organizations.

Primary social systems are noted for their face-to-face association and co-operation among the members. They serve individuals and, at the same time, these individuals are fused into a common whole. Means and ends become intimately tied to one another within a primary system. Secondary systems, by contrast, stand out as opposite but also complementary to primary group systems. Secondary group systems represent a larger whole with an emphasis upon contractual, formal, and rational convenient relationships. People are linked with each other; nevertheless their involvement remains specialized and limited. Most striking, these systems function separately and apart from the individuals involved. Secondary settings, in contrast to primary ones, are not an end in themselves but represent means to other ends (Resnick, 1980).

Secondary orientations–such as formality, rationality, and structural emphases–find less favour in primary systems. In secondary systems, correspondingly, primary orientations such as spontaneity, informality, and personalization cause strain and are a sign of dysfunction. It is essential then to identify and discriminate between the respective variables and demands of primary and secondary groups.

Variations in Emotional Demands

The expression of emotions in primary systems is expected and encouraged. Group members are expected to convey affect and to be emotionally supportive of each other. In secondary groups a different norm is operative: emotional neutrality. The latter requires a withholding of personal emotions and relies upon an inconsequential acceptance of others. Emotional expression may deplete energy and lead to a diminishing involvement, or it may be transformed into obstacles for necessary cooperation. The norms of both systems create potential complications. In organizational settings, the demand for emotional neutrality is easily experienced as coolness or disinterest. The latter may lead to a reduction of energy input and to "merely attending to one's work."

It is no wonder that workers deeply involved in the care of children find much personal satisfaction in their practice but they are simultaneously pulled by the need for neutrality and some may even consider deep emotional involvement as "improper professional" behaviour. Other workers with greater emotional restraints are astonished to find children in care being less personally responsive to their semi-neutral behaviours, even though such workers seemingly attend to all details of group living. The administration rarely questions the performance of emotionally neutral workers' practice, but emotionally expressive co-workers may criticize such care-giving performance as being "cold" and "uncaring." We observe that some workers attend *personally* and *affectively* to the children, deeming that fulfilling *care* requirements is central to group care practice; others conscientiously attend most judiciously to *service* demands, expressing harmonious caring within the organization. Such competing expectations create an ever-present strain in primary systems that have an organizational mission, as highlighted by Wolins and Wozner (1982):

> The logistic requirements of the well-oiled bureaucracy negated the demands of close, intimate interactions–the essence of people-changing activity. . . . The recipients of care become objects of the bureaucrat's manipulations and are denied control or participation in decisions that affect re-claiming activity. (p. 54)

As Goffman (1961) contended, the bureaucratic model is antithetical to reclaiming.

STANDARDIZATION IN OPPOSITE DIRECTIONS

Primary group systems depend essentially upon *particularistic* standards. Only the person within each situation will know in which way a rule is applicable. It all depends upon the particular circumstances and the individuals involved. These notions are applicable to face-to-face interactions. In contrast, secondary group systems build upon *universalistic* standards. Rules apply to all in order to be fair to each. Uniformity in standards assures clarity, order, and authority of standards. Either particularism or universalism may lead to complications for its respective system. Standards purely adaptable to each situation may eventually obviate all standards, while an insistence upon general standards will deny individual requirements. This may be carried to the extent where uniform rules may eventually have little relevance for the person involved, rendering uniform regulations ridiculous. In organizational life, particularistic considerations are immediately perceived as a threat to law and order or favouritism unbecoming to an organization. In primary group life, universal rules are quickly resented as obstacles to individual initiative and differences. In group care practice, much energy is invested in working out applicable rules or standards for each living unit and child. These struggles, whether or not a set of rules is actually fair and applicable, can be understood by Parsonian concepts. Arguments for uniform getting-up time, for instance, are supported for their fairness, orderliness, and universal clarity for *all*. Counter-arguments could justify adaptive wake-up procedures citing fairness to particular children's circumstances or individual worker's preferences.

Scope of Interest

Primary group systems, like kinship systems, serve *manifold* interests. This multi-dimensional interest or preoccupation with many details, forges a homogeneous group prototype (i.e., a family, a commune, a friendship association, or a congenial living unit). Secondary systems, in comparison, concentrate upon *specific* interests in well-defined areas while serving a wide spectrum of purposes. It is not surprising that, in a case presentation for example, the organization-oriented workers can explain *typical work* with specificity and technical detail. On the other hand, clinically-oriented persons will likely preface their remarks with the explanation that their account is "atypical." They are apt to lose their audience through their mixture of details spiked with generalizations, unless their clinical accounting establishes a profile or constellation– that is, a viable case report. A valid case presentation, by the way, evolves out of an interlinking of details into a generalized explanatory whole.

In another area of practice, we note that diffusion of worker or agency interests is frequently augmented by specific interests such as an all-out push for greater physical order, for individual tutoring, or for reliance upon group meetings. Each push tends to distort the program towards the selected, more narrowly specified area. In addition, while undergoing such "purges," workers and children tend to become classified according to their performance in selected spheres of interest. It is no wonder that group care programs blossom or shrivel under specialized program reforms. Much depends upon whether program changes include both inherent group care realities: primary and secondary system demands.

Status Alignment

A preference for *ascription*–the qualities owned by persons according to their positions in life–adds stability to primary group life. This is true so long as these qualities actually define the nature of face-to-face interactions. The following instances are a few of many variations: older and experienced workers are more competent; younger or new members of staff require added guidance. Sex, ethnic, and other genuine differences are significant so long as they do not perpetuate stereotypes but represent real affirmative differences. In organizational and primary systems, achievement or accountable competence defines status. Definition of status and change of status for organizational and primary systems have relevance in relation to system strains (Resnick, 1980) and contemporary struggles over changing societal norms (Maier, 1969, 1974). In group care practice, a continuous internal conflict exists as to how members' status is to be measured in their *ascribed* roles within their primary group position. For children, an example would be eldest, youngest, leader. For workers, seniority, job classification, or personal achievements may apply.

Competence requirements seem to encroach more and more upon primary as well as secondary group demands (Maier, 1974). Then, too, awareness of sexism and racism in traditional primary group life–where reliance upon ascriptive values also perpetuated discriminatory practices–has furthered a shift towards secondary system practices. To put it another way, there has been a shift to award status by actual competence and achievements. This leaning towards competence rating in primary settings brings with it the danger of "hollow existence" for staff and residents alike. Are children and workers appreciated because they are familiar in one's life experience, because they are part of one's heritage, or because of their accomplishments and deeds (Resnick, 1980, pp. 40-42)?

A study of the foregoing variables highlights the dynamic tension that is inevitable in both types of systems. Tension and repeated requirements of adaptation are particularly germane to group care settings where organizational service demands basically rely upon face-to-face interactions. System stresses, then, call attention to either adaptation towards organizational maintenance or clearer emphases upon children's and workers' primary care requirements. In either event, system strains can be viewed as dynamic rather than stultifying forces.

Two Orders of Primary Group Systems

Children and workers are frequently admonished to adhere to group norms "for the sake of everyone" or "for the sake of the group." Frequently, it is not clear whether "everyone" pertains to the group members or refers to the persons associated with the group's sponsorship, the group's *supra-system*. On the other hand, "for the sake of the group" might be a shorthand expression used for the well-being of the individual group members as persons. Another possibility could be "for the sake of the maintenance of a group" as a sub-unit of a larger system (Maier, 1978, 202-05). Each of these appeals serves different demands and different masters. Group care workers have to be clear in knowing with which primary group they are aligned at various points of their "practice."

If the group focus and concern of the moment pertain directly and personally to the individuals making up the group, then the interactions serve essentially the individuals' capabilities, enhancing interpersonal relations and self-verification. Care workers then have to deal with the group members' effectiveness in communication, interpersonal negotiations, and power juggling. Workers' group building efforts serve, essentially, as a source of individual identity formation. In practice, this would mean that a group planning session for an evening of fun would have to include an opportunity for *all* group members to share their wishes and expectations, searching for common denominators and give-and-take negotiations with regard to expectations which cannot be accommodated on that particular evening. Above all, the evening of fun has to stand as a joint group accomplishment so that members may verify that "I had a part in our having fun." In short, "for the sake of the group" in this context reflects individual group members' investments as well as a sense of group achievement.

In contrast, when concerns revolve around group building tasks that seek to maintain and to enhance the group as part of a larger whole, then efforts serve primarily a supra-system of which the immediate group is a part. An example would be care workers and children engaged in establishing their "citizenship" credibility, posing their group as a viable unit within a larger group care centre. Concerns will typically reflect the mechanisms of control, establishment of norms, and value aspirations which are in tune with the larger system's expectations. Adaptation occurs not so much in tune with individual members' readiness to change but instead to the degree that everyone can stretch in adapting to the group's standards. Workers and children are challenged to find a fit. The group forgoes personal whims, shaping up in order that *the group* might gain or maintain a favourable place within a larger scheme.

Care Workers' Strains

The foregoing discussion of natural system uncertainties and differential but interlocking group-building factors may explain the many worlds in which group care workers operate. Yet an explanation never resolves day-to-day practice dilemmas. A *care* worker within an organizational context exists always in a dual world–in two contradictory systems. No wonder that "burn-out" is a rather common occurrence (Mattingly, 1977). Burn-out, rapid staff turnover, a high degree of personal frustration, perplexing diffusion in job descriptions, as well as expectations can be traced to these contradictory work conditions. The work circumstances have inherent systemic difficulties; they have to be surveyed for their organizational facets rather than for signs of human frailties (Mattingly, 1977; Pines & Maslach, 1980). These complications emerge for all human service workers who are employed or engaged voluntarily to help individuals within the context of a service organization. In everyday family life, a parent comes close to such a dilemma when she or he shares in a child's discouragement or delight over school requirements. Is the parent subsequently to respond as a partner and spokesperson for the child and family or the school system? Moreover, the group care worker is continuously required to function as the clinical (*individual care*-oriented) worker *and* as the agency's (organizational *service*-oriented–bureaucratic) worker. Nevertheless, solutions for some of these vexing situations may be possible.

POTENTIAL SOLUTIONS TO THE STRAINS BETWEEN CLINICAL AND ORGANIZATIONAL SERVICE DELIVERY

Child and youth care within an organizational context does not necessarily have to lurch in different directions, frustrating either clinical or organizational operations. Clinical and organizational requirements do demand different efforts. They can be conceived as dialectic rather than counter-productive forces at the point where the pull of either system constitutes a partial investment rather than a negation of the other system. In other words, clinical demands for continuous flexibility and basic care decisions in the hands of the group care workers can be recognized and carried out as basic organizational procedures.

Organizational uniformity is established through decentralization of power and responsibility. Management and organizational supervision are called upon to ensure that care workers fulfill *clinical* obligations to their clientele. At the same time the care workers can operate amongst themselves with a high degree of variation in style within agreed care and treatment plans.

Parallel to such a clinical/organizational conceptual shift is an organizational stance that demands an overall program policy and requires care workers and others to formulate concrete and communicable care and treatment programs. Such programs need to identify specific outcomes expected (objectives) as well as the actual care and treatment activities to be pursued with individual children and their respective families. Care workers and their supervisory staff have then the opportunity and the challenge of defining their own territory and particular operations *within* these actual spheres of work (Bakker & Bakker-Radbau, 1973). Many instances of organizational interference with child and youth care decisions can be traced to an absence of clarity about the precise nature and boundaries of group care practice, in addition to the tendency of organizational requirements to permeate uniformly across all parts of the service. Clear enunciation of care and treatment objectives and procedures could establish the extent to which group care operates as a vital part of the organizational machinery.

The above suggestion to define primary care or clinical work within a secondary system or bureaucratic operation is consistent with an organizational perspective that views the various parts as a dialectic whole. But the purpose here is not to give greater credence to bureaucratic considerations but rather to call attention to the organizational context which constitutes the *supra-system* within which clinical work is carried out. Group care workers may feel even greater commitment to their work with the children and, hopefully, a true identification with practice rather than yielding unnecessarily to bureaucratic demands. In reality it is the wider context–the organizational factors–that ultimately shapes and determines the nature of group care practice. Consequently, group care work has to be formulated, operated, and evaluated from an organizational perspective. It is within such a perspective that personal (clinical) care and treatment can fully proceed and flourish within a well-organized agency programme.

Responses to Children's Emotional Demands

We postulated earlier that quality practice in group care demands close intimate interactions–the essence of people-changing activity–while bureaucratic practices are antithetical to care and treatment efforts (Wolins & Wozner, 1982, p. 54). Group care workers tend to be caught between these opposing demands such as being fully engaged with *all* children and being especially attentive to children who require individual adult involvement. The daily worker's dilemma is well known: provide a very personal "good night" to all and also provide quality involvement with a few individuals. These difficult time-chores are inherent in all responsive caring and do not represent inadequacy in the organization or staff.

The organizational question is: In which way can staff be assisted to assure more quality time with the children or young people *plus* added time with some? Simultaneously, one needs to recognize as appropriate the children's wish for more attention and the workers' disappointment in not being able to deliver to everyone's satisfaction. Organizationally and clinically, caring efforts have to be objectively reviewed for the possibility of additional or alternative opportunities for personal, intimate interactions between the children and their daily care-givers. Clinically and organizationally, efforts have to be directed towards finding new opportunities for intimate and varied interaction between children and workers. For the latter, this kind of searching may lead to such practices as provision for intimate conversations before bedtime rather than a mere get-together snack period, reading a story rather than a TV hour, a quick tussle, or other special quality time with workers. Another example would be the worker being available in the morning as a person for protests or laughter rather than as an organizer of chores and a manager of the long day ahead.

Bureaucratically, *individualized nurturing care* has to be conceived as the central ingredient of group care work with children who have experienced many separations and disruptions in their lives. Nurturing is not only required out of compassion or a humanistic belief that children and young people need love and affection, it is also based on scientific knowledge that children and young people want and will learn to care for and to love others when they have experienced genuine care themselves (Kobak, 1979; Maier, 1982). Organizationally, then, emotional involvement has to be defined as part and parcel of the work commitment for care workers. It has to be explicitly identified in each job description as an integral part of the daily ingredients of group care practice.

Another practice dilemma stems from the continuous personal and emotional demands placed upon workers in the face of administrative expectations that they must not get too deeply involved emotionally in their work. This admonition seems to originate from organizational demand for objectivity. Emotional involvement, at the same time, is the group care worker's specialty (Bames & Kelman, 1974; Maier, 1984). In many ways, group care workers find themselves in the same situation as parents who are overtaxed by children's never-ending and frequently incomprehensible demands. In fact, care workers–in a different way–find themselves akin to "abusive parents" who, as Durkin (1982a) observed, "are chronically overstressed and under-supported, have incompatible demands made on them, and are alienated and relatively powerless to control their fate" (p. 5).

In tune with Durkin's pointed analysis, desired change cannot be accomplished by a frontal attack on the quality of a worker's involvement. Instead, personal stress can be reduced through institutional support and the establishment of manageable working conditions. In concrete terms, this would mean established working hours with periodic rest breaks in a location that assures separation from the work place. Also, it is essential to work out concrete, achievable care objectives rather than vague care expectations. A vague objective like "to help the children to manage well throughout the day" is absurd when these same youngsters can barely manage sufficient concentration to lace up their shoes. Above all, it means providing care workers with support and supervision for their *care* work rather than their managerial work *per se*, so that their emotional involvement enhances rather than deters nurturing care. Such practices are psychologically sound, make clinical sense, and can be logically as well as bureaucratically arranged, managed, and appraised.

Standardization in Apparently Opposite Directions

Clinical processes and organizational processes, as has been re-counted earlier, commonly proceed in opposite directions as if the two should never meet. Maybe a conceptual shift can link the clinical neces-sity to deal with individuals and small primary units in terms of their re-quirements with the organizational mandate for universality. In group care practice, workers tend to stress vehemently the special needs of in-dividuals and their separate living units, as if these needs were so un-usual. Actually, individual requirements of people within their particular primary groups are derived through membership and are not particu-larly special. They represent merely the facts of life.

Our difficulties are not so much from the children's special needs as from our inability to formulate, communicate, and organize these re-quirements effectively. Teachers have lesson plans and curricula. Nurses have charts and nursing procedures (Krueger, 1981). Social workers, psychologists, and psychiatrists have case summaries, assess-ments, and treatment plans with step-by-step intervention objectives and evaluations. What do other group care workers have? They have, at best, generalized statements, specifying acts of close control, unending patience, or the mandate of providing loving care. In some settings, group care workers do have precise directions about how to award points and tokens for specific behaviours, but workers are left on their own to decide how they deal with the children and their group in gen-eral. These widely varied expectations are topped by the organizational expectation to maintain an orderly, smoothly run, contented group care centre. The fact remains that from a clinical point of view there is no doubt that group care workers must have a *program* or intervention plan for each child in care as well as for the management of their unit-as-a-whole.

To augment general schemes, workers and their supervisors have to set up *personal care programs* akin to curricula in education. Such un-dertakings must be the *universal* practice of the service. The organiza-tion has to see to it that this kind of framework is maintained in order to assure fair and consistent care objectives for all. At the same time, the collective of children in care will be guaranteed, in principle, life-fulfill-ing activities according to idiosyncratic requirements. *Personal care* programs would then take up plans in the way educational plans specify the events of the day as a curriculum. In so doing, the entire nature of present definitions of childcare work in a residential programme . . . the grind of supervising kids ends. We are with them both individually and as they mesh together in the group. Control issues vanish and are replaced with content issues, highly relevant pieces of the total curriculum. (Bames & Kelman, 1974, p. 19)

Bureaucratic verification of individualized care and treatment can be further refined by the very fact that every service receiver has individual requirements. The service deals with ordinary growth and developmental phenomena which for all children is anchored in the *interpersonal* interactions between care-givers and care-receivers (Maier, 1984). Children are children, regardless of whether they receive family care or not. This truism is particularly relevant for the transmission of macro-systems values. "Children learn particular cultural values and particular moral systems only from those people with whom they have close contact and who exhibit that culture in frequent relationships with them" (Washington, 1982, p. 105).

Moreover, an extensive study of children treated successfully and unsuccessfully highlights that the most salutary change occurred when consistency existed in meeting clients according to their particular situations and their current understanding. Such results can be obtained even though it creates for the casual onlooker situations of uneven, inconsistent behavioural handling (Division of Youth and Family Service of the State of New Jersey, 1978).

Interests on Different Ends of the Continuum

As outlined earlier, clinical considerations encompass a wide spectrum of the residents' lives. In fact, the more the styles of workers interacting in a child's life are diffused, the more efficiently workers carry out their care obligations. However, it is also true that organizationally a group care service has to be clear about its service mission and the ways in which it uses resources. Rigid adherence to a bureaucratic service mission, however, tends to stifle all those responses that seem appropriate in a creative clinical care and treatment programme for children.

There seems to be a pull in two opposite directions. In one direction there is an effort to expand and deal with more when more is needed; in the other there is a gravitation towards holding the line within the province of the available resources, that is, to manage with that which is actually at hand. In holding to their respective directions both group care workers and organizational administrators are doing their respective jobs. In fact, at times the workers in the group care centre themselves become administrators, and they themselves are apt to limit the use of resources in order to have enough to go around. But whatever the circumstances this struggle will be evoked between human and humane desires for an abundance of life and the bureaucratic necessity to control and to make do with that which is given in an economy of scarcity.

The organizational managers are commonly those who have the actual knowledge and control over the boundaries between agency and the community (just as in the living units, the group care workers have their sway). The organizational team are the "gatekeepers" and the ultimate controls are without question in their hands. Having made a realistic acknowledgement of these factors, it is then important that group care workers relate themselves to the requirements of their practice and see to it that provision is made for those things they deem necessary for the children's development and enriched living experience. They are the ones who know what is needed. Organizational limitations, never-ending demands, public relations, and limited budgets are all legitimate pressures, and clearly enunciated reminders of these issues may be offered at periodic intervals, yet the necessity for additional resources, unexpected requirements, alterations and expansion in activities, as well as unforeseen circumstances are also legitimate reasons for service delivery. All these demands would remain unnoticed and unattended by the service unless clearly articulated by care personnel.

Foremost, group care workers have to operate throughout as the representatives of care, ever ready to interpret the care requirements of children. Organizational wishes and restraints will always become readily known due to indigenous power contained in supra-system demands. Workers' faithful and unchallenged acceptance of this power renders them "good servants" of the organization but diminishes their value as group care workers. The workers' pronouncements on the necessities for "their" children, including apparent luxuries, make them into responsible child or youth care workers and thereby into effective members of the organization. The distance between management and care practitioners must be shortened in order to make known and to secure what is needed for a life similar to that afforded to children in their own homes.

Moreover, to follow Pina's poignant assessment, workers on the front lines are the ones who discover innovative solutions. Their concerns can no longer be treated as exceptions when, in reality, they offer continuing reminders about the need for novel and urgent solutions (Pina, 1983, p. 3).

Status Alignment

Employment on the basis of ascribed or achieved qualifications presents a dilemma either way. Group care as a profession or as a craft (Eisikovitz & Beker, 1983; Maier, 1983) demands training and competency achievement in terms of clinical *and* organizational work. The ascribed value of "being part of the children's lives" is another essential feature. The care-givers' role as vital participants in the residents' life development–to be the children's or young people's primary care persons in their everyday life–becomes a decisive variable in terms of staff selection, work, or time-off scheduling and the workers' place within the centre.

In ascribed terms, care staff *own* their place in the organization while the quality of their work has to be prescribed and appraised on the basis of actual achievement in providing interpersonal care services. This achievement is colourfully described by Durkin (1982b), who claimed that "one of the greatest joys of being a child and youth care worker is that what you are as a unique configuration of personality traits, interests, skills, hobbies, and how you have fun–that is, what you are as a person–gets full use on the job" (p. 16).

And it can be added that such personal qualities are used to meet the life requirements of the children as developing persons and members of a residential living-unit group. Then the group care worker will be a full professional within a bureaucratic organization: Personal satisfaction can be found, using her or his own creativity as a professional.

CLOSING COMMENTS

Provision of individualized (clinical) child or youth care work within a group care (organizational) setting has been reviewed using a Parsons and Resnick "thinking screen." The latter explains the counter-pulls of primary and secondary system variables and processes. Resnick's conceptual analysis (1980) has been employed to understand some of the strains inherent in group care practice pursued as a clinical endeavour and, by contrast, as an organizational model.

Our purpose has been to conceive of group care practice as primary care or a clinical enterprise. *Primary care* is the essence of a group care worker's activities, implementing the children's developmental requirements (Maier, 1984) to obtain a close attachment with the children in care and, lastly, in order to foster a sense of permanency in the children's lives (Maier, 1982). The care-givers' work is defined as *clinical*, because their focus has to proceed on the basis of each child's individual requirements rather than to deal sociologically with the children as a class or group.

At the same time, we must be mindful of the fact that such care is not being provided within a primary group system: the family, commune, or kinship network. Instead, it occurs in a socially engineered group care setting, a secondary organizational group. Organizational features place primary care in a different context and bring organizational demands in conflict with clinical realities.

In the second half of this chapter we have attempted to seek out potential ways and possible solutions for accepting inter-system strains as necessary ingredients of nurturing care within an organization. In fact, for many of these inter-system strains we neither have a solution nor want to provide solutions. The system strains seem to be part and parcel of the nature of contemporary living in modern, technological societies. Moreover, while the mutual "system wheels" turn, the partial inter-meshing can be conceived as dialectical control processes which "grind" out a viable whole of ill-meshing but salutary encounters. Organizational demands may offer their own legitimate characteristics, such as minimizing or guarding against depletion of workers' own individual energies by yielding to children's endless personal requirements.

The introduction of interpersonal neutrality within an organizational context may assist staff to maintain satisfactory work relationships with co-workers and supervisors while they are intensely involved with the youngsters in care. An ancient proverb can be paraphrased here: Give to the children what *is* the children's and to the organization what *belongs to* the organization! In the spheres of standard setting and diversity of interests, the strains of the system or dialectic envelopment might include a scenario that can neither be accounted for nor resolved by workers or the organization. Indeed, this kind of tension may be representative of future life experiences anywhere. It is important for workers to deal with these events as part of a child's life experience. It is to be hoped that workers can transmit skills to children which allow them to reframe their experiences or at times to adapt to them rather than by-pass or flatly accept restraints. This can be powerful intervention in group care practice.

Finally, this chapter brings together two spheres of life experience and two disciplines of knowledge that are rarely studied, viewed, and dealt with as one joint enterprise. This way of thinking requires that separate system-partners, by virtue of their division of labour and allegiances, become cooperators in their naturally conflict-ridden, joint enterprise. These highly distinctive work approaches necessitate additional working orientations in order to incorporate the other system's realities (Resnick, 1983). In other words, personal care work within an organizational context demands more than appreciating and co-operating with other systems' demands. Viable group care practice may also require an evaluation and expansion of one's own theoretical orientation and practice procedures.

The next step is to find bridging concepts and linking practices with the immediate and wider worlds of which every child, young person, or worker–indeed every living-unit however securely fenced off–and each service organization and their respective communities, are a part.

NOTES

1. The major ideas underlying this chapter build upon Talcott Parson's formulation on "Pattern Variables" (1964), and in particular, Professor Resnick's lucid development of Parson's formulation (1980). I am personally indebted to my colleague Professor Herman Resnick for teaching me this rich material on primary/secondary system strains.
2. "A class of people" is here used sociologically–an empirically defined category of people as a distinct unit which is separate from other classes.
3. This factor is clearly visible in a number of highly applauded and well-known residential treatment programmes which are operated akin to the norms of former feudal societies. We can list among others, Bettelheim's Orthogenic School (Bettelheim, 1950, 1955; Neill, 1960; Mayer, 1960; Phillips, Phillips, Fixsen, & Wolf, 1973).

REFERENCES

Bakker, C., & Bakker-Radbau, M. K. (1973). *No trespassing: Explorations in human territorially.* San Francisco: Chandler and Sharp.

Barnes, F. H., & Kelman, S. M. (1974). From slogans to concepts: A basis for change in child care work. *Child Care Quarterly, 3*(1), 7-23.

Bettelheim, B. (1950). *Love is not enough.* New York: Free Press.

Bettelheim, B. (1955). *Truants from life.* New York: Free Press.

Bronfenbrenner, U. (1979). *The ecology of human development.* Cambridge, MA: Harvard University Press.

Division of Youth and Family Service of the State of New Jersey. (1978). *The impact of residential treatment.* New Brunswick, NJ: Institute for Criminology Research, Rutgers University.

Durkin, R. (1982a). *The crisis in children's services: The dangers and opportunities for child care workers.* Banff, Alberta: 2nd National Child Care Workers' Conference. Unpublished paper.

Durkin, R. (1982b). Institutional child abuse from a family systems perspective: A working paper. *Child and Youth Services Review, 4*(1), 15-22.

Durkin, R. (1982c). No one will thank you: First thoughts on reporting institutional abuse. *Child and Youth Services Review, 4*(1), 109-13.

Durrant, M. (1993). *Residential treatment: A cooperative, competency-based approach to therapy and program design.* New York: W. W. Norton.

Eisikovitz, Z., & Beker, J. (1983). Beyond professionalism: The child and youth care workers as craftsmen. *Child Care Quarterly, 12*(2), 93-112.

Fewster, G. (1990). *Being in child care: A journey into self.* New York: The Haworth Press, Inc.

Fulcher, L. C. (1983). *Who cares for the caregivers? A comparative study of residential and day care teams working with children.* Unpublished doctoral dissertation, University of Stirling, Great Britain.

Gabarino, J. (Ed.). (1982). *Children and families in the social environment.* New York: Aldine.

Gabarino, J., & Stocking, S. M. (1980). *Protecting children from abuse and neglect.* San Francisco: Jossey-Bass.

Garfat, T. (1998). The effective child and youth care intervention. *Journal of Child & Youth Care, 12*(1/2), 1-168.

Garfat, T., McElwee, N., & Charles, G. (in press). Self in social care practice. In N. McElwee & P. Share (Eds.), *An Irish social care text.* Dublin, Ireland.

Goffman, E. (1961). *Asylums.* New York: Doubleday.

Kerins, M. (1995). Caring for the caregivers. *The Child Care Worker, 13*(1), 7-8.

Kobak, D. (1979). Teaching children to care. *Children Today, 8*(2), 6-7, 34-5.

Krueger, M. (1981). *Some thoughts on research and the education of child care personnel.* Unpublished manuscript, Milwaukee: University of Wisconsin.

Krueger, M. A. (1991). Coming from your center, being there, meeting them where they're at, interacting together, counselling on the go, creating circles of caring, discovering and using self, and caring for one another: Central themes in professional child and youth care. *Journal of Child & Youth Care, 5*(1), 77-87.

Litwak, E., & Szelenyi, I. (1969). Primary group structures and their functions: Kin, neighbors, and friends. *American Sociological Review, 34*(4), 465-81.

Maier, H. W. (1969). When father is no longer the father. *Journal of Applied Social Studies, 1*(1), 13-20.

Maier, H. W. (1974). A sidewards look at change and what comes into view. In *Social Work in Transition: Issues, Dilemmas and Choices.* Seattle, WA: School of Social Work, University of Washington.

Maier, H. W. (1977). The child care worker. In J. B. Turner (Ed.), *Encyclopedia of social work.* New York: National Association of Social Workers.

Maier, H. W. (1978). *Three theories of child development* (3rd edition). New York: Harper & Row.

Maier, H. W. (1979). The core of care. *Child Care Quarterly, 8*(3), 161-73.

Maier, H. W. (1981). Essential components in care and treatment environments for children and youth. In F. Ainsworth & L. C. Fulcher (Eds.), *Group care for children: Concepts and issues.* New York: Methuen/Tavistock.

Maier, H. W. (1982). To be attached and free: The challenge of child development. *Child Welfare, 61*(2), 67-76.

Maier, H. W. (1983). Should child and youth care go the craft or the professional route? *Child Care Quarterly, 12*(2), 113-18.

Maier, H. W. (1987). *Developmental group care of children and youth: Concepts and practice* (pp. 119-120). New York: The Haworth Press, Inc.

Maier, H. W. (1991). Developmental foundations of residential care and youth care. In Z. Eisikovitz & J. Beker (Eds.), *Knowledge utilization in residential care practice.* Washington, DC: Child Welfare League of America, 25-48.

Maier, H. W. (1994). A therapeutical environmental approach. *Research and Evaluation, 3*(2), 3-4.

Mattingly, M. A. (1977). Sources of stress and burn-out in professional child care work. *Child Care Quarterly, 6*(2), 127-37.

Mayer, M. F. (1960). The parental figures in residential treatment. *Social Services Review, 34*(3), 273-85.

Neill, A. S. (1960). *Summerhill: A radical approach to child rearing.* New York: Hart Publishing.

North American Consortium of Child and Youth Care Education Programs. (2002). *Curriculum content for child and youth care practice: Recommendations of the task force of the North American Consortium of Child and Youth Care Education Programs.*

Osler, K. (1993, September). Diagnosing organisational conflict: Key questions to ask. *The Child Care Worker, 11*(9), 15.

Parsons, T. (1964). *The social system.* New York: Free Press.

Peters, D. L., & Madle, R. A. (1991). The development of effective child and youth care workers. In J. Beker & Z. Eisikovits (Eds.), *Knowledge utilization in residential child and youth care practice* (pp. 297-299). Washington, DC: Child Welfare League of America.

Phillips, E. L., Phillips, E. A., Fixsen, D. L., & Wolf, M. M. (1973). Achievement place: Behavior shaping works for delinquents. *Psychology Today, 7*(1), 74-80.

Pina, V. (1983). Comment: Isolationism is dead. Survival mandates flexible systems. *Newsletter of the Child Care Learning Center, 5*(2), 3.

Pines, A., & Maslach, C. (1980). Combating staff burnout in a day care center: A case study. *Child Care Quarterly, 9*(1), 5-16.

Redl, F., & Wineman, D. (1957). *The aggressive child.* New York: Free Press.

Resnick, H. (1980). A social system view of strain. In H. Resnick & R. J. Patti (Eds.), *Change from within.* Philadelphia: Temple University Press.

Resnick, H. (1983). The political dimension in social welfare organizations: The missing ingredient in social work education. Unpublished manuscript, School of Social Work, University of Washington, Seattle.

Ricks, F. (1989). Self-awareness model for training and application in child and youth care. *Journal of Child & Youth Care, 4*(1), 33-42.

Ricks, F. (1992). A feminist view of caring. *Journal of Child & Youth Care, 7*(2), 49-57.

Smith, M. (2002, February). Caring for the carers. *CYC-Net*, Issue 37, retrieved from *http://www.cyc-net.org/cyc-online/cycol-0202-smith.html*.

VanderVen, K. (1982). Principles and guidelines for child care personnel preparation programs. *Child Care Quarterly, 11*(3), 221-49.

VanderVen, K. (1993). Advancing child and youth care: A model for integrating theory and practice through connecting education, training, and the service system. *Child and Youth Care Forum, 22*(4), 265-283.

Washington, R. (1982). Social development: A focus for practice and education. *Social Work, 27*(1), 104-09.

Whittaker, J. K. (1979). *Caring for troubled children*. San Francisco: Jossey-Bass.

Wolf, M. M., Phillips, E. L., Fixsen, D. L., Braukmann, C. T., Kirigin, K. A., Wither, A. G., & Schumaker, J. (1976). Achievement Place: The Teaching-Family model. *Child Care Quarterly, 5*(2), 92-103.

Wolins, M., & Wozner, Y. (1982). *Revitalizing residential settings*. San Francisco: Jossey-Bass.

Chapter 6

Developing a Shared Language and Practice

Stephen F. Casson

SUMMARY. The provision of a coherent "parenting," "teaching," and "developmental" program is a complex undertaking. It has all the makings of an organizational, managerial, and therapeutic nightmare when different types of workers, with marked differences in personality and values, become responsible for different children with a variety of problems in a living-learning environment. Without an action plan to help engender a shared language for practice, the needs of both children and staff are at risk. *[Article copies available for a fee from The Haworth Document Delivery Service: 1-800-HAWORTH. E-mail address: <docdelivery@ haworthpress.com> Website: <http://www.HaworthPress.com> © 2005 by The Haworth Press, Inc. All rights reserved.]*

KEYWORDS. Group care, residential care, residential treatment, group homes, youth work, youthwork, group work, at-risk youth, direct care

---

Address correspondence to: Stephen F. Casson, The Miller's Cottage, Whitley Mill, Hexham, Northumberland, NE46 2LA, UK.

[Haworth co-indexing entry note]: "Developing a Shared Language and Practice." Casson, Stephen F. Co-published simultaneously in *Child & Youth Services* (The Haworth Press, Inc.) Vol. 27, No. 1/2, 2005, pp. 117-149; and: *Group Care Practice with Children and Young People Revisited* (ed: Leon C. Fulcher, and Frank Ainsworth) The Haworth Press, Inc., 2006, pp. 117-149. Single or multiple copies of this article are available for a fee from The Haworth Document Delivery Service [1-800-HAWORTH, 9:00 a.m. - 5:00 p.m. (EST). E-mail address: docdelivery@haworthpress.com].

doi:10.1300/J024v27n01_06 *117*

REFLECTIONS AFTER TWENTY YEARS ABOUT DEVELOPING A SHARED LANGUAGE AND PRACTICE

In the social care profession what is it that stands the test of time, or what has changed through fashion, through ineffective results, or through political dictates? It is a sobering experience to re-read what one wrote 20 years ago. It is also both satisfying and encouraging to conclude that most of the questions asked and the arguments made are still highly relevant for 2005.

The thrust of my 1985 chapter was that, in order to provide an effective service to groups of children and young people, it was incumbent on top leadership to first examine the shape of each of the jigsaw pieces and how they interlink. Then we were talking about group care action planning. The current jargon is about customers, stakeholders, quality management, and assuring quality and excellence, but the key themes remain very similar. The rhetorical quip of "A failure to plan is a plan for failure" is more relevant today as managers are judged by the speed of their implementation of new services—within budget—now that individual performance management holds sway. The key arguments in 1985 were as follows:

1. The larger the number of staff involved in a direct service to children and young people, the stronger must be the staff cohesion around team responses and approaches to be used by staff. Without this the result will be a regime or even cult where the different personalities of child or youth care workers rule supreme depending on who is on shift or who is managing.
2. It is beneficial to design different kinds of youth care cultures or child and youth care regimes around the developmental traits and needs of specific children. To match the regime to the child or young person requires first that an assessment can be made of the child(ren) and the results can be translated into the kind of environment that would work best for that young person. Then those working with that young person are able to consistently and constantly radiate that matched environment and the necessary approaches.

The 1985 chapter articulated the Conceptual Level Matching Model with the research that supported such an approach. Today, the request would be that no child or youth care culture or regime is designed without first finding evidence to support details of that design. Without doing so there is basic irresponsibility: We would be experimenting with children and young people without first being assured that particular approaches and cultures are supported by outcomes-based research.

3. Once the design of the child or youth care establishment is decided for specific categories of young people, then staff can be recruited with the basic values that would support such a design. Training into the approaches to be used is central, including being familiar with necessary policies and procedures. All of this ensures that the rationale of the service is understood and staff members have the wherewithal to consistently implement the approaches and deal effectively with eventualities.

In addition to points raised in the 1985 chapter, child and youth care workers, managers, and policy makers should today also consider the following points if quality outcomes for children and young people are to be realistically achieved:

1. Identify all the groups that have a stake or interest in the specific child or youth care setting, e.g., young people, relatives, neighbours, the commissioners of the service.
2. What are those stakeholders' particular expectations, requirements, and fears?
3. How can the aspirations of disparate stakeholders be addressed whether at face value or reframed in such a way as to make them workable (Casson & Manning, 1996)?
4. Clarify the means by which all these stakeholder needs can be met: the regime/culture and approaches to be used by all staff.
5. Specify the means by which there is regular and routine internal and external managerial monitoring of whether the setting is adhering to its philosophy and approaches. In addition, what more infrequent professional audits will be used to ensure that practices are up to date, professionally acceptable, and the results are effective (George & Casson, 1994)?
6. Highlight the improvement culture where all staff members have the obligation to identify what is not working, what almost went wrong, or what could be done more efficiently or more effectively. Let those who lead the service emphasize their commitment to obtaining the quality improvement ideas of staff, who may also be the conduit for ideas for change coming from young people and other stakeholders (Casson & George, 1995).

7. At particular intervals, perhaps annually, have a detailed review of all the components of the service to assess the extent to which it is delivering the vision, identifying where to make radical changes, and where to make minor amendments. The effectiveness of such fundamental reviews should be based on demonstrated openness by various levels of leadership and a culture of evidence-based development as opposed to defensive obfuscation or window-dressing. Such a review is all the more powerful when the views of the various stakeholders are known and incorporated into any performance review.

8. Finally, the morale, wellness, and energy of staff is pivotally important in facilitating changes in children or young people since it is through the basic minute-by-minute transactions between young persons and staff members that, as a child's confidence develops, new perspectives are gained and internal controls start being exercised. With low staff morale, high turnover, absenteeism, and disillusionment within the staff group, the quality of relationships and transactions between staff and young people are likely to be harmed.

These eight additional points are essential elements in any organisation where assurance of quality outcomes is important or where the views and involvement of the stakeholders are taken seriously and used to maintain relevance in a rapidly changing world. These themes are also precursors to the pursuit of excellence within any organisation.

MORE THAN A JOB–A POUND OF FLESH

It is 3:45 p.m. Jerry, a group home worker, is responsible for twelve adolescent boys and girls, ranging in age from 15 to 18, who are returning from work or school. His colleague, who should have been on duty, has just called in sick. This colleague predicts she will be away from her work for seven days. Two residents are preparing a sandwich, another is watching television, one is getting ready to go out, and two of the others are doing nothing in particular. Jerry knows he has to take care of all that happens until two other group home workers arrive at 8 a.m. the next day. He calculates that there are 16 hours left as the minutes start ticking by interminably slowly.

Jerry keeps his fingers crossed that tonight the residents will behave themselves, perhaps watch television, go out to a disco, or just do anything that interests them. If all goes well, he will write up some case records, bring some financial accounts up to date, and generally be helpful. He will make his mark on this shift so at the staff meeting people will recognize the hard work he has put in to get the paperwork up to date. He might even have time to watch the film on television at 8 p.m. If there are only three or four residents in the building, it might be a pleasantly quiet evening.

> *Commentary:* What is the purpose of Jerry coming to work? What should he do with the residents until they go to bed? How should Jerry or any group home worker spend his time with a group of adolescents? To what extent does he organize activities for them, arrange transport, and travel? What would be the point of it? Should he go and rent a couple of video films to entertain a sizeable number of boys and girls and thereby probably encourage them to stay in? Should he have a heart-to-heart conversation with the two residents with whom he gets on best to help them straighten out some of their problems (is this counselling?)? On the other hand, should he do nothing at all, as this would be a good preparation for the residents to learn how to fill up their own time, to work out for themselves how to spend the evening, and be a bit realistic about life in the big wide world?

A social worker for Julie, aged seventeen and four months pregnant, drops in to talk about Julie and her plans for the future. She wants a private talk with Jerry in the office. Jerry wishes she had more sensitivity about how the establishment works and realized he should be amongst the boys and girls as they return home from school. Perhaps she might telephone next time to make an appointment. What is the point of talking to her anyway? He is not interested and has too much to do. At least she might spend an hour with Julie, which will keep her quiet.

The phone rings, and it is an assertive auditor saying he is coming tomorrow morning to go through the books. The group home worker explains that tomorrow there is a staff meeting. The auditor states that he only needs an hour from the senior worker in the establishment, and that will not cause too much disruption to the staff meeting. He will arrive at 10:30 a.m. Jerry feels a surge of anger that this outsider, probably in a suit, takes no notice of him and intends to interfere with an important meeting. There will be less time for discussion about four residents due for in-depth reviews. Oh well, the interminable conversations about residents get nowhere, so an hour less might be a good thing.

Commentary: Where does Jerry stand with an unscheduled visit from a social worker and insensitive high pressure from an auditor? Should he tell them both to come at a time convenient to the establishment, or should the establishment constantly shuffle its operations like a small pack of cards to maintain the good will and co-operation of outsiders? Whatever Jerry decides, how will he know whether or not he is doing the right thing? If he means to ensure outsiders come at convenient times, how will he go about influencing the social worker and auditor to cooperate? If what he does succeeds will he be looked upon as a competent and mature person and, if there are complaints, what will it be that he has done wrong?

Charles, an aggressive sixteen-year-old who recently left school, throws himself into the office complaining that he will not spend an hour longer at the Youth Employment Programme where he has been working. Someone has accused Charles of stealing money. He tells Jerry what to do with the job and, what is more, he will not be looking for another one. The group home worker feels embarrassed to be the subject of such an outburst in front of the social worker. He wonders what she is thinking about him, allowing this verbal aggression and all these interruptions, when he is meant to be talking with her. Jerry thinks, "If only I had more time and there was someone else working with me, then things would be different."

Jerry nods to the social worker to let her know that he has not forgotten his business with her, while he reassures Charles that he realizes he must have a lot of strong feelings about what has just happened at work. "However, I will spend time with you later," says Jerry, "because I am talking to the social worker about an important matter just now."

Charles shouts at Jerry that if that is the way he feels about his being called a liar and a thief then it is not important to Jerry; he will go out and break into somebody's home and it will all be Jerry's fault. In his own head Jerry believes he should be talking with Charles, yet why does he receive the blame? He is only doing his job.

Commentary: What is the optimum approach to working with Charles? What kind of person is he? Can he be described or assessed in such a way that Jerry is immediately aware of how to deal with this anger and hurt? Should Jerry immediately stop what he is doing with the social worker and turn all his sympathy to Charles? Should he model to Charles the social skill of holding an emotion in check until the right time to let it out? Should he be very mat-ter-of-fact in his approach to Charles? Should he let him know that it is Charles' problem and although he might help Charles work out what to do, the solution rests with Charles? Should he immediately act on Charles' behalf, call the Youth Employment Programme, sort things out, and try to get him another chance? How can a group home worker know what response to give Charles apart from an intuitive guess about what might work or, on the other hand what might not? If his response does not help, then his com-petence is undermined in his own eyes and those of his colleagues.

At that moment the doorbell rings and in walks a man delivering nu-merous food provisions for the next seven days. He comes into the of-fice to get a signature and to explain why the provisions delivered are different from what was ordered, how certain missing items will be de-livered next week, and how this will not affect the bill, as . . . Jerry signs the order form and makes a few notes at the bottom about next week's order. Charles and the delivery man leave the office.

The social worker talks about Julie's pregnancy with Jerry as he fin-ishes his note about the provisions. She wants to know what Julie thinks about adoption. Jerry, who has not seen Julie for some time and has never talked to her about adoption, shows his impatience. He has sud-denly remembered that the agency's local maintenance crew has not yet unblocked the drains from the first-floor kitchen and toilet, although someone telephoned them five hours ago with an urgent request. Jerry apologizes to the social worker and excuses himself, suggesting that she return when Julie's key or primary worker is on duty and, together, she and the social worker can plan the next stage. He inwardly curses the time and energy he has expended on this irritating woman.

Jerry telephones the maintenance service and finds that there is no chance that they will arrive before tomorrow afternoon. He telephones the supervisor but gets no reply. He looks through the Yellow Pages for emergency drain cleaning numbers and makes arrangements for one company to visit within the next two hours. Just as he is congratulating himself on solving the problem, he hears shouting in the passage. He looks out and finds Mark being accosted by a middle-aged man and a younger woman. He has never seen them before. Jerry tries to put his stamp of authority on the scene. "What is going on?" he demands. The older man, smelling of alcohol, says he is Mark's father and this is his new wife. He is not leaving without Mark, as he is having to pay a sizeable proportion of his wages to keep his son in this den of iniquity. "Look at those two," he says, as he points at two girls reclining on a settee, one with a dress slid halfway up her thighs and the other with her mouth open and her tongue provocatively aggravating Mark's father.

He walks up to Jerry and, standing only three feet away from his face, demands that Jerry should tell Mark to pack and that he should hand over all Mark's money, medical card, and so on.

The group home worker's blood is thumping through his body. His mouth is dry. Jerry tells Mark, his father, and the new wife that he is not going to carry on an argument like this in front of everybody. If they want to discuss it then they can come into the office. In the office Mark's father stands over Jerry as he sits in a chair and shouts belligerently. Mark tells his father to stop it. Jerry informs all three parties that if Mark leaves the building, the police will be called and he will be reported as an absconder.

Mark solves the problem by telling his father that he will not go with him. He has never given him any breaks in life and, therefore, he does not want anything to do with him now. He storms out of the group home. The father blames Jerry and threatens him. Twenty minutes later the father leaves with his new wife, telling Jerry they will be back to get their revenge.

> *Commentary:* What is the optimum approach Jerry could use to reduce the turmoil with Mark, his father, and new wife? Should he be confronting, reflective, directive, or permissive? Is a belligerent response or reduced tension a matter of chance or is it connected to Jerry's response? Do workers deal with this sort of situation in an idiosyncratic way that reflects their personality? Is it possible to weigh up the characteristics of the children, the characteristics of the group home worker, and the characteristics of the setting to come up with a recipe that will work for everyone in this situation at that time with those particular people? Or does one recruit workers on the basis that, in their own indomitable way, the right personalities can deal with all comers? Does a person who can deal with all comers and all situations do anything other than enforce a spirit of calm, order, and control on an establishment whether or not this has anything to do with development and growth for children? Will one energetic worker operate in a unique and different way from other persevering staff?

Jerry goes into the main living area to welcome back three residents who have been working. He is about to ask them how their day has gone when the emergency drain cleaners arrive. Jerry shows them what is blocked and leaves them to it. A couple of girls, immaturely and with much noise, follow the workmen around making loud whispers about their looks and how they are not likely to be worthy of their attention because of their menial job as drain cleaners. The two men respond in kind and Jerry attempts to move the girls elsewhere. They are abusive to him and resistive, seemingly finding satisfaction in being the centre of attention. Jerry gives up, returning to the kitchen, feeling embarrassed that he has so little power and influence with residents.

He finds a couple of boys unearthing fruit and biscuits from the boxes of supplies. He reacts angrily as he has not yet checked the produce that has been left. He starts the inventory of those provisions to ensure everything is there. He makes a note that they are four pounds short of butter. He asks a resident to put the supplies away for him.

It is now 6:30 p.m. The boy and girl responsible for preparing and cooking the evening meal for everybody have not returned from school. Jerry asks Fiona and Marian if they will do it, but they refuse. Jerry debates in his mind whether to force the issue and tell them they have got to do it. Instead, he asks another resident, John, who says he might but only if Jerry gives him three cigarettes. They end up in an argument about people only doing things if they are paid for them. Jerry becomes more irate and starts peeling potatoes and preparing vegetables himself.

> *Commentary:* Are there some common attributes or strategies that can make an impact on provocative adolescent girls or residents who refuse to help out with the overall functioning of the establishment? If people will not give a hand, is it best to let people go hungry or should the group home worker do it himself? After all, the worker is responsible for the nutritional needs of the adolescents. Is bribery or cajoling people with future reinforcement relevant here? Is it preferable to let the attention-seeking girls work it out with the drain-cleaning crew or is intervening strongly more appropriate?

The two drain cleaners tell Jerry they have finished, he signs the work order, and they leave. Jerry checks the toilets and showers and finds them working adequately. At that moment the drain cleaners return and state that a wallet has been taken from a jacket in the van outside. The crime must have been engineered by a resident from the home. Two of the residents immediately start arguing with the cleaners, saying that in no way are they thieves, and how dare they blame poor unfortunates who live in residential care. The men shout back and insults are thrown to and fro. Jerry tells the cleaners he has no evidence about who took the wallet and they ought to call the police. The telephone call is made.

Forty minutes later two policemen arrive and interview the two men, Jerry, and all the group home residents who were around at the time. Jerry has to sit in on each interview with the residents. The police, no further on, leave at 8:50 p.m. No evening meal has been cooked. The two residents who should have prepared dinner have still not returned. Jerry thinks about when to report them as missing.

By this time eight people are hungry and are waiting for a meal. They criticize Jerry for not being a proper youth care worker since he has not provided adequate food and nutrition. Jerry calls them all into the lounge. He states he is not prepared to do the work, and unless he has some volunteers who will make the meal, everyone will go hungry. Jerry has doubts about whether this is right.

Three residents volunteer to do the cooking. Jerry discusses with the two girls their provocation of the drain cleaners. When he asks what they were trying to achieve, they laugh. He tells them in strong, cutting terms that their behaviour is unacceptable and that they have given the home a bad name. This could mean that in retaliation service companies may provide only a second-rate service in the future.

> *Commentary:* Jerry's head is pounding. For five-and-a-half hours there has been turmoil. It will be another eleven hours before he is relieved by other workers. "All my hard work is merely stopping this place from disintegrating," he thought. "Surely this is not why I applied for this type of work." Jerry feels alone. He has no idea what he will do if the residents are uncooperative tonight and give him a hard time. Other jobs and professions suddenly seem more attractive.

Reflection on the foregoing incidents with Jerry, the apocryphal and yet surprisingly real group home worker, leaves one with a sense of chaos, a state of affairs characteristic of this line of work now that the so-called profession of residential and day care has come into its own. The profession's foundations have been built on shifting sands of change. Until the last decade or so, many child and youth care establishments were run on the notion of a husband or wife or both managing a group of children virtually singlehanded as houseparents with the assistance of cleaning staff, laundry maids, and the occasional relief worker.

The philosophies, ideologies, and values of child and youth care were integrated within that husband and wife as houseparents or in some particular individual who worked virtually every hour of the week. Thus, while the philosophies, ideologies, and values used by the houseparents might be judged by others to be right or wrong, simple or complex, rigid or flexible, the essential merit in this arrangement was that each resident was confronted with a single set of attitudes and values that were both consistent and enduring.

When these particular philosophies and attitudes were in tune with and matched the needs and characteristics of a particular child, then progress was likely to be seen. Where there was a mismatch, the successes were less common and transfers to other centres were a frequent result. Group home facilities such as these were advocated in the United Kingdom in 1946 by the Curtis Committee, which envisaged the establishment of family group homes, preferably run by a married couple, where children could be closely in touch with the experiences of everyday life.[1] The woman was expected to "play the part of a mother to the children, while the man must play the father . . . [pursuing] out of door recreational activities rather than physical care of the child" (Report of the Care and Children Committee, 1946).

Today, with the vast increase in numbers of child and youth care staff and supervisors working in group care settings, there is some comfort in knowing that somewhere amongst the differing philosophies and attitudes of staff, a child is likely to find understanding and someone who is on his or her wavelength. On the other hand, the provision of a coherent parenting, teaching, and developmental programme is a complex undertaking with, for instance, twelve young people and six youth care staff. The exercise becomes an organizational, managerial, and therapeutic nightmare! More often than not, what happens is that a collection of different types of workers, with marked differences in personality and values, become responsible for a collection of different types of young people with a variety of problems. Together these two groups interact in an environment where all too frequently the philosophies, assumptions, approaches, and styles have not been clearly determined. This problem is the curse of residential and day care services for children and young people and, indeed, the curse of the helping professions when several different persons have to work together to provide therapeutic interventions for a child or young person and family.

DISPARITY AMONGST WORKERS

Senior managers in residential and day care services frequently comment on the number of people who apply to them for employment in settings for children, young people, the elderly, mentally handicapped, or mentally ill people, even when no vacancies have been advertised. At interview these job applicants will emphasize that what has motivated them is their interest in working with people; they have something to offer to residents. They have always got on well with children, adolescents, elderly or handicapped people, and they want to do something meaningful with their lives. In the main, the majority of these people are untrained. As the interview progresses, it is common practice to ask for specific information about how the applicant would view a particular situation and what his or her response might be. A typical answer is, "It depends on the circumstances and what I find to be best at that particular moment of time. It will depend on who is involved, what is the background to the problem, and what is expected in that particular establishment." A response such as this suggests that the applicant is interested in using personality, beliefs, attitudes, and intuition to help persons less fortunate than him or herself. Personality and beliefs are in their own right a product of personal background, upbringing, and experience. It may be that the applicant wants to apply his or her own skills and knowledge, relationship abilities, and uniqueness to work intensively with a particular group of children using the programme elements available at the centre.

But, in more sophisticated language, the applicant will be expected to use personality–still the product of genetic make-up and upbringing–in interactions with children or young people whether these have an impact or not.

When recruiting and employing staff for group care settings, what is being looked for? Consideration will be given to values, personality, mixture of rigidity and flexibility, dogged control versus negotiation, permissive approaches versus detailed surveillance, and so on. Without a definite profile of the type of person best suited to working in a particular group care centre or agency, then recruitment involves an intuitive and possibly prejudicial approach to hiring staff, and decisions are based more on the characteristics of the person doing the hiring than on the traits of the employee. Some recruitment officer's track records for selection are excellent, while others' records are abysmal when considering the length of service of those they hire, the candidates being able to manage the job, and their ability to work as team members. Some people are good at hiring men but do a poor job with women. Some are excellent with basic grade workers but second-rate at employing supervisors.

Thus, in group care settings there will be a range of staff from different backgrounds with varied values, parenting experiences, religious principles, sexual mores, hygiene habits, dressing and grooming practices, nutritional ideals, and eating habits. In summary, an establishment with six workers will tend to be a place where six individual workers come together to work with a group of children or young people with a spectrum of philosophies, practices, and behaviours that will be varied in at least six different ways.

If one person had been responsible for hiring these six workers, then it may be easier to detect a pattern in their characteristics; it is more likely that one would find people with certain similarities included and those with other traits excluded. The frequent pattern is that several persons have had the responsibility over months or years for hiring staff for a particular establishment or group of establishments. Thus, the differences and heterogeneity will probably be greater and values, ideology, and morals will frequently be in conflict amongst workers at the shop floor and at the level of shop floor supervisors.

It can be argued that the attitudes, energies, and optimism of each staff member are the critical influences for maintaining "good order" in an establishment, for stimulating children or young people to interact with each other, staff, and outsiders in a positive way, and for making definite progress in a planned direction. Based on these unique personality features, the group care worker assesses the crucial elements of treatment, makes decisions about the children's group and specific treatment plans for individual young people, and imposes sanctions on behaviour within a given set of procedures. This personality quagmire–the coherence or lack of coherence between staff members–would seem to be the main element that influences the success or failure of routines, intervention methods, and planned activities that surround a child or young person's total working day.

Unless staff members have organized themselves into a cohesive team with an integrated climate that absorbs the different ideologies, values, and philosophies, then the energies of workers may go into surviving or just competing with each other, virtually ensuring that no treatment is accomplished.

Taking into account the complexity of practice and the number of personalities involved, let us return to the picture of Jerry doing battle in his group care centre. Immediate questions that are posed include:

- How can a centre deal with a host of unanticipated eventualities in a way that is predictable and planned?
- How can a group of staff, working shifts with no more than one or two workers on duty at any time, maintain a particular intervention approach for a particular child whatever the circumstances?
- To use Henry Maier's (1981) imagery, how can the best or ideal rhythm for a specific child be learned and practised by the group care worker in all interventions resulting in the unity of rhythm between staff member(s) and child?
- How can a centre draw together a diverse group of workers into a cohesive team that can affect the lives of a diverse group of children?

Some of these questions can be answered by having a clear statement of intentions within a specific group care establishment. The following sections examine a step by step approach to formulating an action plan for group care practice.

DEVELOPING AN ACTION PLAN: STRATEGIC AND PRACTICAL CONSIDERATIONS

An action plan seeks to define a care and treatment programme with children or young people. It details specific actions and establishes clear boundaries within which certain types of action will take place. It describes the children or young people with whom the centre works and the norms and culture of the staff. Logic first dictates a clear knowledge of the people for whom the programme is intended. Thus, prior to the development of any residential or day care setting, it is essential to know something about the existing children or young people and those anticipated in the future.

When group care workers are asked to describe the residents with whom they work, some of the most frequent responses include sex, age, criminal offence, active/passive, cooperative/uncooperative, violent/victim, clever/stupid, runaway, impulsive, thief, cheat, substance abuser, liar, fearful, untrustworthy, intimacy problems, not being successful, not being sane or well, or not being happy. Frequently these descriptions revolve around a child or young person's behaviour. There might be half-a-dozen positive descriptions and a dozen negative descriptions concerning any one young person.

Psychological, psychiatric, and educational reports produce some other descriptions for the same child. Labels such as these, however sophisticated, frequently have little bearing on the day-to-day interactions between staff members and children. Indeed, with twelve children in a residential unit there would be an overload on any one worker if she or he were to remember all the assessment statements concerning all the young people who live there. Such statements and the implied responses are seldom helpful in a window-smashing episode, a refusal to go to bed, a scapegoating incident, or a situation involving damage to a staff member's car. At such times the group care worker's natural, intuitive, and personality-induced responses come to the fore. If the problem is resolved then the worker will be looked upon as being competent, whether or not the diagnostic description and implied treatment strategy have been adhered to in any way.

Hoghughi (1980) described the usefulness of a diagnosis and treatment description for problem children as being subservient to alleviating a child's problems. Hunt (1972) wrote about the same problem experienced by teachers in schools. Hunt (1966) proposed a set of conditional statements indicating the environmental conditions thought appropriate for a child of a specified state in order to produce a sequence of change aimed towards a desired state. The crucial issue is whether workers are able to make use of such information on most occasions and under most circumstances.

This is quite different from the diagnostic approach that a psychotherapist might hold in mind at a bi-monthly outpatient clinic. Here, the psychotherapist is likely to be in charge and his or her background, uniqueness, and idiosyncrasies are integrated with an approach to treatment, put into practice every two weeks. When more than one person is involved in the therapy then approaches need to be understood by each participant so that each worker's response is integrated with shared attitudes, philosophies, and practices.

Brill (1977), using the Conceptual Level Model, demonstrated that in some situations group care environments can be designed to give children differing amounts of structure. Conceptual Level is based on a theory of personality development (Harvey, Hunt, & Schroder, 1961) where the stage of development for a person, whether maladjusted, delinquent, or normal, may be assessed. Where a person is located on this developmental continuum indicates his or her conceptual level made up of cognitive complexity (differentiation, discrimination, and integration) as well as interpersonal maturity (increasing self-responsibility). A person with a higher conceptual level is thought to be more structurally complex, more capable of responsible actions, and more capable of adapting to a changing environment than a person at a lower Conceptual Level.

Brill's research was based on the conceptual level of each child placed in two different residential units. These units were designed with different amounts of predictability, consistency, staff control, order and organization, tangible reinforcements, opportunity for expressiveness, emphasis on personal problems, autonomy, and so on. Children of very low conceptual level did better in the more highly structured residential facility and had fewer problems in terms of time being spent in detention or absconding from the programme.

These results compared favourably with the results of children with very low conceptual level placed in a unit where the environment was less "structured" and less organized by staff. Those children whose conceptual level was low as compared with very low did slightly better when the amount of structure was reduced in small quantities. In short, the mismatched, low conceptual level boys in residence had more than twice the problem behaviour incidents as those matched to the programme in which they were placed in terms of unit precision, consistency, directiveness, and structure. Also the time spent "out of programme" (in their room or elsewhere) because of unacceptable behaviour or because of absconding was three-and-a-half times greater for the mismatched children than for those matched.

Brill and Reitsma (1978) further discovered that if the conceptual level of the primary worker (the key person in charge of coordinating the care and treatment plan for a young person and providing most counselling time with him) is one stage above that of the child, then development was apparently heightened and change in a positive direction was most obvious. In addition, Brill and Reitsma found that according to Interpersonal Maturity Level (Grant, Grant, & Sullivan, 1957), if the primary worker was matched by personality to the needs and characteristics of the child, then progress in a residential establishment was significantly greater than for those children not matched or completely mismatched (Palmer, 1967, 1968, 1972).

In short, Brill and Reitsma found that when there was an optimum match between the resident and the key or primary worker, then residents spent one-third less time in residential care and had one-half the rate of problem incidents than when there was a mismatch between resident and primary worker. Yet again, when the primary worker was matched to the child, according to Palmer's Interpersonal-Level matching criteria, these residents had one-eighth of the problem incidents and only two percent of their time in residence was spent out of programme. This compared favourably with the mismatched primary worker where residents had eight times as many problem incidents and 25 percent of their time in residence was spent out of programme.

The importance of this is that both the Interpersonal Maturity and Conceptual Level Models provide typologies from which to develop differential treatment environments for different children. A great deal is known about which type of staff member will work best with which type of children and in what type of programme. There is also a good deal known about what basic techniques are best used with different children.

In summary, our starting point was the chaotic set of crises encountered by Jerry the care worker. It is possible for Jerry to achieve greater clarity as to how he should deal with each situation that confronts him. It is possible to know more clearly the type of residents normally placed in his unit, with the obvious implications this has for any type of intervention. Appropriate recipe(s) for particular groups of young people can help maintain Jerry's sanity and motivation while assisting the children themselves to progress on to more complex and responsible behaviour. Then the dynamic characteristics of practice in a unit necessitates the monitoring of children's progress to keep track of what developmental changes take place during their placement in group care. As the make-up of the resident group alters over time, so the Action Plan of the care establishment needs to change in fairly precise ways, because of the characteristic patterns of interaction between particular children and particular environments to produce planned results. Hunt (1972) stated, "The issue is not which environment is best but rather which environment is best for a particular person to produce a specific effect" (p. 17).

In the same way that a child's developmental stage is regularly assessed, so it is equally important to monitor what is happening between staff and children and between different children. It is necessary to assess whether the action plan is really being put into practice or whether aberrations and numerous exceptions are the order of the day. Finally, the tasks of monitoring child and centre characteristics should be balanced against an evaluation of the programme as a whole. Here the results may be compared with evaluations from other places using the same practice language concerning young people, care and treatment environments, and programmes. Frequently the central question involves asking, "What kinds of children are participating in the group care service, under what circumstances, and what does that imply for management and treatment?" (Warren, 1973).

In what follows, an outline is provided for use in compiling a programme Action Plan. Those seeking to use this outline simply use the different headings to start compiling an informative statement of their service and service objectives. An interim Action Plan is best reviewed on a 3 to 6 month basis during the first year and then on a twice yearly basis thereafter.

Section I: Social Policy Mandate and Philosophy of the Centre

The Definition of Centre Mandate

So many are the variables concerning children, staff, programmes, strategies, and even length of time in care, the arguments so recurring about what approaches work best that, optimally, many decisions about programme design, general philosophy, and methods of working may need to be taken outside the group care unit. The leaders and those already working in a setting make representations to managers or administrators about their views on child assessment, prescribed actions, and broad outlines of intervention. It is clearly advocated that decisions such as these about mandate should not rest only with the team leader and immediate staff group.

Frequently such important decisions are left to team leaders because an agency has no coherent way of describing young people or staff programmes as an integrated whole. Care and treatment goals are frequently written in vague, fuzzy terms (Kushlik, 1975; Mager, 1972) such as "realising a child's potential," "broadening experience and skills," "increasing self-confidence and ability to make relationships," or "to aid insight into self-defeating processes."

What is unhelpful is the realization that most group care centres adopt such statements as basic beliefs or as an accepted part of their service claims. The British Association of Social Workers (1977), in the opening pages of its document defining "The Social Work Task," offered an example of how fuzzy language (Mager, 1972) was adopted by a professional body. A mandate written in such global terms, with words likened to a belief system, is not helpful for a team of workers who require clarity of expectations about the fundamental direction and ethos of their programme. A mandate written in global terms can lull an agency into the false impression that it actually has detailed direction for its various programmes. However, when many programme descriptions are examined closely, frequently one finds that no integrating formula holds the scheme together: neither the care and treatment strategies for particular young people, the characteristics and traits of staff needed, nor methods for systematically monitoring and evaluating change.

To summarize, chaos and disillusionment are more likely to exist and be in evidence unless there is a statement of policy expectations or mandate about what kind of young people the programme will serve and general ideas about the treatment strategies expected. Those working in group care programmes might well ask themselves: (1) What is the policy mandate for our present work setting? (2) Who decided these expectations? and (3) What are the concepts that underpin the policy mandate and assumptions used to integrate young people, staff, and programme? Asking staff to write down their individual answers to these three questions and then asking the staff group to examine their replies during a team meeting provides its own revelation of similarity, difference, and confusion.

When setting up a new service, a team leader may well have the luxury of working out key areas of the programme prior to hiring staff. If the staff group are already in post, as happens in most cases, an effective tactic that can assist staff to develop their work occurs naturally through the developmental process which an action plan employs. It evolves from within the staff group, under the clear leadership of the team manager, and seeks to use the aspirations of each staff member.

Minimum requirements are that the team leader has knowledge of group dynamics and the workers should not be totally inexperienced at working in staff groups where at different times the members may be challenging, confronting, intimate, or revealing. If the majority of a team have little knowledge of group dynamics and the steps through which groups develop and regress, then the action plan exercise may get bogged down with interpersonal problems that get in the way of its primary task. Menzies (1977) referred to this as anti-task activity. If it happens, then the team leader needs to acquire (or needs to be instructed about) guidance in group dynamics, sensitivity training, or something similar.

Philosophy of the Unit

To be realistic, it must be remembered that an Action Plan provides detailed statements on the whole variety of features concerned with group care practice: a centre's rules, resident group culture, staff, and so on. It is not a solution and decision-making print-out of every variable likely to confront a worker in the course of a shift. The Action Plan is used to clarify issues about the establishment's philosophy and beliefs, the principles underlying client management practices, communication approaches and aspirations. When these issues are clearly articulated and written so as to be understood and endorsed by all who work in the centre (or in association with a centre), so there develops the basis for a shared approach to practice. Real differences and individual preferences amongst staff members will be highlighted during what can become a drawn-out process of coming to a negotiated agreement about a shared language of practice. Conflicts emerging in relation to different orientations, backgrounds, experiences, beliefs, level of commitment, and lifestyles are essential steps in the development of an Action Plan.

At least three questions need to be asked of staff as they engage in this step of the Action Plan process. It is comparatively easy for all workers to give initial responses to these questions separately and in writing, in a 5-10 minute task. Staff members are asked:

1. What are the guiding principles that underlie the work of this centre, its work with young people, staff, neighbours, and other professionals?
2. What ideas or concepts are used to explain the unit's work with young people?
3. Describe in a few words the communication or interpersonal approach used in interactions between staff and young people, between young people, and between staff?

This kind of written exercise is frequently a stimulus for people to take such a fuzzy or ideological question seriously. Responses from staff in different units are given as examples.

In the first case, no responses at all were given, with workers unable to formulate a written statement of philosophy for themselves, let alone a philosophy that might incorporate principles for the whole unit. In such a case, specific instruction, experiential work, and clarity of thinking were necessary in order to get the workers to think in terms of philosophy.

In the second case, clearly articulated statements from individuals were in conflict with the statements of other workers. Such statements were products of the different backgrounds from which the workers had come as compared with a common definition about the resident group.

Third, at different times in a very short period, the same workers answered the three questions very differently, revealing the temporary nature of the centre's philosophy. Statements that are based on the past few shifts of work are often presented in subjective terms.

Fourth, a coherent, systematic response was obtained from a fourth team, indicating the successful completion of important groundwork which was necessary in order for workers to perform with a shared approach to practice.

Section II: Child Development and Orientations to Group Living

Child and Youth Development

This section outlines the particular features involved and events that take place in the centre that give the setting a uniqueness. This involves such items as:

1. influencing young people's group culture;
2. transmitting values to young people;
3. young people's rules and procedures;
4. young people's meetings.

The team leaders are encouraged to make certain that in thinking of child and youth development, the sub-headings of an Action Plan will reveal important norms that may be distinctive features of the centre. Not everything taking place with children or young people needs to be mentioned, otherwise the Action Plan document will be so large that it cannot be used as a staff guide or handbook.

Like the process described above, benefit can come from asking individual workers to spell out in writing what they consider to be the ideal culture initiated and enacted by staff with young people in the centre. Writing this up on large paper and posting it around the wall (wallpapering) offers an insight to everyone about the common and divergent attitudes held by staff members towards the young people. If the unit is already functioning with young people, each worker can also be invited to write how they assess the present youth group culture. Comparisons between the ideal and present group cultures are important and frequently result in productive discussion.

Different strategies for influencing and having an impact on youth group culture are readily available. Jones (1968) advocated a participative approach, Vorrath and Brendtro (1974) outlined a peer responsibility approach, while Brown and Christie (1981) and Pizzat (1973) have offered social learning approaches to practice. The basic philoso-

phy of the centre, already completed, must be compatible with and reinforce the key interventions planned with a group of residents. Feedback
from workers who have struggled with these two sections in an Action
Plan revealed that these sections are frequently the least tangible of the
lot. They are the most difficult to sort out and yet the most important,
because all other aspects of the Action Plan build from a coherent statement about the centre's philosophy and its orientation to the youth population it serves.

Values and Attitudes to Child or Youth Behaviour

Once the basic orientation to work with young people is clear and the
workers have clarified major expectations that they have for the young
people, then a series of more specific questions need to be asked. A
highly relevant but seldom asked question for all workers is: "What are
the specific values that we want the young people to learn?"

In practice this question can be considered with staff using an exercise similar to that described earlier. At a staff meeting, workers can be
asked to "Write down six basic values you want children or young people to learn." Such an exercise can demonstrate, in a reasonably relaxed
way, the important differences in social background that exist between
workers and, therefore, different priorities given to teaching children.
The individual value preferences can be wallpapered around the wall,
giving staff an opportunity to note whether their recommended values
are acknowledged. As group care workers have engaged in such an exercise, several responses occur:

- Some staff members have similar values.
- Some values may be wrapped up in a personal language that dis-
  guises the basic value and to which several other values can be im-
  puted. Many workers hold the value, for example, that "residents
  should attend a dentist every six months." Here the value is not
  seeing the dentist but perhaps ensuring that a child keeps his or her
  teeth for a lifetime or maintains his or her good looks. Alternatively the worker may be saying, "I don't want you to have to suffer a lot of dental work; therefore it is better to do something each
  day than it is to wait until your teeth rot." In other words: a stitch in
  time saves nine.
- Some values held by workers are total absolutes, such as always
  telling the truth or telling the truth in certain circumstances. Does
  telling the truth mean truthful replies only when asked a question?

And does it include voicing opinions when someone expresses dislike or revulsion, as when seeing a dirty intoxicated man asleep in a chair? Such absolute values, and how they should be applied in a given setting are opened for debate amongst workers.

Workers tend to find absolutes and procedures easier to recall than to identify values that they might find helpful to reinforce with young people in day-to-day practice. Group care teams are encouraged to refine a half-dozen social values that the workers' group can reinforce over and over again during any shift, whether events go well or badly. In so doing, a group care team helps to promote consistency and enable children or young people to assimilate learning through repetition time and time again. This is especially relevant for egocentric, impulsive youths whose interests are solely in the present. It is also helpful for those who have surges of emotion that dominate mind and actions.

When value orientation has been considered, some workers on both sides of the Atlantic have objected to the notion of filling children's minds with a particular set of ideals. Such an approach has been thought contradictory to the notion of individual freedom. These workers want to emphasize values where children are allowed to pick and choose for themselves and change their own values. To counter such arguments, proponents of the Conceptual Level Matching Model have shown that a large proportion of residents in some centres have not become dependent on any clearly defined norms or values.

For this reason, until personal values become part of a young person's pattern of functioning, it is neither appropriate nor possible for that young person to start being independent or commence working out one's own beliefs. Brill (1979) highlighted the importance of flexibility in negotiation and expressiveness in work with children and young people who had internalized personal values. However, approaches such as these have often been misused with young people who are physically mature but whose egocentricity is extreme and whose interpersonal maturity is low. Brill and Reitsma (1973) demonstrated that significant behaviour problems come about as the result of staff wanting young people to work out their own value systems. Such findings serve to reinforce the argument that group care workers all too frequently use idiosyncratic approaches in their direct care practices.

Relevant values for egocentric children or young people might include the following:

• Stop and think (before acting or responding).
• Listen to what others say.

- Do unto others as you want them to do to you.
- Face up to others.
- Face up to problems.
- Your views and ideas are important.

Group care workers seem to have little difficulty considering what these values might involve in practice. They also tend to support decisions about using all events, positive or negative, to emphasize these value prescriptions with direct suggestions about their importance. After frequent use and practice, the workers may start to use indirect suggestion by telling stories or using metaphors which contain these values (Grinder & Bandler, 1979; Lankton, 1979).

Rules and Expectations

Workers will have to decide what to include in this section and, more importantly, what to leave out. A statement of all rules and expectations will be so huge and overpowering that it will alienate most young people, staff, and others. Procedures and rules can include the daily routine or timetable with specific indications as to when events occur. Important expectations and rules can also be included, especially those that are fundamental to the smooth functioning of the establishment along certain lines. Some rules come to the forefront because of contravention on a regular basis, and others because these rules, when broken, cause difficulties for staff. Basic expectations can be spelled out around daily living routines, including:

- Chores, details, or daily jobs.
- Leaving the centre, weekend or holiday absences, absconding, and so forth.
- Formal or informal counselling sessions.
- Pocket money and other.

Rules might include statements such as:

- No violence against any person.
- No drugs or alcohol.
- No visiting each other's bedroom after 9 p.m.
- No sex on the premises.

No matter how much effort workers put into spelling out rules, most of them are likely to be written in negative terms. Some centres have stated the penalties that will be imposed for non-compliance with expectations or violation of the rules. Other centres have tended to reinforce daily compliance. Still other centres have been known to bring violations to a regular group meeting.

Putting only basic rules and expectations down on paper often results in the claim made by some outsiders that more rules and expectations should be written into an Action Plan. Ultimately, the decision about what to include will necessitate each group care worker listing all the rules and expectations as they see them in the centre and then everyone rank ordering the importance of these. The revelation that comes from workers through such an exercise is that different staff view norms, rules, and expectations differently. Some rules and expectations might apply with some members of staff, while others might operate quite differently. For example, it may be discovered that some workers have a rigid approach to ensuring that young people go to bed at the stated time. Others, however, may allow television to be watched until the end of a programme or until activities have been completed. The smaller the unit with fewer staff working alongside each other, the more likely it is that very different procedures will evolve for different shifts. Again using the evidence supplied by Brill and Reitsma (1978) and Hunt (1972), the more egocentric and immature the child or young person, the more learning approaches should emphasize systematic and consistent interactions throughout his/her wakeful day.

The very fact of consolidating rules and expectations in workers' minds will force them to clarify particular demands or prohibitions used in their centre. The end result for an Action Plan is that while numerous agreements will be made concerning basic prompting and general compliance from residents during certain events, only a few rules will actually need to be written down. Otherwise, the list becomes never-ending and forever-changing. A crucial function at staff meetings is to review and update rules and expectations at regular intervals for everyone's benefit.

Section III: Links with Family, Peers, and Significant Others

Family Development

Here, workers are invited to consider the attitudes that are held towards involving parents in the life of the programme. For instance a particular group home had a clear objective about intensive work with parents. This objective was written into their social policy mandate by the agency that funded them. Basic expectations concerning work with families were stated, involving at least two contacts with the family by each worker each week, with at least one of these meetings being at the group home. A specific contract was to be negotiated with the parents at the time of referral. Any home visits would be followed up by detailed discussion so as to examine how the visit had gone. Parents were actively encouraged to use the same techniques with their young person at home as the group care workers were using, most frequently a Behaviour Modification approach.

In other establishments, contact with families may be less intensive. Whatever the level of contact, it is important that practices carried out with families are clearly stated and workers know what actions are expected of them in this respect. If the philosophy and attitudes underpinning practice are to ensure that parents become partners in helping (Whittaker, 1979), then the methods used to engage parents as partners will need to be stated. Ainsworth explores this practice issue further at a later stage in this volume. It is worth remembering the evidence supplied by Taylor and Alpert (1973) who found that, more than anything else, the determining factor about future adjustment following an institutional care placement is the frequency of contact between parents and their child.

Involvement of Peers and Others

The friends and associates of children or young people will inevitably have contact with a group care centre. Whether school friends or work mates are concerned, the Action Plan should make a basic statement about how these involvements should be managed. Parties in the early morning hours, under-age drinking, or sexual involvements are some issues that might develop. Involvement with other "outsiders" should also be noted whether these include health and social service workers, police, neighbours, shop deliverymen, volunteers, or others. This subsection of an Action Plan is rarely complete. Rather, workers are required to constantly upgrade their involvements with others in practice.

After-Care

Centre workers are asked to consider their relations with young people who have left the centre and gone elsewhere. Any contact that is planned or engineered to provide continuing encouragement and support for ex-residents should be stated. Sinclair (1971) and Moos (1975) argued that basic adjustment to living outside a group care centre is correlated with the after-care environment that a person will be living in. The implication is that a young person is more likely to succeed with any social skills learned in a group care centre if those prompting these skills in an after-care environment include the people who have struggled with him or her in close proximity during previous weeks and months. Of course, if this is to happen, it may only be possible when those using a centre live in close proximity and have few problems concerning transportation. This step in the Action Plan process enables numerous changes and adjustments to be made and identifies practical ideas about after-care which could become part of the service.

Section IV: Staffing and Staff Development

A summary statement about how the staff group functions together as a team, including reference to the consultation and supervision available, is very different from the statements made in the child and youth development areas. In itself, this section can be brief. There is opportunity for a team leader and team members to expand or contract the Action Plan headings to suit the particular orientation of the centre. The issues referred to here give an illustration of what could be expected in some settings.

It is interesting to note how people identify subjectively with the notion that what happens within the staff group is often reflected back in what happens with the young people. Thus, the level of energy available in a team, its commitment to interpersonal and intra-personal development, the workers' orientation to staff meetings, and availability of consultation and supervision all contribute to the morale, satisfaction, and effectiveness of group care workers.

In writing on this matter and use of the Group Environment Scale (Moos, Meel, & Humphrey, 1974) to assess team climates, Brill indicated that a moderate level of leader control appeared to be a necessary but not all-sufficient condition for effective team functioning. It would seem that leader control should be combined with (a) a high level of organization and clarity around daily norms, expectations, and routines, and (b) teamwork to minimize workers' loss of energy through frustration and anger and to maintain a high task focus. Under such conditions, it is expected that staff morale would be higher and rates of turnover considerably reduced (Brill, 1979, pp. 120-123).

The corollary to this is that inefficient staff meetings, no predictability around consultation and supervision, or a lack of clarity about who does what, when, and how are likely to be reflected in low morale amongst residents, more behaviour that is out-of-control, and more complaints about the handling of different situations. Thus it is that a brief section about care for the caregivers is an important feature of any Action Plan. As Maier (1977) argued, "It is inherent that the caretakers be nurtured themselves and experience sustained, caring support in order to transmit this quality of care to others" (p. 17).

Staff Meetings

Some statement should be made about the frequency of staff meetings and who is obliged to attend. This would influence the rostering of staff. If different people attend for different sessions this is likely to alter the way in which meetings can be conducted. Action Plans can spell out expectations for staff meetings using short statements concerning the organization of each meeting and how this reinforces the philosophy of the unit. Increased efficiency and positive feedback about how time spent in meetings has become more productive is the consistent response from workers using this approach. Workers seem to be especially pleased with the increased cohesion reported in relation to work with residents and in planning for the future.

Staff Consultation and Supervision

The Action Plan should note how an establishment stands with regard to the team leader providing a formal consultation and supervision service. If a unit is committed to such a service, the Action Plan needs to spell out how it will be conducted. This contrasts dramatically with a team leader holding staff meetings simply because of a perceived obligation and without clarity of purpose and organization. Such ad hoc, unplanned meetings waste time. The system of staff consultation and supervision, spelled out in an Action Plan, might involve:

1. a review of previous decisions;
2. a review of key worker activity;
3. the health, job satisfaction, and morale of workers;
4. fulfilling the tasks of the job;
5. any other business;

6. a summary of decisions taken; and
7. an evaluation of the meeting.

The Action Plan might make formal note of the importance of consultation by specifying a minimum number of meetings per month and obligations associated with taking notes at meetings. An alternative route is to ensure that a meeting is never adjourned without setting a date for the next session.

Section V: Key Worker Responsibilities

An aspect of group care practice that is becoming increasingly common involves a direct-care worker coordinating all aspects of care and treatment for a particular child or young person. Such a worker also disseminates information about that young person to all other staff. In some places this person is termed the "primary worker" while in other places such a person is called the "key worker." If such a system operates, then the basic responsibilities of a key worker need to be spelled out in the Action Plan. This might include planning care and treatment activities, report writing, liaison concerning job finding or school attendance, formal counselling sessions, working with family, and so on. An Action Plan seeks formally to incorporate this feature into the overall service.

Section VI: Evaluation of Staff Performance

Another important area in the Action Plan involves specification of how performance and actions of each worker will be monitored and evaluated. An Action Plan with clear philosophy and procedures will be a waste of paper unless there is clarity around evaluation of staff performance. It is important for a team leader to be involved in setting up a recording system that can monitor how each worker is performing. Thus, a clear record of performance can be used to focus discussion on actual practices at staff meetings, individual consultations, and during in-service training sessions. Without this section being clearly articulated, there is no definite reason for workers to conform to the Action Plan. A useful exercise involves staff being asked to identify in writing those practices they believe are going well, those that are unproductive, and those likely to need oversight in order to guarantee consistent performance. It is a frequent cause for surprise that many workers request an inspectorial approach so as to improve their own individual performance and to enforce changes in the performance of others.

Section VII: Programme Development and Evaluation

This final section is oriented toward examining what happens over the course of time with children or young people, the group care workers, and the setting. Whatever the major interests of the team, these will be reflected in the information collected.

Resident Change

Some centre teams are oriented towards looking at criminal activity, violence, and problem incidents while the child or young person is in residence. If this is so, then the Action Plan should state how the required information is collected. Such information might also include the rate with which children or young people are unfavourably discharged or removed from the centre. Others might be interested in overall changes experienced by a child or young person during his or her time in receipt of services, so diagnostic testing at the beginning of the stay would be replicated at pre-determined intervals. The increased demands for care and treatment accountability make this issue of service evaluation a very important consideration in any Action Plan for practice.

Unit Environment

Only a few programmes look at evaluation measures concerning a centre's environment. The environment scales developed by Moos (1974, 1975) can be used to assess the environment of group care along nine comparative dimensions, including the *Relationship* dimensions of involvement, support and expressiveness; the *Personal Development* dimensions of autonomy, orientation, and achievement; and *System Change* dimensions of order and organization, clarity of expectations, and control. This is done by using a questionnaire completed separately by each worker and resident. The information obtained from such an environmental analysis enables future development of the service.

For instance, with low conceptual-level adolescents in an institutional setting, certain environmental profiles would seem to enable the establishment to run most smoothly (Brill, 1979). If more mature people are in residence, then other profiles are necessary. Chase (1973) correlated certain environmental patterns that went with a reduction in absconding, where less absconding was found in environments with reasonably high staff control and a high emphasis on expressiveness by both staff and residents. Such findings further emphasize the importance of systematic evaluation in group care practice. It is on this basis that the Action Plan and future development of the service can proceed.

Information About Staff

Finally, it is important to consider the information about staff that might interest a centre. The rate of staff sickness in a centre is an important consideration. In recent years there has been a growing interest in job satisfaction and staff morale and changes or trends in satisfaction and sickness which take place over time. If these issues are important to workers, then a monitoring of basic information about staff attendance and performance may help to reduce the amount of sick leave in a centre. High levels of sick leave frequently put heavy demands on other workers who can have their hours increased with little warning. This, in itself, can influence job satisfaction amongst team members, as demonstrated in a study of group home staff (Johnson, Rusinko, Girard, & Tossey, 1978) where those working in excess of fifty hours per week were more likely to report symptoms of burn-out and feelings of despondency. The opposite results may be found in teams where workers concentrate on staying well and dealing with practice issues as they emerge.

CONCLUSIONS

A shared language for practice in group care has been suggested through the development of a centre Action Plan. It is not intended that all the features suggested here should be dogmatically adhered to by those seeking to develop an Action Plan for the first time. Rather, they are offered as examples which illustrate the action planning framework. A range of exercises have also been suggested which can enable workers to produce a coherent statement about how their service will operate.

Certain assumptions have been made throughout this chapter about the importance of a common theme that draws together the disparate characteristics of children or young people, treatment environment, and intervention strategies. The Action Plan is intended to be a negotiated statement of common themes that tie people and programmes together. In so doing, an Action Plan can help workers to reduce the level of conflict, competition, or despair that can all too easily develop in daily practice. Since the development of an Action Plan involves a team process, it is likely to increase the clarity of focus expected for each worker. The completed document is also useful in public relations with other professionals and referral agencies.

NOTE

1. Family group homes of the same nature were quickly adopted in New Zealand as well and continue to operate there with little modification nearly 60 years later.

REFERENCES

Brill, R. (1977). *Implications of the conceptual level matching model for the treatment of delinquents.* Paper presented at Conference of the International Differential Treatment Association, Rensselaerville, New York.
Brill, R. (1979). *Development of milieux facilitating treatment* (Final Report No. 4). Montreal: Universite de Montreal, Groupe de Recherche sur L'Inadaptation Juvenile.
Brill, R., & Reitsma, M. (1978). *Action research in a treatment agency for delinquent youth* (Final Report No. 1). Montreal: Universite de Montreal: Groupe de Recherche sur L'Inadaptation Juvenile.
British Association of Social Workers (1977). *Report of working party on the social work task.* London: BASW Publications.
Brown, B. J., & Christie, M. (1981). *Social learning practice in residential child care.* Oxford: Pergamon Press.
Casson, S., & George, C. (1995). *Culture change for total quality: An action guide for managers in social and health services.* London: Pitman Publishing.
Casson, S., & Manning, B. (1996). *Total quality in child protection.* Lyme Regis, Dorset, England: Russell House Publishing.
Chase, M. M. (1973). *A profile of absconders.* New York: New York State Division for Youth, Research Department.
George, C., & Casson, S. (1994). *Care sector quality: A training manual incorporating BS5750 (Social Services Training Manuals).* Brighton, England: Pavilion Publishing.
Grant, J. D., Grant, M. Q., & Sullivan, E. D. (1957). The development of interpersonal maturity: Applications to delinquency. *Psychiatry, 20,* 272-83.
Grinder, J., & Bandler, R. (1979). *Frogs into princes.* Utah: Real People Press.
Harvey, O. J., Hunt, D. E., & Schroder, H. M. (1961). *Conceptual systems and personality organization.* New York: John Wiley.
Hoghughi, M. (1980). *Assessing problem children: Issues and practice.* London: Burnett Books.
Hunt, D. E. (1966). A conceptual systems change model and its application to education. In O. J. Harvey (Ed.), *Experience structure and adaptability.* New York: Springer.

Hunt, D. E. (1972). *Matching models in education.* Toronto: OISE.

Johnson, K. W., Rusinko, W. T., Girard, C. M., & Tossey, M. (1978). *Job satisfaction and burn-out: A double-edged threat to human service workers.* Washington, DC: Academy of Criminal Justice Science Meeting, March.

Jones, M. (1968) *Social psychiatry in practice.* Harmondsworth, England: Penguin.

Kushlik, A. (1975, December). Some ways of setting, monitoring, and attaining objectives for services for disabled people. *British Journal of Mental Subnormality, 21*(41).

Lankton, S. R. (1979). *Practical magic: The clinical application of neuro-linguistic programming.* Cupertino, CA: Meta Publications.

Mager, R. F. (1972). *Goal analysis.* Belmont, CA: Fearon Publishers.

Maier, H. (1977). *The core of care.* Stirling, Scotland: Aberlour Child Care Trust, The First Aberlour Trust Lecture.

Maier, H. (1981). Essential components in care and treatment environments for children. In F. Ainsworth & L. C. Fulcher (Eds.), *Group care for children: Concept and issues.* London: Tavistock.

Menzies, I. E. P. (1977). *Staff support systems: Task and anti-task in adolescent institutions.* London: Tavistock Institute of Human Relations.

Moos, R. H. (1974). *Evaluating treatment environments: A social, ecological approach.* New York: John Wiley.

Moos, R. H. (1975). *Evaluating correctional and community settings.* New York: John Wiley.

Moos, R. H., Meel, P. M., & Humphrey, B. (1974). *Combined preliminary manual: Family, work and group environment scales.* Palo Alto, CA: Consulting Psychologists Press.

Palmer, T. (1967). *Personality characteristics and professional orientations of five groups of community treatment project workers: A preliminary report of differences among treaters.* Sacramento, CA: Community Treatment Project.

Palmer, T. (1968). *Rating inventory for the selection and matching of treatment personnel.* Sacramento, CA: Community Treatment Project.

Palmer, T. (1972). *Differential placement of delinquents in group homes, final report.* Sacramento: California Youth Authority and the National Institute of Mental Health.

Pizzat, F. (1973). *Behavior modification in residential treatment for children.* New York: Behavioral Publications.

Report of the Care and Children Committee (The Curtis Report). (1946). Cmnd 6922. London: HMSO.

Sinclair, I. (1971). *Hostels for probationers.* London: HMSO.

Taylor, D. A., & Alpert, S. W. (1973). *Continuity and support following residential treatment.* New York: Child Welfare League of America.

Vorrath, H. H., & Brendtro, L. K. (1974). *Positive peer culture.* Chicago: Aldine.

Warren, M. Q. (1973). *Community corrections: For whom, when, and under what circumstances? What the research tells us.* Sacramento, CA: Community Treatment Project.

Whittaker, J. K. (1979). *Caring for troubled children.* San Francisco: Jossey-Bass.

Chapter 7

Creating and Sustaining a Culture of Group Care

Frank Ainsworth
Leon C. Fulcher

SUMMARY. Group care centers are established to provide a range of living, learning, treatment, and supervisory opportunities for children and young people who, for a variety of reasons, need alternative, supplementary, or substitute care. It is important, therefore, that group care centres establish an organizational climate, ethos, or culture of caring that is consistent with these objectives. This is achieved through internal organizational design, administrative routines, maintaining the physical environment, and support for staff team functioning, including attention to specific work methods. *[Article copies available for a fee from The Haworth Document Delivery Service: 1-800-HAWORTH. E-mail address: <docdelivery@haworthpress.com> Website: <http://www.HaworthPress.com> © 2006 by The Haworth Press, Inc. All rights reserved.]*

KEYWORDS. Group care, residential care, residential treatment, group homes, youth work, youthwork, group work, at-risk youth

---

Address correspondence to: Frank Ainsworth, School of Social Work and Community Welfare, James Cook University, Townsville 4811, Queensland, Australia.

[Haworth co-indexing entry note]: "Creating and Sustaining a Culture of Group Care." Ainsworth, Frank. and Leon C. Fulcher. Co-published simultaneously in *Child & Youth Services* (The Haworth Press, Inc.) Vol. 28, No. 1/2, 2006, pp. 151-176; and: *Group Care Practice with Children and Young People Revisited* (ed: Leon C. Fulcher, and Frank Ainsworth) The Haworth Press, Inc., 2006, pp. 151-176. Single or multiple copies of this article are available for a fee from The Haworth Document Delivery Service [1-800-HAWORTH, 9:00 a.m. - 5:00 p.m. (EST). E-mail address: docdelivery@haworthpress.com].

TWENTY YEARS LATER: A REFLECTION

This chapter focuses on conceptual building blocks that shape the organizational and practice culture of any group care centre. These building blocks provide the foundation for an organizational climate of caring required to effect changes with children and young people placed in such centres. Whether contemplating institutional care facilities, smaller 24-hour group living units, or day centres in health care, education, social welfare, or criminal justice systems, parallel considerations apply. Looking back after twenty years, the framework and language used to describe these building blocks for an organizational culture of group care still resonate. The concepts remain centrally important to all concerned with developing and sustaining responsive child and youth care practices.

Such an assertion becomes clear when reviewing the questions found at the end of section and exploring answers to these questions in the light of current practices. These questions need to be addressed by programme managers and direct care workers to ensure that the organizational cultures of their group care programmes are consistent with service expectations and are responsive to the service needs of their client populations. The responses to each question need to address both direct and indirect caring methods and skills noted in Chapter 1 as well as approaches used by those working with families as highlighted in Chapter 4.

New questions may, of course, require consideration not least of all because of population changes amongst children and young people now being referred to group care centres. Questions also need to be asked about whether new features require addition to this framework. For example, drug use amongst young people placed in group care programmes is now more prevalent than it was 20 years ago as is the prevalence of young people living as HIV-positive. Do group care programmes now require specialist drug counselling services as an integral part of their programme? The increasingly specialised therapeutic focus of many group care services may prompt thinking in such directions. Furthermore, given the increased specialisation services, what pre-employment training and qualifications may now be required and what expectations might have changed about the ongoing professional education of group care workers?

Yet another question arises from the advances in neuroscience, psychology, biochemistry, and psychotherapy that now influence each other more directly than ever before, providing new knowledge about how the structure of the brain evolves after birth and how emotions and relationships are shaped by brain chemistry and social interactions (Gerhardt, 2004). How might such new knowledge reshape group care methods and skills, including continuing developments with family work? It is also worth noting the research findings that show how group care programmes are not all bad and that, when used appropriately, they are actually very effective (Ainsworth, 2001).

Might changes in the population served and the potential new roles for more specialised group care services require a systematic review of the knowledge base identified 20 years ago or that the building blocks of organizational cultures of group care centres need reformulation? Or might contemporary service developments add new dimensions to the original framework? On reflection we think not. Such developments may add new content to the framework but do not radically alter it. Responsive group care programmes still require that specific attention to be given to:

* child and adolescent development
* structural features of a group care (social structure, norms, language, and values)
* organizational design (dependence, independence, and support)
* design of the physical environment
* team functioning and group development
* the role of the individual worker

All of these features retain their significance and remain equally vital to the delivery of developmentally enhancing services for children and young people.

Frank Ainsworth
Leon Fulcher

INTRODUCTION

In what follows, a number of features associated with creating and sustaining a culture of practice in group care centres are explored as these relate to services for children and young people. First, we outline the developmental conditions in which young people learn and develop most effectively. Next, the organizational culture of group care is considered, highlighting the social structure, language, norms, and values associated with responsive practice in a centre. Third, issues of programme design are addressed, highlighting complex relationships that exist between interpersonal dynamics and organizational contexts in group care practice. Attention then turns to a consideration of the physical environment and to ways in which the siting and physical design of a centre influences the culture of practice that develops there. Team functioning and youth group development are next considered since group dynamics are fundamental characteristics of practice in the group care field. Finally, attention returns to the role of individual workers, exploring the extent to which individuals can support development and learning for particular children or young people.

Institutional care, residential group living, and day services exist to provide a range of "living, learning, and treatment opportunities" (Ainsworth, 1981, p. 223) for children or young people who, for a variety of reasons, need alternative, supplementary, or substitute provision (Davis, 1981) of a type usually available within the context of family life. This is the *raison d'etre* for the existence of group care. Therefore it is important for group care centres to create an ethos and organizational culture that is consistent with the above objectives. This is accomplished through reference to a centre's internal programme design, its administrative routines, its physical environment, and characteristics of staff team functioning in the programme, including reference to specific work methods. Such factors are influential in shaping the practice culture of a centre, irrespective of whether it is located within health care, education, social welfare, or criminal justice systems.

When considering factors that influence the culture of group care, due account has also to be taken of knowledge about how children learn and develop. It is argued that knowledge such as this should guide decisions about events in the life of a group care centre rather than being dependent on administrative expediencies and organisational decision making, as noted by Maier in Chapter 5. It is argued that the cultural integrity of a centre can be achieved only by monitoring decisions related to the organization and physical environment of a centre and an evaluation of whether these decisions support growth and development for young people. Only in this way can workers confirm whether the culture of group care in a centre provides living, learning, and treatment opportunities that reinforce growth-enhancing processes for children. It is all too easy for these processes to be disrupted if well-intentioned group care personnel fail to consider the implications of particular actions carried out with children in their care. Growth-diminishing experiences are, unfortunately, common features of group care practice with children and young people, in spite of good intentions.

DEVELOPMENTAL CONDITIONS

Few authors have written about child and adolescent development in a manner that allows contemporary research findings to be immediately useful to group care workers and retain a central place in group care practice. For that reason, it is worth reviewing those conditions that provide the most favourable opportunities for learning and development. Our focus is on interpersonal structures (Bronfenbrenner, 1979) and processes (Maier, 1981) that provide the conditions for responsive group care. Our argument is that, until recent years, such knowledge has not been grounded sufficiently in an understanding of contextual influences on child and adolescent development.

In attempting to move towards a clearer appreciation of these matters, Bronfenbrenner (1979) provided a series of core definitions and hypotheses that sought to spell out the optimal conditions under which learning and development take place. These definitions associated with the ecology of human development refer to various elements that contribute to human activity in particular settings including activities, roles, and interpersonal relations. Attention is particularly drawn to those definitions and hypotheses that clarify the contributions made by interpersonal relations in developmental processes with young people. Such a narrowing of focus here should not be taken to imply a downgrading of the other elements simply to draw attention to the particular characteristics of group care practice, nor a failure to recognize how all the elements interact together.

Bronfenbrenner (1979) defined a relation as that which "obtains whenever one person in a setting pays attention to, or participates in, the activities of another" (p. 56). Three different types of relation were identified, each of which applies to group care practice with children or young people. The first of these involves situations where someone engages with a young person to observe a particular activity such as when a worker and child pay attention to each other's activities during the first days of placement in a centre.

By acknowledging the part that each plays in such an observational process, the minimal conditions for learning are enacted and the stage is set for a second type of youth-adult relations. Here the focus is on shared participation in related but not necessarily identical tasks, such as when a worker and young person wash the dishes after a meal. The emphasis in this type of relation is the reciprocal nature of the activity through which the emotional dimension of a relationship develops. This leads to a third type of youth-adult relations where enduring feelings develop between one and the other that influence the thoughts and behaviours of each. In such instances, a relationship can be said to exist even when the parties are no longer together.

These formulations may help one to understand better the influence of interpersonal relations in life-long learning. For group care workers engaged with children and young people, they offer special possibilities, taking as "the theatre for their work the actual living situation as shared and experienced by the child" (Ainsworth, 1981, p. 234). As a result, group care workers are in an ideal position to engage continuously and deliberately in relations of the type described above and in so doing provide contexts for learning. Throughout every hour of every day, group care workers are presented with opportunity events in which they can engage in all three types of relation and thereby help young people to grow and develop. Bronfenbrenner (1979) hypothesized that maximum achievable impact occurs when a worker and child engage in all three types of relation simultaneously (p. 60). If a relation is characterized by mutual antagonism then it is disruptive of learning, emphasizing the point that learning and development are most likely to be achieved when a close relationship exists between workers and the young people with whom they work.

While Bronfenbrenner helped to clarify the types of relation workers need to create in their work with young people, Maier (1981) highlighted the importance of attachment and the experience of dependency that are part of the intimate process of forming relationships. Maier noted how temperamental differences, even among very young children, can influence the rhythms of interaction which develop with those who provide care. It is important for workers to understand these facts so as to respond to any antagonism that may enter into and disrupt their relationships with young people, thereby restricting learning opportunities. Group care practice involves sensitive engagement with young people in a manner that is compatible with each child's needs and avoids the disruptive pitfalls that limit development.

Maier (1981) addressed the importance of establishing vital attachments between workers and young people that offer opportunities for a good experience of dependency, the pursuit of which may be clouded by difficult and demanding behaviours. Maier encouraged group care workers to view such phenomena afresh by placing these aspects of development in a normal sequence of daily life events. Dependency need not be viewed as a sign of weakness or psychopathology. Through attachment relationships, young people obtain the necessary prerequisites for learning and development. Rather than being fearful of the implied demands associated with attachment relationships, group care workers need to encourage these processes so that children will eventually "be free" (Maier, 1982a) to assume responsibility for themselves in later life. Such freedom cannot, however, be forced into existence. It develops instead through the experience of a secure attachment to another person and a growing sense of safe dependence on them.

Better than most writers, Bronfenbrenner and Maier help group care workers to see how to engage in the task of encouraging developmental processes with children. Bronfenbrenner did this by clarifying the type of interpersonal relations that must develop, while Maier provided a detailed understanding of the events which facilitate such relations. In so doing, both writers also highlight how dysfunctional institutions need not exist provided that they are restructured to allow practices outlined above. Wolins and Wozner (1982) echoed this view, highlighting the extent to which "theoretical, philosophical, and ideological determinants" influence the culture of a group care centre (Fulcher & Ainsworth, 1981, p. 83). In this respect, it may be helpful to pose a number or questions which workers might wish to ask about their own group care centres.

- To what extent are all three types of interpersonal relations in your centre actively considered, including observational relations, shared activity relations, and emotional attachments?
- How does your centre acknowledge the importance of and facilitate opportunities for children or young people to experience dependency? Or is dependency frowned upon and seen only as a negative feature of practice and relationships that develop between workers and young people?
- In what ways can it be said that your centre accepts the need for workers and young people to develop attachment relationships or is attachment and personal relationships viewed with suspicion?
- To what extent does your centre allow for differences in the temperament of children and the different patterns of interaction that are required as a consequence?

THE CULTURE OF PRACTICE

It is perhaps helpful to clarify the notion of culture that is being used here. All participants in a group care centre interact within a system that contains a language, values, norms, and social structure of its own (Eisikovitz, 1980). Culture therefore accounts for the totality of experiences in a centre, enabling one to consider whether some aspects of a centre's culture may be at variance with the culture of the surrounding community. In this respect, the culture of a group care centre warrants careful examination because variance between the internal and external cultures may provide evidence that the original learning and development goals have been compromised and the centre's service integrity undermined. This helps to explain why consideration must be given to the provision of cultural safety for all residents admitted to a centre (Fulcher, 1998). Failures to address cultural safety can emerge as the result of concerns associated with the wider service system or because of unrealistic community expectations imposed through a confused "social policy mandate" (Fulcher & Ainsworth, 1981, p. 78).

Much has been written, although not necessarily in the field of child welfare, about efforts in therapeutic communities to create an internal culture that facilitates personal growth and change amongst members (Hinslelwood & Manning, 1979; Jansen, 1980; Kennard, 1983). In such instances, variance between the culture of a group care centre and that of the wider community may be justified. On the other hand, purely institutional cultures must be evaluated critically, given the negative evaluations that have come from the health care (mental health and mental handicap) and criminal justice (prison and reformatory) systems. These studies have provided support for the notion of institutional dysfunction (Jones, 1967; Jones & Fowles, 1984), seriously questioning the integrity of some of the oldest and now least attractive group care centres. Indeed, much of the thrust towards normalization of resident experiences (Wolfensberger, 1972) was stimulated by attempts to reduce differences between group care cultures and promote more culturally normative conditions.

The culture of practice is, of course, the product of a multiplicity of factors, some of which are to be found in interactions between young people and workers within the centre and some with those outside it. Other interactions are also influential in shaping services in the group care field, and the culture of practice can only be fully understood through consideration of both "interpersonal dynamics and organizational contexts" (Ainsworth & Fulcher, 1981, p. 2).

Twelve structural variables associated with a differential assessment and evaluation of group care programmes were identified elsewhere (Fulcher & Ainsworth, 1981; Fulcher, 2001, pp. 417-435), and included:

Comparative Variable 1:   Duty of Care Mandate to Deliver
Child and Youth Care Services

Comparative Variable 2:   Siting and Physical Design of the
                           Centre

Comparative Variable 3:   Personnel Complement and
                           Deployment of Staff

Comparative Variable 4:   Recurring Patterns in the Use of
                           Time and Activity

Comparative Variable 5:   Admission and Discharge Practices

Comparative Variable 6:   Social Customs and Sanctions

Comparative Variable 7:   Social Climate of the Centre

Comparative Variable 8:   Links with Family, School, and
                           Community

Comparative Variable 9:   Criteria Used for Reviewing and
                           Evaluating Performance

Comparative Variable 10:   Theoretical, Philosophical, and
                           Ideological Determinants of Care

Comparative Variable 11:   Opportunity and Social Cost-Benefit
                           Ratios in the Delivery of Group
                           Care Services

Comparative Variable 12:   The Public Policy Environment and
                           Organisational Turbulence External
                           to the Centre

Two of these variables–theoretical or ideological determinants and social policy mandate–were noted earlier in this chapter. Other variables such as siting and physical design of a centre, personnel complement and deployment, and recurring patterns in the use of time and activity are considered below to show how they further shape the culture of practice in group care. Variables such as social customs and sanctions, social climate of the centre, links with family, school, and community, criteria for reviewing and evaluating performance, and cost factors also influence the culture of practice but receive only limited reference here. With inclusion of a twelfth variable–the external organization environment–it is worth noting that all twelve structural variables can be clustered under the four themes of social structure, language, norms, and values that make up the culture of practice in a centre, shown in Table 1.

The task of mapping interactions between all these variables to see how each feature is influenced by the others remains to be done. Anthropological research methods offer some possibilities in regard to this complex task. An anthropological perspective is compatible with the social ecology orientation (Apter, 1982; Whittaker, 1975) and, to some extent, that of a systems perspective (Hunter & Ainsworth, 1973; Polsky, 1963). Each of these frameworks encourages one to view group care centres as dynamic entities and to think of the constituent parts of a whole being in continuous interaction and change. As one part changes, so it interacts with other parts, resulting in a new equilibrium.

These perspectives pose direct implications for supervision, service monitoring, service planning, or management of personnel within group care centres and in the broader service system. This is because many of group care personnel view their duties as that of maintaining boundaries (Miller & Gwynne, 1972) between the constituent parts of a centre and the wider service system and including attempts to balance conflicting demands. Because the cultural perspective enables group care workers at all levels to see how an action at one point impacts on events in other parts of a centre, it also has direct practical relevance for children, because it allows workers to think of a wider range of interventions that might be used to achieve learning and development outcomes.

Interventions cannot therefore focus solely on interactions with children. Interventions at some point in the physical environment and organizational or administrative systems may also be required so as to improve learning and developmental opportunities for children. Of course, this does not in any way limit the importance of work undertaken directly with children or the importance of direct practice skills

TABLE 1. Structural Features That Shape the Culture of Practice in Group Care

SOCIAL STRUCTURE
- Siting and Physical Design of Centre
- Personnel Complement and Deployment of Staff
- The Public Policy Environment and Organisational Turbulence External to the Centre

LANGUAGE
- Recurring Patterns in the Use of Time and Activity
- Social Climate of the Centre
- Criteria Used for Reviewing and Evaluating Performance

NORMS
- Admission and Discharge Practices
- Social Customs and Sanctions
- Links with Family, School, and Community

VALUES
- Duty of Care Mandate to Deliver Child and Youth Care Services
- Theoretical, Philosophical, and Ideological Determinants of Care
- Opportunity and Social Cost-Benefit Ratios in the Delivery of Group Care Services

that this entails. A further set of questions that workers might use to explore the validity of arrangements established in their centre include:

- How far is the culture of your centre consistent with that of the community that immediately surrounds it?
- What opportunities are provided for the growth and development of young people in your centre?
- What would have to be changed so that children or young people acquire cultural experiences similar to those available to families elsewhere?
- What reasons are given for the special cultural features found operating in your centre?
- To what extent are special cultural features in your centre primarily for the convenience of staff or for the wider service system instead of young people and their families?

It is anticipated that answers to these questions will vary depending on the occupational identity of workers asking the questions: nurses, teachers, child and youth care workers, social workers, or staff in correctional facilities. The location of the centre within health care, education, social welfare, or criminal justice will also influence the answers to each question since language, a key feature of culture, tends to differ across each of the four systems.

ISSUES OF ORGANIZATIONAL DESIGN

A supportive organizational design and a sympathetic administrative ethos are, of course, necessary prerequisites if group care workers are to create and exploit interpersonal processes that promote learning for children and young people. Regrettably, there is evidence to suggest that the conventions of large organizations often take over and inhibit far-sighted therapeutic environments (Canter & Canter, 1979). There is also evidence that senior administrators, prone to making elegant policy statements, may do very little to translate these statements into organizational systems that protect the developmental aims of group care centres (Raynes, Pratt, & Roses, 1979).

A partial explanation for this can be found in the way that large public and private organizations are controlled by external sources (Pfeffer & Salancik, 1978). For example, managers may carry functions that are largely symbolic and that interest groups ultimately determine the resources available to an organization. In this way such external bodies actually control the way it functions. Such an analysis poses many implications for group care workers since, in order to survive, centres have to obtain resources and support from the controllers of social policy, whoever such controllers may be.

Some consequences of inappropriate organizational design and administrative structures were illustrated in a comparative study of residential facilities for the adult mentally handicapped in the British health care system (Raynes, Pratt, & Roses, 1979). This study showed how complex and inappropriate divisions of responsibility, rigid hierarchies, poor communication between managers and direct service workers, and limited feedback from direct workers up through the organization to managers resulted in reduced quality of service, limiting the developmental opportunities available in group care centres. Resource factors (the state of the facility, staffing complement, and operational budgets) as well as non-resource factors (qualifications of staff, quality of teamwork, and staff attitudes) were critical influences on a centre's capacity to provide services (Davies & Knapp, 1981; Fulcher, 1983).

Factors such as personnel complement and deployment, state of the physical environment, equipment, food and consumables, staff attitudes, characteristics of the social environment that surrounds a centre, experience of residents prior to admission, and so on were all highlighted as important. Raynes, Pratt, and Roses (1979) found that inappropriate divisions of responsibility limited the authority of the unit leader, making it impossible to control resource and non-resource issues. This, in turn, prevented unit leaders from delegating authority to direct care workers in continuous contact with residents, preventing them from executing their caring tasks in a manner compatible with residents' needs.

If group care workers working directly with children and young people are to make maximum use of the interpersonal relations and processes that enable learning and development to take place, then they require sufficient authority to ensure that such opportunities are made available. As noted earlier, Bronfenbrenner highlighted ways in which learning and development are facilitated when children engage in increasingly complex activities with someone towards whom they have established a strong emotional attachment and "when the balance of power shifts in favour of the developing person" (1979, p. 61). This implies that a unit leader needs to guarantee protection of and support for individual workers whilst struggling to create developmental conditions for young people. It also implies that a unit leader needs to offer delegated authority. This may involve allowing a shift in power and responsibility for certain actions from workers to young people, whenever this is appropriate.

However, such transfers of authority need to occur when young people are ready for enhanced responsibility and not simply because it is administratively convenient or organizationally safe. Having said this, it should be noted that human service organizations find it difficult to tolerate such flexibility, since it runs counter to the managerial control and formality of procedures adopted by most social service bodies (Kakabadse, 1982).

The search for models of organization in keeping with views about how young people learn and develop is not entirely without hope. It is worth examining the systems model developed by Miller and Gwynne as the result of an action research study of residential institutions for the physically handicapped and young chronic sick (1972).[1] This model places great store on providing opportunities for residents and workers to engage in the type of reciprocal activities and power sharing that are critical to child and adolescent development. In addition to an overall centre management function, this model identified three internal systems that cater respectively for the needs of residents and workers to have psychological and physical dependence, independence, and support (Miller & Gwynne, 1972, p. 190).

The centre management function was conceived in terms of giving a centre legitimacy with the external community, exercising control over admission and discharge practices, and maintaining the integrity of and balance between the three internal systems. A dependence system is concerned with personal caregiving roles that ensure physical safety and security as well as emotional safety and security. An independence system is concerned with personal growth and the promotion of social competencies aimed at preparing a young person for semi-independent living elsewhere. The support system, meanwhile, is concerned with managing internal and external boundaries between, for example, a young person's daily life in the centre and their connections with family members, peers, and significant others through activities that promote ongoing learning and development.

In an interesting discussion of this model, Miller and Gwynne (1972) suggested that it differs substantially from that which is normally found operating in many group care centres. They pointed out the need for clarity around the aims of group care centres and also noted that a dependent culture was prominent whenever unit leaders had insufficient authority to control the external boundary between the centre and other parts of the larger organization. In those centres where the unit leader had significantly more authority to control the external boundary and to limit or enhance resources moving between the centre and the wider organization, it was far more likely that an independence culture was found between residents and workers, thus supporting learning and development for residents and workers alike.

While lacking in detail about implementation of their model, Miller and Gwynne (1972) offered important insights into issues that concern group care workers dealing with children and young people. It provided an organizational framework that encourages workers to remain child-centred in their practice, promoting appropriate relationship dependency, as well as facilitating and supporting independence and promoting social competencies. Links can also be made between this model and material contained in the parallel literature on therapeutic communities that emphasizes the importance of participatory styles of decision-making and power sharing (Hinslelwood & Manning, 1979; Jansen, 1980; Kennard, 1983). This literature also draws attention to therapeutic communities that have failed to survive in the formal resource systems of health care, education, social welfare, and criminal justice. Generally speaking, the practical implications associated with implementing therapeutic communities were found to be overwhelming in traditional and hierarchically structured systems where control of resources and decision-making are expected to remain in the hands of senior personnel.

The search is likely to continue for ways of making the organizational structures and administrative routines associated with group care services reflect appropriate levels of participative decision-making and power sharing between workers and young people. Until such time as clearer solutions are found, workers are advised to continue using techniques of internal advocacy and change designed to make service systems more human and humane (Brager & Holloway, 1978; Resnick & Patti, 1980; Weisman, 1973). Indeed, it may be that internal advocacy and the pursuit of more humane services require more concerted attention by group care workers wishing to improve the learning and development opportunities available for young people in their centres. Given the way that organizational design influences the culture of practice in group care centres, workers may find it helpful to contemplate a further set of questions.

- How does the organizational structure of your centre influence the work undertaken with young people?

- What administrative routines operate within the centre that encourage workers to initiate activities and promote children's best interests and social competencies?
- What systems of accountability respect the need for workers and young people to engage in joint activities and power sharing?
- How does the organizational structure and the administrative routines in the centre promote a culture that encourages learning and developmental opportunities for workers and young people?

THE PHYSICAL ENVIRONMENT

At first glance it may seem that focusing on the physical environment of a centre detracts attention away from relational elements that shape the culture of practice in any centre. There is an unfortunate but commonly held view that, given sufficient commitment and imagination, workers can overcome poor siting and physical design features in their centres. Such a view was even promoted by an influential British government publication on care and treatment environments for children (Her Majesty's Stationary Office, 1970). That publication claimed that "unsuitable buildings may affect adversely the easy workings of a community home even though they do not prevent good staff from operating well" (p. 41). This belief, without evidential support, runs contrary to the experience of many group care workers who know only too well that important limitations are imposed on their practice by the physical environment in which they work.

Yet, surprisingly, very little has been written directly about designing group care centres and the importance of the physical environment of care. Bettelheim (1974) wrote about a "Home for the Heart," giving testimony to the importance of environmental symbolism, spatial messages, and territoriality. Redl and Wineman (1957) are credited with the familiar statement that group care practice with children requires "a home that smiles, props that invite, and space which allows" (p. 42). Fortunately, more attention has been given since the 1990s to the importance of physical environments (Anglin, 2003; Canter & Canter, 1979; Ward, 1998; Webster, 1997). Environmental psychologists such as Sommer (1969), Proshansky, Ittleson, and Rivlin (1979) and Hayduk (1983) have given increasing attention to the importance of personal space and the physical environment. Germain (1981) attempted to address this issue as it relates to social work practice, while Maier (1982b) called attention to ways in which "the space we create controls us" in group care practice.

Views expressed by each of these writers serve to emphasize the extent to which the culture of group care is heavily influenced by the siting and physical design of a centre. While it is possible for workers to influence and adapt to some physical design limitations, countless other design features remain out of their control. The siting and physical design of a centre may represent in bricks and mortar the ideas of earlier generations of practice. This architectural history serves to inhibit the development of new and more contemporary approaches. Many workers have referred to their facility as a "purpose-built unit with the wrong purpose built in," even when their centres are comparatively new. The location of a centre can reduce the opportunities for workers and children to engage in ordinary life tasks through which learning by observation and shared activity might be achieved (Rivlin & Wolfe, 1979). The uninviting external appearance of a centre, including the fenced or walled, fortress-like image of an institution can inhibit valuable contacts being made with adults and children living in the immediate neighbourhood.

Slater and Lipman (1980) identified several concerns associated with spatial design in group care practice. First, it is worth examining the amount of choice that a building allows for workers and children in terms of private, public, and social spaces. Second, attention is drawn to the question of whether a building encourages independence. The extent to which centre design offers convenience provides a third consideration which workers should address. A fourth concern involves the extent in which privacy is permitted and encouraged by the way the facility is designed. Finally, workers might consider the extent to which the design of a centre is comprehensible in terms of quickly finding one's way around the building and feeling safe there. In so far as resources for group care centres are likely to remain limited in the foreseeable future, workers are advised to consider a range of potential pressure points in their work that are aggravated by poor design features. It is ironic that workers may need to call in builders rather than employing new care staff, since this may be a more effective use of resources.

The recent development of comprehensive assessment schedules for sheltered care environments (Anderson & Davison, 2003; Moos & Lemke, 1979) enables group care workers to evaluate their centres along a number of dimensions including physical and architectural features, staff-resident characteristics, policy and programme resources, and social environments. Such measures offer those with responsibility for group care centres the possibility of pinpointing key features which place added stress on workers and restrict their effectiveness in direct work with children. At the very least, workers need to recognize the importance of space and physical arrangements if they are to make the best possible use of available space.

The protection of limited private space and concern about the physical condition of furnishings can do much to make an unsympathetic environment more welcoming and comfortable to live in. Often very basic issues such as whether children have access to all parts of a centre, whether they have personal space allocated to them which is theirs alone, and whether children may retreat into their own private spaces have a profound impact on the culture of a group care centre (Maier, 1982b).

Writing about group care centres for the elderly, Davies and Knapp (1981) drew attention to a number of indicators of good centre design. These features apply also to living and learning environments for young people where the language of space and physical arrangements are especially powerful (Maier, 1981). *Ownership and original function* of the centre are worthy of consideration, as is *size, general centre design*, and the *internal scale* (relations between rooms). The location of bedrooms, sitting rooms or spaces, dining facilities, bathrooms, and toilets are all worthy of attention. A rich variety of social interactions take place in corridors, halls, and passageways, these "spaces between the rooms."

Space for social events such as parties, games, or meetings are important considerations as are the stereo, billiard table, and minibus. Micro-design features, such as lighting, full-length mirrors, and lockers are design elements that can be easily ignored. Availability of accommodation for workers, including its location and size relative to space occupied by children represents another important consideration. Finally, in addition to the siting of a centre, its age, general state of repair and decor are all influential in the culture of practice that develops there.

All of these issues were highlighted in one particular centre that did not have a room large enough to contain seating for all the workers and children who lived and worked there. This had a profound impact on the culture of the centre. A total community meeting could not be held, with the consequence that opportunities for shared decision-making were restricted. In evaluating the effectiveness of the centre's work with children, this physical constraint was not even considered. Instead, the centre's limited effectiveness was attributed entirely to lack of skill on the part of the unit leader and to inadequate training on the part of other workers. This example illustrates how "the space we create does indeed control us" and how evaluations of group care practice may ignore the influence physical environments can have on care and treatment outcomes with young people.

Workers might usefully consider a further set of questions to explore ways in which the physical environment of their centre supports a culture that promotes learning and development objectives.

- To what extent does the geographic location of your centre restrict or enhance opportunities for young people to learn and develop?
- How does the internal layout of the centre facilitate interactions between young people and workers?
- To what parts of the centre can young people have access at any time and what personal spaces are available into which they can retreat?
- To what extent does the physical design of your centre support workers in the task of creating developmental opportunities for young people?

TEAM FUNCTIONING AND GROUP DEVELOPMENT

Group care practice with children is preeminently team practice. Since group care services are provided from a discrete centre of activity, primarily (although not exclusively) through the medium of a group, so there is created a life-space in which daily events are shared between workers and young people (Ainsworth & Fulcher, 1981). A group culture is also reinforced as workers operate in a public arena and share responsibility with others for the growth and development of individual children or young people. Most exchanges are open to observation by others, and over the course of weeks and months, it is inevitable that work with individual young persons or groups will be shared by several workers.

As members of a team, group care workers are required to simultaneously engage in work with individual young people and a group of many children. This often requires changing focus quickly from the needs of one young person to the needs of another while at the same time ensuring that the needs of the total group of children are not neglected (Elliott, 1980). This is a particularly difficult aspect of group care practice and highlights the complex task which workers are expected to perform. It is rarely possible in group care practice for one person to claim responsibility for successful interventions with young people. In the same way, individual workers are rarely to blame for a centre's failure with a child. The occupational stresses associated with group care practice are not unrelated to the complexities of work in this field, and practice is almost always observed by others of similar status (Mattingly, 1981). Further stresses are associated with the inevitable closeness that develops between workers and children.

The literature on these features of practice, teamwork in particular, is not extensive. More often than not, when teamwork has been addressed, it has been examined from a managerial perspective (Payne, 1982; Payne & Scott, 1982). Less attention has been given to the occupational focus of group care that underpins a team approach to practice. Fulcher (1981) identified six issues that are worthy of consideration when addressing the problem of team functioning in group care practice (pp. 194-195). These issues involve who the team members are, how the team carries out its work, where team members are assigned for duty, when team members are expected to work, what orientations different members have in the team, and for what reasons teamwork objectives receive support.

Later Fulcher (1991) highlighted ways in which these six issues interact to shape patterns of team functioning in group care over time, reinforcing the need to consider recruitment and deployment issues carefully to achieve comparative balance along gender lines, age distribution, social and cultural characteristics, and training.

Leadership and decision-making are invariably addressed by writers about group processes (Douglas, 1979) from outside the field of group care. This is because there is agreement that identity formation and group cohesion are of central importance in team or group development strategies. Moreover leadership styles that involve open discussion and shared decision-making are more supportive of group development than authoritarian styles. Most writers on group or team development, therefore, seem to favour a style of leadership that encourages reciprocity, mutuality of positive feelings, and shared decision-making amongst the members of a group. In essence, this parallels the type of developmental conditions outlined by Bronfenbrenner (1979) in which children have optimal opportunities for learning.

In highlighting the parallels between conditions that optimally promote team or group development and those that promote individual learning and development, a cautionary note is indicated. While having a responsibility for its own development and that of its members, a group care team has the primary task of providing learning and development opportunities for young people placed in its centre. A careful balancing of needs and responsibilities has to occur if workers and young people alike are to achieve satisfactory experiences during their engagement with a group care centre. Balance needs to be encouraged between task performance with young people and the maintenance of team cohesion and collaboration between team members. Without such balance, the primary task cannot be performed and team morale is likely to suffer (Adair, 1983; Fulcher, 1991).

This problem conveniently illustrates the relationship between individual and group-oriented objectives, drawing attention to an issue that is very real for those engaged in group care practice. Workers are regularly faced with the dilemma of needing to assist an individual child with personal learning and development issues when, at the same time, having to give attention to a group of young people. In this respect, it is worth noting the relationship that Maier (1978) has drawn between individual and group-oriented objectives, as adapted and shown in Table 2. It can be seen how the individual and group objectives identified by Maier (1978) might refer to both children and workers in a group care centre.

Whichever the case, it shows how individual and group needs must be accommodated simultaneously. In this respect a dilemma is addressed which group care workers often feel is at the heart of their practice. It also emphasizes the culture of practice by identifying aspects of group development associated with social structure, language, norms, and values. It underlines the socialization influence offered by the culture of any centre, assisting individual young people to enhance their social competence and engage in acceptable cultural roles.

Issues associated with team functioning and group development pose a further set of questions which workers might consider with respect to their own particular centres.

- What do you mean by the notion of "team" and in what sort of team are you involved?
- How does the style of leadership used in your team influence the way the team works?
- By whom are decisions made in your team?
- What sort of messages do young people get when they look at the way your team works?

- What parallel processes might be recognized when comparing the functioning of your team with what might be happening in the children's group?
- To what extent does the group culture in your centre assist young people with individual learning and developmental needs?

THE INDIVIDUAL WORKER

This chapter has been concerned throughout with the significance of interpersonal relations and processes considered essential for learning and development in children and young people. As such, the focus on interactions between individual young people and group care workers is inevitable. A strong, pervasive culture that consistently reinforces the work carried out in a group care centre is essential if learning and development is to be achieved for young people in these settings. Factors thought to influence the culture of practice in group care have included organization design, administrative routines, the physical environment, team functioning and group development, as well as roles carried out by individual workers.

Ainsworth (1981) highlighted the importance of mentoring relationships based on work in the field of adult development (Levinson, Darrow, Klein, Levinson, & McKee, 1978). Mentoring that focuses on group care practice with children and young people includes the following roles:

- to act as a teacher to enhance a young person's skills and intellectual development
- to serve as a sponsor and use influence to facilitate a young person's advancement
- to be a host and guide who welcomes a young person into new situations and the social world, acquainting a child with the values, customs, resources, and cast of characters
- to act as a role model of virtues, achievement, and ways of living that a young person can admire and seek to emulate
- to provide counsel and moral support in times of stress
- to support and facilitate a young person's development and realization of personal goals

All of the roles referred to above can be said to reinforce the culture of practice in group care for children and young people. As our under-

TABLE 2. Developmental Objectives for Individual and Group Intervention

Individual Objectives	Group Objectives
Self-realization	Clarity in group norms and values
Personal competence	Tolerance of individual differences
Competence in relating to and identifying with others	Group cohesion
Competence in problem solving	Division of labour and clarification of group roles
Meeting cultural role expectations	Shared decision-making and group continuity

standing of child and adolescent development increases, it may be possible to identify additional dimensions of the mentoring role that group care workers fulfill with young people. This is especially important given that reciprocal activity and mutuality of feeling between a young person and worker is necessary if a gradual transfer of power from one to the other is to be achieved.

In the systems that contain group care centres, workers are referred to by titles such as nurses, teachers, child or youth care workers, social workers, or corrections officers. Because of their training backgrounds and occupational allegiances, group care workers may not see or describe their primary task in developmental terms and may use different languages to describe their work. The nurse may think primarily of therapeutic interventions, the teacher about teaching, the youth care worker or social worker may think of caring, while the youth justice officer may think in terms of supervision. Such differences in language highlight, to a greater or lesser extent, the unequal status that exists between workers and young people rather than reciprocal interactions, mutuality of feeling, and shared decision-making. The lack of reciprocal interaction is likely to result in increased social distance rather than encouraging closeness where workers and young people are side by side observing each other, doing things together, and jointly influencing each other's thinking and behaviour.

This developmental focus and the mentoring roles that group care workers fulfill with children and young people need to be supported and promoted by the culture of practice in any given centre. Some further questions may be posed to enable workers to assess the extent to which this operates in their centre.

- How are group care worker's roles described in your centre?
- To what extent are workers encouraged to get closely involved with a child or young person, or how is such close involvement interpreted?
- To what extent does the formal language of your centre, for example, job titles or descriptions of daily tasks, emphasize learning and development for children or young people?
- In what ways might it be said that closeness between workers and particular children or young people is nurtured and protected or actually disrupted?

CONCLUSION

In this chapter, we have explored various aspects associated with the culture of practice in group care for children and young people. First, the developmental conditions in which young people learn and develop most effectively were outlined. Next, the organizational culture of practice in group care was considered, emphasizing the social structure, language, norms, and values associated with practice in a centre. Third, issues of organizational design were addressed, highlighting the relationships that exist between interpersonal dynamics and organizational contexts in group care practice. Attention then turned to a consideration of the physical environment and to ways in which the siting and physical design of a centre influences the culture of practice which develops there. This led on to a consideration of team functioning and group development, since group dynamics are an integral part of practice in the group care field. Finally, consideration returned to the role of the individual worker, exploring the extent to which individuals can support development and learning for individual children or young people. Whether referring to the culture of practice in health care settings, educational settings, social welfare settings, or criminal justice settings, group care practice is likely to require treatment, teaching, nurture, and supervisory control in order to assist children and young people towards learning and development objectives.

NOTE

1. Miller and Gwynne have noted how the diagrammatic presentation of organizational systems was developed by A K Rice (1963, pp. 16-25) and Miller & Rice (1967, pp. 32-42).

REFERENCES

Adair, J. (1983). *Effective leadership.* London: Pan Books.

Ainsworth, F. (1981). The training of personnel for group care with children. In F. Ainsworth, & L. C. Fulcher (Eds.), *Group care for children: Concept and issues* (pp. 225-244). London: Tavistock.

Ainsworth F. (2001). After ideology: The effectiveness of residential programs for "at risk" adolescents. *Children Australia, 26*(2), 11-18.

Ainsworth, F., & Fulcher, L. C. (Eds.). (1981). *Group care for children: Concept and issues.* London: Tavistock.

Anderson, E. W., & Davison, A. J. (1993). *Applying the Children Act (1989) in boarding and residential environments.* London: David Fulton Publishers.

Anglin, J. P. (2003). *Pain, normality, and the struggle for congruence: Reinterpreting residential care for children and youth.* New York: The Haworth Press, Inc.

Apter, S. (1982). *Troubled children–Troubled systems.* Oxford: Pergamon Press.

Bettelheim, B. (1974). *A home for the heart.* London: Thames & Hudson.

Brager, G., & Holloway, S. (1978). *Changing human service organisations, politics, and practice.* San Francisco: Free Press.

Bronfenbrenner, U. (1979). *The ecology of human development.* Cambridge, MA: Harvard University Press.

Canter, D., & Canter, S. (1979). *Designing for therapeutic environments.* Chichester, England: Wiley.

Davies, B., & Knapp, M. (1981). *Old people's homes and the production of welfare.* London: Routledge & Kegan Paul.

Davis, A. (1981). *The residential solution.* London: Tavistock.

Douglas, T. (1979). *Group processes in social work.* Chichester, England: Wiley.

Eisikovitz, R. (1980). The cultural scene of a juvenile treatment center for girls: Another look. *Child Care Quarterly 9*(3), 158-174.

Elliot, D. (1980). Some current issues in residential work: Implications for the social work task. In R. Walton & D. Elliot (Eds.), *Residential care: A reader in current theory and practice.* Oxford: Pergamon Press.

Fulcher, L. C. (1981). Team functioning in group care. In F. Ainsworth & L. C. Fulcher (Eds.), *Group care for children: Concept and issues* (pp. 170-197). London: Tavistock.

Fulcher, L. C. (1983). *Who cares for the caregivers? A comparative study of residential and day care teams working with children.* PhD Thesis. Stirling, Scotland: University of Stirling.

Fulcher, L. C. (1991). Teamwork in residential care. In J. Beker & Z. Eisikovits (Eds.), *Knowledge utilization in residential child and youth care practice* (pp. 215-235). Washington, DC: Child Welfare League of America.

Fulcher, L. C. (1993). Yes Henry, the space we create does indeed control us! *Journal of Child & Youth Care, 8*(2), 91-100.

Fulcher, L. C. (1998). Acknowledging culture in child and youth care practice. *Social Work Education, 17*(3), 321-338.

Fulcher, L. C. (2001). Differential assessment of residential group care for children and young people. *British Journal of Social Work, 31*, 417-435.

Fulcher, L. C. (2004). Learning metaphors for child and youth care practice. *Journal of Relational Child & Youth Care Practice, 7*(2), 19-27.

Fulcher, L. C., & Ainsworth, F. (1981). Planned care and treatment: The notion of programme. In F. Ainsworth & L. C. Fulcher (Eds.), *Group care for children: Concept and issues* (pp. 71-88). London: Tavistock.

Gerhardt, S. (2004). *Why love matters: How affection shapes a baby's brain*. London: Brunner-Routledge.

Germain, C. B. (1981). The physical environment and social work practice. In A. N. Maluccio (Ed.), *Promoting competence in clients: A new/old approach to social work practice*. New York: Free Press.

Hayduk, L. A. (1983). Personal space: Where we now stand. *Psychological Bulletin, 94*(2), 293-335.

Her Majesty's Stationery Office (1970). *Care and treatment in a planned environment*. London: Home Office Advisory Council on Child Care.

Hinslelwood, R. D., & Manning, N. (Eds.). (1979). *Therapeutic communities: Reflections and progress*. London: Routledge & Kegan Paul.

Hunter, J., & Ainsworth, F. (Eds.) (1973). *Residential establishments: The evolving of caring systems*. Dundee, Scotland: Dundee University, School of Social Administration.

Jansen, E. (1980). *Therapeutic communities*. London: Croom Helm.

Jones, K. (1967). *New thinking about institutional care*. London: Association of Social Workers.

Jones, K., & Fowles, A. J. (1984). *Ideas on institutions*. London: Routledge & Kegan Paul.

Kakabadse, A. (1982). *Culture of the social services*. Aldershot, Hampshire: Gower Publishing.

Kennard, D. (1983). *An introduction to therapeutic communities*. London: Routledge & Kegan Paul.

Levinson, D. J., Darrow, C. N., Klein, E. G., Levinson, M. H., & McKee, B. (1978). *The seasons of a man's life*. New York: Alfred Knopf.

Maier, H. W. (1978). *Three theories of child development* (3rd edition). New York: Harper & Row.

Maier, H. W. (1981). Essential components in care and treatment environments for children. In F. Ainsworth & L. C. Fulcher (Eds.), *Group care for children: Concept and issues* (pp. 19-70). London: Tavistock.

Maier, H. W. (1982a). To be attached and free: The challenge of child development in the eighties. *Child Welfare, 61*(2), 67-76.

Maier, H. W. (1982b). The space we create controls us. *Residential Group Care and Treatment, 1*(I), 51-59.

Mattingly, M. (1981). Occupational stress for group care personnel. In F. Ainsworth & L. C. Fulcher (Eds.), *Group care for children: Concept and issues* (pp. 151-169). London: Tavistock.

Miller, E. J., & Gwynne, E. G. (1972). *A life apart*. London: Tavistock.

Miller, E. J., & Rice, A. K. (1967). *Systems of organization*. London: Tavistock.

Moos, R., & Lemke, S. (1979). The *multiphasic environmental assessment procedure, preliminary manual*. Palo Alto, CA: Stanford University Social Ecology Laboratory.

Payne, C., & Scott, I. (1982). *Developing supervision of teams in field and residential social work*. Paper No. 12. London: National Institute for Social Work.

Payne, M. (1982). *Working in teams*. London: Macmillan.

Pfeffer, J., & Salancik, G. R. (1978). *The external control of organisations: A resource dependence perspective.* New York: Harper & Row.

Polsky, H. W. (1963). *Cottage six–The social system of delinquent boys in residential treatment.* New York: John Wiley.

Proshansky, H. M., Ittleson, W. H., & Rivlin, L. G. (Eds.). (1979). *Environmental psychology: Man and his physical space.* New York: Holt, Rinehart & Winston.

Raynes, N. V., Pratt, M. W., & Roses, S. (1979). *Organisational structure and the care of the mentally retarded.* London: Croom Helm.

Redl, F., & Wineman, D. (1957). *The aggressive child.* New York: Free Press.

Resnick H., & Patti, R. J. (1980). *Change from within: Humanizing social welfare organizations.* Philadelphia: Temple University Press.

Rice, A. K. (1963). *The enterprise and the environment.* London: Tavistock.

Rivlin, I. G., & Wolfe, M. (1979). Understanding and evaluating therapeutic environments for children. In D. Canter & S. Canter (Eds.), *Designing for therapeutic environments.* Chichester, England: John Wiley & Sons.

Rommer, R. (1977). *The end of imprisonment.* Oxford: Oxford University Press.

Slater, R., & Lipman, A. (1980). Towards caring through design. In R. Walton & D. Elliott (Eds.), *Residential care: A reader in current theory and practice.* Oxford: Pergamon Press.

Sommer, R. (1969). *Personal space: The behavioural basis of design.* Englewood Cliffs, NJ: Prentice-Hall.

Ward, A. (1998). *Intuition is not enough: Matching learning with practice in therapeutic child care.* London: Routledge.

Webster, R. (1997). *Feng shui for beginners: Successful living by design.* St. Paul, MN: Llewellyn Publications.

Weisman, H. W. (1973). *Overcoming mismanagement in the human service professions.* San Francisco: Jossey-Bass.

Whittaker, J. K. (1975). The ecology of child treatment: A developmental educational approach to the therapeutic milieu. *Journal of Autism & Child Schizophrenia 5*(3), 223-37.

Wolfensberger, E. (Ed.). (1972). *The principle of normalisation in human services.* Toronto: National Institute on Mental Retardation.

Wolins, M., & Wozner, Y. (1982). *Revitalizing residential settings.* San Francisco: Jossey-Bass.

Chapter 8

Resident Group Influences
on Team Functioning

Gale E. Burford
Leon C. Fulcher

SUMMARY. Research has documented important interplays between
the diagnostic characteristics of residents in group care centers and the
functioning of staff teams responsible for the delivery of services. Factors
that impact on the quality of working life satisfactions and frustrations are
variable over time and may originate from within the team, the resident
group, the service organization, or the social policy environment external
to the centre. Outcomes may draw team members together or promote destructive levels of turbulence, maladaptation, or anti-task behavior with
significant consequences for all concerned. *[Article copies available for a
fee from The Haworth Document Delivery Service: 1-800-HAWORTH. E-mail address: <docdelivery@haworthpress.com> Website: <http://www.HaworthPress.
com> © 2006 by The Haworth Press, Inc. All rights reserved.]*

KEYWORDS. Group care, residential care, residential treatment, group
homes, youth work, youthwork, group work, at-risk youth, teamwork

Address correspondence to: Gale E. Burford, Department of Social Work, University of
Vermont, 443 Waterman Building, Burlington, VT 05405.

[Haworth co-indexing entry note]: "Resident Group Influences on Team Functioning." Burford, Gale E.,
and Leon C. Fulcher. Co-published simultaneously in *Child & Youth Services* (The Haworth Press, Inc.) Vol.
28, No. 1/2, 2006, pp. 177-208; and: *Group Care Practice with Children and Young People Revisited* (ed:
Leon C. Fulcher, and Frank Ainsworth) The Haworth Press, Inc., 2006, pp. 177-208. Single or multiple copies
of this article are available for a fee from The Haworth Document Delivery Service [1-800-HAWORTH. 9:00
a.m. - 5:00 p.m. (EST). E-mail address: docdelivery@haworthpress.com].

TWO DECADES OF SIGNIFICANT CHANGE, YET SOME THINGS HAVEN'T CHANGED AT ALL!

Reflecting back on the contents of this chapter, one is struck by the particular policy and practice context in which the research was conducted. The 1970s and '80s were of considerable influence for those of us caught up in the excitement of the many developments and innovations in the treatment of young people who come in conflict with the law. And the Canadian Province of Quebec was an exciting place in which to be engaged in child and youth care practice. While the treatment discoveries and innovations were mainly originating in the United States, especially in the California Youth Authority (Palmer & Mc-Shane, 2001), Quebec's Youth Protection Act of 1979–with its distinctions between children and young people and its emphasis on rights and responsibilities–predated similar changes in language and legislation in most developed countries by a decade or more. So many of the assumptions now regarded as general knowledge about community supervision, foster care, group homes, probation, education, treatment, and behaviour management in residential centres and community-based programmes were being formed during that period (Palmer, 1992; Palmer & McShane, 2001).

A new chapter would be needed to fully explore the main policy and practice currents that intersected during that time and to shed light on the learning about what worked, what did not, and what got set aside in the emergence of the neo-liberal state in the United States and Canada. Such a new chapter would have to consider the influence of the various rights movements, including children, women, victims, and indigenous peoples, the rise and declining influence of critical social theory, and the emergence of post-modernism and post-structuralism–particularly in their North American expressions–and of course the devolution of services aimed at rebuilding civil society. The youth development, restorative justice, and community-centred family practice innovations would also warrant discussion.

Yet concerns about treatment of youth offending behaviour have persisted. To paraphrase Warren (1978), whether one frames the work with young offenders as care, supervision, education, or treatment one is always left with the question of whether they will get into trouble with the law again. And, as is now so well understood, the work should not be divorced from considerations about repairing harm to the victims of their crimes and keeping communities safe. During the era in which the research reported here was carried out, victims were at best ignored and at worst vilified or re-traumatized. And work was often carried out without sufficient regard for the safety of communities or the involvement of the families, schools, neighbourhoods, and other groups who would be expected to embrace these young people both during and after interventions. Such themes were perhaps the most glaring omissions of the "rehabilitation" era. There is a lot that is known about how to stimulate positive growth, development, and behaviour change with "deep end" young offenders.

However, such developmental changes do not reliably carry over into post-intervention environments unless parallel changes have been achieved in those environments and adequate supports are provided to support the maintenance of such changes. Without such service supports, youth adaptation to those environments becomes synonymous with relapse. Yet a major omission noted during the rehabilitation era risks being repeated again in the delivery of contemporary services. Policy makers persist with monolithic thinking in the search for single, simplistic, and universal solutions that will work with all young people in all circumstances.

Good youth care policy needs to be holistic and should aim to coordinate and integrate the multiple aims of justice services by offering a range of high-quality services known to yield positive outcomes in residential and community programs, build safety for crime victims and communities, and repair harm. However, contemporary trends show policy makers falling predictably back into one-size-fits-all programming and resource allocation practices that foster competition instead of cooperation.

Therein rests the continued interest on the part of the editors of this volume in the research originally reported in this chapter: the need to illuminate the practical meanings of teamwork in group care practice. This research, while carried out under highly unique circumstances that can no longer be replicated, holds continuing relevance for the field of child and youth care. The original research was carried out as part of a larger study of teamwork (Burford, 1990) which itself was an extension of an earlier study of teamwork in group care (Fulcher, 1983, 1991). In rereading the chapter now, it is interesting to note the various conceptualizations of teamwork that appeared and to draw links to now widely embraced notions concerning partnerships, collaboration, participation in decision-making, and empowerment as antidotes to the highly individualized, expert-driven practice models embraced in previous eras.

In some ways, contemporary enthusiasm for the ethic of empowerment and devolution could be thought of as an expression of those early interests in teamwork and teaming. As the old saying goes, the people at the bottom of the power hierarchies are those who are usually calling for more cooperation than those at the top of such hierarchies who enjoy privileges associated with the status quo. It would be interesting to trace how notions of teamwork have evolved from the days of milieu-therapy on through Trieschman, Whittaker, and Brendtro's assessment of "The Other 23 Hours" (1969), and then the rejection of residential care and treatment during the era of deinstitutionalisation through to the era of restorative justice. An enduring theme, we suspect, would be the need to nurture the capacities of the people who work most closely with children and young people themselves and to develop greater understanding of how to support these workers to provide high quality work over time with those young people who present society's greatest challenges.

And that is, of course, what drove the original question for the particular research reported in what follows. Things go better when everyone on the team is reading from the same page and knows when to face in the same direction. This type of research was made possible only by agreeing to the use of diagnostic classification systems. The research project of which the chapter was a part argued the case for multiple-method approaches to practice and multiple-indicators research into the complex phenomenon of teamwork in group care practice. One of the enduring challenges to carrying out such research involves the ideological struggles between those who do research. In the same way that policy frameworks vie for dominance, so it is that theorists and researchers also clash over how to ask the questions and how to interpret the answers. It has proven to be highly difficult to bring the critical social theorist, the logical positivist or advocate of truly scientific methods, the constructivist, and the symbolic interactionist together, for example, to address the same research questions.

This is made difficult, in part, by the same processes that privilege one policy or practice over another, namely, resource or funding allocation. Some would reject the typologies used in this study altogether. Others would point to the futility of trying to make sense out of phenomenological or ethnographic expressions in order to reliably inform policy with any formal validation. The study of which this chapter was a part argued that all of these perspectives needed to be represented in the interests of sustainable, developmental, and quality policies, practices, and service outcomes.

The proposition remains true that young people who offend repeatedly are different in important ways from their non-offending counterparts. These repeat offenders are also different from one another in ways that have important implications for successful treatment of the problems of offending. These young people require the pro-social, age-appropriate activities that non-offending young people would get and which would help keep these young people from slipping further behind in their development (e.g., education, recreation, employment, and social skills learning opportunities), placement, and behaviour management.

The study offered strong support for the proposition that the *who you work with makes a difference*, that is, the characteristics of the clients interact in significant ways with the character of the responses to them. In re-examining the final recommendations of the chapter, the authors would not change what they asserted twenty years ago. Internally oriented young people do need to have relationships with helpers that go beyond simply managing them. Other young people react badly to such "psychologizing" of the relationships. Younger, more pliable young people should not remain in group care programmes long-term without very good reasons–perhaps unless their violent behaviour cannot be managed in any other way–owing to the strong dependency they form in institutions.

And child and youth care workers engaged long term with power-oriented teenagers are particularly vulnerable to work-related stresses that are different from those working with internally conflicted teenagers. The findings of the chapter have enduring relevance for the choice of placements for young people and the type of supervision needed by the staff who work with them.

INTRODUCTION

This research was carried out between 1977 and 1983 as part of a staff training and development effort with Shawbridge Youth Centres in Montreal, Canada. The study was completed during a time of significant changes in the social policy environment at federal, provincial, and community levels. These changes impacted significantly on child and youth care programs offered by the agency at a time when rapid change and expansion were commonplace.[1] An increase in the number of secure unit beds along with the addition of detention services and the sudden admission of girls into a service traditionally established for boys challenged most care and treatment efforts in the agency. In some instances, rapid change threatened to compromise the agency's own expectations concerning quality of care and education for the children and young people it served. Staff development and training activity was thus initiated around two primary objectives: (1) to support staff in fulfilling the expectations of their job and living-unit programme objectives; and (2) to establish practice standards for child and youth care in the agency as a whole.

The action research project that accompanied staff training and development sought to explore and describe characteristics of staff team functioning as a central component of residential group care and treatment. Between 1968 and the early 1980s Shawbridge Youth Centre employed a differential treatment classification scheme as the diagnostic basis for planning the supervision and treatment of delinquents admitted into its residential, day, and community programs. As such, the agency was ideally suited for a study that explored the interplay between selected diagnostic groupings of residents and the functioning staff teams assigned to work with those residents. Specifically, this study sought to determine what quality of working life satisfactions, frustrations, and/or uncertainties were evident amongst staff teams depending on the diagnostic characteristics of resident groups with whom they worked.

REVIEW OF THE CONTEMPORARY RESEARCH AND PRACTICE LITERATURE

Throughout the 1970s the argument that nothing works was prominently featured in the child and youth care literature based on broad generalizations about a very complex area of study. While policy makers in North America were largely swayed by these arguments, some practitioners, agency managers, and researchers continued to press home the point that selected interventions do work with particular groups of offenders under certain conditions (Gendreau & Ross, 1979; Jesness, 1980; Jesness et al., 1972; Palmer, 1974, 1976, 1978; Ross & Gendreau, 1980; Warren, 1983). Many researchers had noted the masking effect that occurred when all young people, programmes of care and treatment, methods of intervention, types of staff, and patterns of service delivery were grouped together for evaluation purposes (Gendreau & Ross, 1979; Grant & Grant, 1959; Hunt, 1971; Jesness, 1965, 1971; Lukin, 1981; Megargee, 1977; Palmer, 1978; Quay, 1977). Programmes that have used differential methods of assessment and programme planning have contributed much to practice knowledge about what works, with whom and under what conditions.

Practice wisdom has long suggested that in some instances the characteristics of young people placed in a residential centre will influence the functioning of individual staff members and impact on the functioning of caregivers' teams. Any team of workers who have coped with the admission of a difficult resident, whose needs drastically alter the social climate of the centre, would probably reaffirm such practice wisdom. The literature on transference and counter-transference phenomena would suggest that some forms of influence between the characteristics of particular residents and particular staff may be especially subtle and even more enduring (Menzies, 1977). Still, the knowledge available about these influences and dynamics is still largely at the level of speculation or assumptive wisdom.

Some researchers who have used differential assessment methods to control for characteristics of both clients and service providers have concluded that the inappropriate matching of client and worker is among the most important of all child and youth care decisions to be faced. That this should be so important is supported by researchers both inside and outside the child and youth care field. When controlling for differences between types of young people, style of teaching or counseling, and setting, researchers have demonstrated that such a match results in important differences in terms of behaviour management, educational achievement, treatment outcomes, and/or cost-effectiveness (Andre & Mahan, 1972; Brill, 1978; Hunt, 1971; Palmer, 1976; Warren, 1983).

Palmer (1976) found that by matching "internally oriented" workers with "internally conflicted" delinquent young people, it was possible to identify different patterns of rearrest, reconviction, and recidivism. Such differences could be documented up to four years after treatment in community-based projects where a variety of residential programs had been used as backup. While the use of matching was indicated for certain other diagnostic sub-types, none of the results were quite so spectacular as with those involving young people who were diagnosed as internally conflicted. Barkwell (1976) replicated this study in a juvenile probation setting in Manitoba, Canada, finding that the more intensive the contact between worker and client, the more important it became to avoid inappropriate matching between worker style and client characteristics. Worker style was identified as the major variable predicting outcome.

Andre and Mahan (1972) found differences in the performance of students who were matched with the style of their teachers when compared with those who were not matched. The characteristics of preferred teaching plans (including "atmosphere" of classroom), procedures for motivating students, curriculum content, and behaviour management strategies were carefully defined. Students in the homogeneous classrooms did as well as or outperformed students being taught in regular heterogeneous classrooms on all measures. In addition, staff with teaching assignments in the homogeneous classrooms reported higher overall satisfaction with their work.

Beneficial outcomes using the Conceptual Level matching model (Hunt, 1971) have been demonstrated in a variety of settings including for example, classrooms (Tomlinson & Hunt, 1971), group psychotherapy with alcoholics (McLachlan, 1972, 1974), and residential education programs (Hunt & Hardt, 1967). In each instance, students or patients were matched with the level of program structure and/or the conceptual level of their teacher or therapist. Of particular relevance to group care practice was the finding by Brill (1978) that delinquent boys whose diagnosed conceptual levels were matched with that of their primary or key worker evidenced fewer behavioural problems during that placement and for at least six months during follow-up than did a group of mismatched controls.

In separate studies where group care and treatment environments were matched to the type of youngster, Palmer (1972) and Jesness (1971) found benefits for particular types of youngsters ranging from reduced recidivism to decreased management problems. In the former study, the perceived needs of young people were taken into account when one of five group homes was selected and, in the latter, residents were grouped homogeneously according to assessment characteristics. While valuable enough in their own right to beg careful application and further research, these findings were still unable to account for the complex dimension of teamwork long considered a dimension of group care practice with considerable relevance to planning and practice outcomes (Fulcher, 1991).

During the course of a 168-hour week, residents may come into contact with many different types of workers, educators, administrators, volunteers, and other auxiliary personnel. They will also live in close proximity with other residents who are different than themselves. As such, reciprocal influences become more difficult to evaluate, restricting applications of a single-subject research design to examine interactions between different workers and residents. Still the teamwork variable remains something of an enigma. The value of a team approach has become a prominent theme in the group and organizational literature, prompting a plethora of ideas associated with team building, team development, and teamwork, to mention but a few. It has long been assumed that the collective and cooperative actions of staff members were of major importance in group care settings where a number of different workers engage young people or groups of residents through a variety of mediums (Fulcher, 1979). Within the residential centre itself, it has been difficult to evaluate the impact of multiple staff interactions with children around the tasks and meaning of experiences in day-to-day living (Maier, 1981; Mattingly, 1977; Ross, 1983; Whittaker, 1979).

One way researchers have sought to account for the collective actions of staff has been through attempting to measure the degree of program implementation (Scheirer & Rezmovic, 1983). Researchers attempting to control for program design and operation have found that staff frequently work from program designs and/or job descriptions that are insufficiently detailed so as to guide staff interventions at the minimum, let alone satisfy requirements for reliability, validity, or accountability (Quay, 1977). Johnson (1981) found that programs are inclined to drift from their intended practices and that this occurs for a variety of reasons.

The foundations for the notion of team building are to be found in the literature on small group theory and studies of organizational behaviour. The influence of Bales (1950), Homans (1950), Lewin (1952), and others is unmistakable when analysing the daily assumptions made about small groups in the work setting (Fulcher, 1988). Norms, roles, cohesion, interaction, group systems, or sub-systems and group activities are all part of the language taken for granted when discussing the collective of individuals identified as a "team." The metaphor of an athletic team is commonly used when considering the performance of group care workers (Morgan, 1986). Most workers have been introduced to the idea of teamwork as involving two or more members executing a series of linked behaviours aimed at a single outcome.

Expectations about team performance are evident in the illustration of a fifteen-year-old girl placed temporarily in a short-term emergency care unit. While the initial assessment clearly predicted the girl's propensity for seductive behaviour with male workers, some staff during the initial phase overlooked her suggestive comments when alone with her. These escalated into further manipulative behaviour on two or three occasions by "acting as if something forbidden had been going on" when a female worker entered the room where she and a male worker were alone. After an initial period of hostile reaction when all staff challenged her each time she initiated sexual conversation or engaged in inappropriate sexual behaviour, only then did she reveal a history of family incest (later confirmed) that had been concealed previously.

In examples such as this and numerous others in the group care literature, teamwork is easier to define when it does not happen than it is to describe, in a practical way, when found in its optimal state. In his typology of optimal residential environments, Moos (1975) sought to isolate and measure dimensions of social climate thought to influence the behaviour of staff and residents. Moos argued that the satisfactions of both groups may be related to indicators of program quality such as reduced absconding. While this is not the only attempt to relate job satisfactions with outcome measures, in the main researchers prior to the mid-1980s found little support for such conclusions (Argyle, 1972).

Perhaps one of the most valuable contributions Moos gave to the group care field was linking the perceptions of staff members as a group to the residents as a group around three dimensions of social climate: *relationship*, *treatment*, and *system maintenance*. In so doing, the Moos typology received support from practitioners since it stimulated focused discussion between staff members, or between staff members and residents, about whether or not everyone was working together towards shared goals. Hall argued that while job satisfactions vary, particularly in relation to a member's position in the occupational hierarchy, "It is the meeting of expectations that contributes most to job satisfactions" (1969, p. 47). Argyle argued that "job satisfaction is greater among workers who belong to a cohesive group and are accepted by it" (1972, p. 248). On the other hand, job dissatisfaction is seemingly related to factors such as different "types of work, age, sex, and minority group membership" (Hall, 1969, p. 53).

In an attempt to control for the collective variable of group care team, Fulcher (1983) used a measure of self-reported work satisfaction, frustration, and uncertainty (Heimler, 1975, 1979) with individual members of work groups employed in residential and day care centres. By extending Hertzberg's (1968) traditional job satisfaction paradigm to include frustration and satisfaction activities on and off the job (Bronfenbrenner, 1979a, 1979b) and by exploring the functioning of group care teams within a wider "quality-of-working life" paradigm (Davis & Chernis, 1975), Fulcher constructed a "team functioning dimension." The most salient influences on team functioning were found to include siting and physical design of the centre, ratio of female to male workers, percentage of married or cohabiting workers, living in tied accommodation, trade union membership, turbulence encountered in the external organizational environment, and the type of social policy mandate (Fulcher, 1983, 1991).

A COMPARATIVE STUDY:
SAMPLE, MEASUREMENT, AND LIMITATIONS

In this comparative study, an attempt was made to examine whether the diagnostic composition of resident groups and the functioning of staff teams impacted other and, if so, to form hypotheses for further examination into this dimension of group care practice.

An analysis of correlation was carried out for pre-selected resident characteristics in group care services for delinquent young people (independent variables) and staff members providing services (dependent variables) (see Table 1). In addition to including demographic data for both groups, two different diagnostic typologies were used with residents to isolate different psychological characteristics. Two instruments were used with staff members to measure self-reported change (Holmes & Masuda, 1974; Holmes & Rahe, 1967) and quality of working life satisfaction and frustrations (Heimler & Fulcher, 1981).

The Sample

Founded in 1907, the Boys Farm and Training School was renamed Shawbridge Youth Centres during a period of rapid growth and expansion in the mid-1970s. The agency provided a continuum of care for act-

TABLE 1. Pre-Selected Variables–Residents and Staff

Independent Variables: Residents	Dependent Variables: Staff
• Mean Age	• Length of Time in Post
• Median Age	• Mean Age
• Number of Residents	• Ratio of Women
• Numbers of Resident Groups	• Ratio of Staff with Degrees
• Interpersonal Maturity	• Ratio of Unqualified Staff
◻ Level	• Ratio Never Married
◻ Sub-Type	• Ratio of Staff with Their Own Children
• Conceptual Level	• Work Orientation Schedule
	◻ Satisfactions
	◻ Frustrations
	◻ Total Outlook

Source: Data collected at Shawbridge Youth Centres in 1978, 1979, and 1980.

ing-out and delinquent boys and girls between the ages of twelve and seventeen using secure units, campus-style institutional cottages, group homes, and community residence facilities, day care, and fieldwork programmes. All young people occupying a residential bed on 5 September 1978, 15 April 1979, and 15 January 1980 were included in the study. Demographic and diagnostic information was extracted from files in the assessment division under the supervision of the Directors of Treatment and Professional Services.

In every case, the most recent assessment or reassessment data were selected on the young person prior to the calendar date of data collection and recorded separately for each year. All child and youth care and supervisory and auxiliary staff attached to a residential living unit on the calendar dates in question were invited to participate in the study. A team was not included in the sample unless 90 percent of its membership submitted their questionnaires. Resident and staff profiles and resident characteristics are shown in Tables 2 and 3.

Resident Characteristics

1. Demographic data included mean and median ages of residents in each living unit taken separately for each year and included the total number of residents, age range, and number of places or beds in each unit.
2. Interpersonal Maturity Classification System: Juvenile (Warren et al., 1966). While the seven maturity levels in this classification system are theoretical descriptions of interpersonal development around perceptual integration levels, the nine behavioural sub-types were empirically derived from data collected from delinquents found at different maturity levels yielding three diagnostic categories used in this study:
   - Maturity Level (Warren et al., 1966): Research has shown that most delinquents fall into three of the seven maturity levels, with small numbers falling into a fourth. This sample contained only Maturity Level 3 (middle maturity) and Maturity Level 4 (higher maturity) youths.
   - Delinquent Sub-Type (Warren et al., 1966): Of the nine sub-types, only five were found in this sample: the Immature Conformist (CFM), the Anti-Social Manipulator (MP), and the Cultural Conformist (CFC) are middle maturity or level three youngsters (n = 13), and the Neurotic Anxious (NX)

and the Neurotic Acting-Out (NA) are higher maturity or level four youngsters (n = 14). Research has shown that only a small percentage of non-delinquent youth can be described by any of these delinquent sub-types (Harris, 1983).

- Delinquent Sub-Group (Palmer, 1974): These three sub-groupings collapse certain of the sub-types together because of their common characteristics. They are the Internally Conflicted group (Neurotic Anxious and Neurotic Acting-Out sub-types taken together), the Power-Oriented group (Anti-Social Manipulator and Cultural Conformist sub-types taken together), and the Passive Conformists (the Immature Conformist group).

3. Each living unit in the study was rank ordered by the percentage of I-Level classifications (maturity level, delinquent sub-type, delinquent sub-group) taken separately and using the median to divide the resident groups into two sub-groups (fewer/more) which could be used for comparative evaluation.

4. Conceptual Level (Hunt et al., 1978): This assessment involved a six-item sentence-completion test that provided a measure of cognitive complexity. While two final scores were yielded, the CL6 or the combined score for the six items was used for this study. The following scoring ranges were used: Stage A = 0-0.39, Stage AB = 0.9-1.2, Stage B = 1.21-1.5, Stage BC = 1.51 and higher. Stage AB was determined solely for the purpose of this study because so many of the young people fell below 1.0 and yet were above 0.5 on the measure of conceptual complexity. This particular range has been frequently described as a stage of transition, suggesting that the young person was beginning to show some acceptance of rules which indicated minimal conformity. Three categories of Conceptual Level data were thus generated for this study:

- Stage: Each living unit in the study was rank ordered by the percentage of young people in the group in each conceptual level stage taken separately. The median was used to divide the groups into two comparative sub-groupings carried out separately for each year.
- Group Mean: The mean was calculated for each living unit and rank ordered separately for each year, again using the median to divide the groups into two sub-groupings for comparative purposes.

- Group Stage: Each group was classified according to the lowest conceptual level stage to account for one-third of the population of the living unit. For example, if one-third of the group were Stage A young people, the group was classified as a Stage A group and so on in ascending order until a particular stage accounted for one- third of the group.

Staff Characteristics (See Table 3)

1. Demographic data included the number of staff in each unit, mean age of the staff, mean length of time in post (months), percentages of women, members with degrees, unqualified members, those married or single, and those with children of their own.
2. The Schedule of Recent and Anticipated Events (Holmes & Rahe, 1967): Four scores were used from this 43-item measure of past and anticipated change.
   - Past Changes: Total mean change was calculated for each item for each year. Teams were rank ordered and the median was used to divide the teams into two sub-groupings for comparative purposes.
   - Anticipated Changes: Same procedure as for Past Changes.
   - Total Past and Anticipated Changes: Same procedure using the mean for Total Past and Anticipated Changes.
   - Past and Anticipated Changes: Same procedure using the difference between Past and Future Change Means for each team.
3. The Work Orientation Schedule (Heimler, 1970), amended by Fulcher (Fulcher & Ainsworth, 1981): This 55-item measure of quality of working life satisfactions and frustrations was scored as: Yes = 4, Perhaps = 2, No = 0. Mean scores were aggregated for each team yielding the following dimensions:
   - Total Satisfaction Score (BPS): Sum of all "Yes" answers in Work, Finance, Social Life, Home Life and Personal Contract.
   - Total Potential Satisfaction Score (GPS): Same as above with Perhaps responses.
   - Area Satisfaction Scores: Sum of Yes answers taken separately for Work, Finance, Social Life, Home Life, and Personal Contract.
   - Area Potential Satisfaction Score: Same as Area Satisfaction Scores above including Perhaps answers.

- Total Frustration Score (BNS): Sum of all Yes answers in Activity, Health, Personal Influence, Moods, and Habits.
- Total Potential Frustration Score (GNS): Same steps as Total Frustration Score above including Perhaps answers.
- Area Frustration Scores: Sum of Yes answers taken separately for Activity, Health, Personal Influence, Moods, and Habits.
- Area Potential Frustration Scores: Same as Area Frustration Scores above including Perhaps answers.
- Outlook Total: Mean average of raw scores for each team.
- Outlook Sub-Scores: Mean average of raw scores for each team taken separately for Achieved Ambition, Hope for the Future, Meaning in Life, Opportunity for Self-Expression, and Life Is Worthwhile.
- Functioning at Best Score: Ratio of Satisfactions to Frustrations when comparing Potential Satisfactions (GPS) with Certainty of Frustrations (BNS).
- Functioning at Worst Score: Ratio of Satisfactions to Frustrations when Certainty of Satisfactions (BPS) is compared with Potential Frustrations (GNS).
- Positive Swing Score: The difference between Certainty of Satisfactions (BPS) and Potential Satisfactions (GPS) highlighting the amount of uncertainty reported about satisfactions.
- Negative Swing Score: The difference between Certainty of Frustrations (BNS) and Potential Frustrations (GNS) highlighting uncertainties reported about frustrations.
- Average Frustrations: The mean of the Overall Frustrations (MNS) compared with the Overall Satisfactions (MPS) scores.

Measurement

A Pearson Product-Moment analysis of correlation was selected to analyse separately for each year the relationship between resident characteristics and diagnostic information (the independent variables) and staff characteristics and data (the dependent variables). The pre-selected level of acceptance was set at $r > .05$ and $r^2 > .7$ (Knapp, 1978).

TABLE 2. Total Number of Residents by Year

Independent Variables: Residents	1978	1979	1980
Total Number of Residents	100	113	93
Total Number of Resident Groups	10	11	11
Mean Age	16.1	16.3	16.3
Median Age	16	16.3	16.2
Interpersonal Maturity Level			
No. of I3 Level (Other Oriented) Youths	26	24	23
No. of Conforming Youths	17	13	12
No. of Power-Oriented Youths	9	9	8
No. of I4 Level (Self-Other Oriented) Youths	73	88	69
No. of Conflicted Youths	69	81	64
No. of Neurotic Acting-Out Youths	29	44	40
No. of Neurotic Anxious Youths	40	37	24
No. of Other Levels and Sub-Types	5	10	9
Conceptual Level			
No. of Stage A (0.0-0.89)	23	29	28
No. of Stage AB (0.9-1.2)	52	42	39
No. of Stage B (1.21-1.5)	16	26	18
No. of Stage BC (1.51 and higher)	9	14	8

Source: Data collected at Shawbridge Youth Centres in 1978, 1979, and 1980.

TABLE 3. Staff Characteristics by Year

Dependent Variables: Staff	1978	1979	1980
Number of Staff	78.0	59.0	96.0
Mean age (years)	30.2	32.6	32.2
Mean length of time in post (months)	15.4	21.6	20.6
Percentage of women	36.8	37.7	36.3
Percentage of members with degrees	51.8	48.9	50.4
Percentage of unqualified team members	19.0	23.5	22.6
Percentage never married	33.9	21.5	27.1
Percentage staff with their own children	30.3	41.5	38.6

Source: Data collected at Shawbridge Youth Centres.

Limitations

The results of this study suffered from all the flaws associated with research which comes about as an afterthought to practice. Such limitations render the findings unpredictable in so far as they can be interpreted beyond the particular setting in which they were obtained. First, the diagnostic criteria used with residents in this study were very specific to the two assessment typologies in question and validation of those two typologies.

The same is true for the Conceptual Level model. While there may be some temptation to generalize to other cognitive models, Conceptual Level remains a very specific measure with considerable validation work to support it. Second, no attempt was made to actually observe or record in any rigorous way the behaviours or expressions of attitude relative to what satisfied and what frustrated staff. Instead, self-reported perceptions about quality of working life satisfactions and frustrations were used.

A third limitation meant that the data could not be generalized over time since some team members and residents were present during more than one of the years in which the samples were drawn. For the same reason, the data could not be grouped together to form an aggregate sample. While other kinds of statistical analysis might have been used to reduce the suspected bias in this regard, other sources of bias would have been introduced because of the type of data collected in the study. For example, the Work Orientation Schedule permitted only three possible responses: Yes, Perhaps, or No meaning that, by itself, this was not interval or ratio level data that might permit more sophisticated analytical procedures.

By taking the average scores for each team and rank ordering these, it was suggested that data could be yielded of the higher order necessary. However, several researchers consulted on this point disagreed. Finally, neither the young people nor the staff members were randomly assigned to living units. Instead they were assigned on the basis of clinical assessments–as well as the frequently occurring need to place a given resident in a vacant bed and to assign a staff member to a vacant position. Nevertheless, in spite of these four limitations, the data still lend themselves–in their present form–to some reasoned interpretations within the framework outlined above.

RESULTS

The relationships between resident group composition and patterns of team functioning at Shawbridge Youth Centres between 1978 and 1980 are summarized below. See Tables 4-8 for specifics.

1. The teams of employees working in living units with more Passive Conforming young people reported higher satisfactions in the Home Life Area.
2. The teams of employees working in living units with more Neurotic Anxious young people reported fewer satisfactions in the Social Life Area.
3. The teams of employees working in living units with higher Conceptual Level stage young people reported higher Work satisfactions; fewer frustrations in the Habits Area; and less frustration overall.
4. The teams of employees working in living units with a higher proportion of Stage A (Low Conceptual Level) young people reported more frustrations in the Habits Area.
5. Teams of employees working in living units with more Maturity Level Three (I3 or middle maturity) youngsters reported higher satisfactions and less uncertainty about satisfactions.
6. Teams of employees working in living units with more Power-Oriented youngsters reported fewer potential frustrations in the Habits Area. These teams reported much less uncertainty in the Habits Area although about the same amount of frustration overall as other teams.
7. Teams of employees working in living units with more Passive Conforming youngsters reported higher satisfactions in the Social Life Area, higher overall satisfactions, and less uncertainty about their life satisfactions.
8. Teams of employees working in living units with more Maturity Level Four (higher maturity) youngsters reported fewer satisfactions in the Social Life Area, fewer overall satisfactions, and greater uncertainty about satisfactions.
9. Teams of employees working in living units with more Conflicted youngsters reported fewer satisfactions in the Social Life Area, fewer satisfactions overall and greater uncertainty about satisfactions, greater frustrations in the Personal Influence Area, and greater uncertainty about frustrations overall.
10. Teams of employees working in living units with more Neurotic Acting-Out youngsters reported fewer satisfactions in the Home Life Area.
11. Teams of employees working in living units with more Neurotic Anxious youngsters reported fewer potential satisfactions in the Finance Area; more potential frustrations in the Activity Area; greater frustration in the Health, Moods, and Habits areas; more

frustrations overall; higher Functioning at Best scores; lower Functioning at Worst scores; and highest Average Frustration scores.

12. The teams of employees working in living units with higher proportions of Maturity Level Three (I3–"other-oriented" or middle maturity) young people reported fewer frustrations in the Personal Influence Area.

13. The teams of employees working in living units with higher proportions of Passive Conforming youngsters reported less uncertainty about overall satisfactions, less potential frustration in the Personal Influence Area, and fewer Frustrations overall.

14. The teams of employees working in living units with higher proportions of Power-Oriented youngsters reported more potential frustrations in the Moods area.

15. The teams of staff working in living units with higher proportions of Neurotic Acting-Out youngsters reported less certainty of satisfaction in the Home Life Area.

16. The teams of staff working in living units with higher Stage Conceptual Level residents reported greater certainty of Satisfactions in the Home Life Area.

Maturity Level

The proportion of I-Level Three youths (I3)–lower maturity and "other-oriented"–was predictive of higher staff team satisfactions (Social Life, 1979), lower team frustrations (Influence, 1980), and greater certainty about satisfactions (Positive Swing, 1979). The proportion of I-Level Four Youths (I4)–higher maturity and "self-other oriented"– was predictive of lower satisfactions (Social Life and Overall Satisfactions, 1979) and greater uncertainty about satisfactions (Social Life and Positive Swing, 1979) amongst the staff teams investigated.

Delinquent Sub-Type

The Neurotic Acting-Out Sub-Type young people accounted for lower team satisfactions (Home Life, 1979 and 1980) and reduced certainty about satisfactions (Home Life, 1979) amongst staff teams. The Neurotic Anxious Sub-Type young people accounted for lower team satisfactions (Social Life, 1978) and higher uncertainty about satisfactions (Finance, 1979); higher team frustrations (Health, Moods, Habits, Overall Frustrations, and Average Frustrations, 1979) and more uncertainty about frus-

TABLE 4. Correlations Between Resident Data, Staff Satisfactions, and Staff Frustrations, 1978

Statistical Correlations Highlighted Between Resident Data (Iv) & Staff Reported Satisfactions (Dv) 1978 (Pearson R^2)

	BWork	GWork	BHome	GHome	BSocial Life
Conforming			0.71	0.81	
NXs			(0.016)	(0.004)	−0.72
CL Stage	0.71	0.71			(0.015)
Stage A	(0.017)	(0.016)			

Statistical Correlations Highlighted Between Resident Data (Iv) & Staff Reported Frustrations (Dv) 1978 (Pearson R^2)

	BHabits	GHabits	Worst	Avg. Worst
Conforming				
Neurotic Anxious (NXs)	−0.75	−0.79	−0.75	−0.72
CL Stage	(0.010)	(0.005)	(0.010)	(0.014)
	−0.72	−0.75		
Stage A	(0.015)	(0.010)		

Source: Shawbridge Youth Centres–Statistical Significance listed in brackets (x)
Note: B Active, B-G Health, G Moods all correlated with significance tests of 0.62 or better (0.033, 0.037, 0.025, 0.033)

trations (Activity, Health, Moods, Habits, Potential Frustrations, 1979); as well as the highest ratio of frustration to satisfaction (Functioning at Best and Functioning at Worst, 1979). The Immature Conformist Sub-Type youngsters accounted for higher team satisfactions (Home Life, 1978; Social Life and Overall Satisfactions, 1979) and greater certainty about satisfactions (Home Life, 1978; Social Life, 1979; Positive Swing, 1979), lower team frustrations (Personal Influence, 1980), and greater certainty about frustrations (Personal Influence, 1980). Because of the comparatively small numbers of Cultural Conformist and Manipulator Sub-Type youngsters in the study, these two groups were evaluated together under the Power-Oriented heading for Delinquent Subgroups.

Delinquent Sub-Group

The Conflicted sub-group accounted for lower team satisfactions (Social Life and Overall Satisfactions, 1979) and greater uncertainty about satisfactions (Social Life and Positive Swing, 1979). The findings for the

TABLE 5. Statistical Correlations Highlighted Between Resident Data (Iv) and Staff Reported Satisfactions (Dv) 1979 (Pearson R^2)

Type of Residents	Gross Negative Score	Basic Social Life	Potential Social Life	Basic Home	Potential Home	Basic Positive Score	Positive Swing
I3s		0.80 (0.008)	0.84 (0.005)				−0.86 (0.003)
Power/ Conforming		0.88 (0.002)	0.93 (0.000)			0.70 (0.026)	−0.87 (0.002)
I4s			−0.83 (0.006)			−0.72 (0.023)	0.92 (0.000)
Conflicted		−0.80 (0.008)	−0.82 (0.007)	−0.80 (0.009)	−0.81 (0.007)	−0.78 (0.011)	0.93 (0.000)
NAs	−0.70 (0.028)	−0.77 (0.012)					
NXs		0.72 (0.023)					
Sub-types			0.72 (0.022)			0.75 (0.016)	−0.88 (0.002)

Note: BPS .6919 (0.29)

TABLE 6. Statistical Correlations Highlighted Between Resident Data (Iv) and Staff Reported Areas of Frustration (Dv) 1979 (Pearson R^2)

Type of Residents	Activity & Fatigue	Potential Health	Personal Influence	Moods & Anxiety	Potential Habits
I3s Power					−0.73 (0.021)
Conform I4s Conflicted			0.70 (0.028)		
NAs NXs	0.74 (0.018)	0.72 (0.022)		0.87 (0.002)	0.97 (0.000)
Sub-types			−0.71 (0.023)		

Source: Shawbridge Youth Centres

TABLE 7. Statistical Correlations Highlighted Between Resident Data (Iv) and Staff Reported Total Frustrations (Dv) 1979 (Pearson R^2)

Type of Residents	Frustration Uncertainties	Frustration Certainties	Potential Frustrations	At Best	At Worst	Average Frustrations
I3s Power						
Conform I4s Conflicted	0.70 (0.028)					
NAs						
NXs		0.85 (0.003)	0.85 (0.003)	0.84 (0.004)	0.74 (0.018)	0.80 (0.009)
Sub-types						

Source: Shawbridge Youth Centres

Passive-Conforming sub-group were the same as for the Immature Conformist Sub-Type. The Power-Oriented Sub-Group accounted for higher team frustrations and uncertainty about some frustrations (Moods, 1980) but less uncertainty about other frustrations (Habits, 1979).

Conceptual Level Stage

Low Conceptual Level, Stage A youngsters accounted for higher staff team frustrations (Habits, 1978) and greater uncertainty about frustrations (Habits, 1978).

Conceptual Level Group Mean

Accounted for no significant changes.

Conceptual Level Group Stage

Higher Conceptual Level Stage groups accounted for higher team satisfactions (Work, 1978; Home Life, 1980), less uncertainty about satisfactions (Work, 1978); less team frustrations (Habits and Average Frustrations, 1978), less uncertainty about frustrations (Habits, 1978) and a higher ratio of satisfactions to frustrations (Functioning at Worst, 1978).

TABLE 8. Correlations Between Resident Data, Staff Satisfactions, and Staff Frustrations, 1980

Statistical Correlations Highlighted Between Resident Data (Iv) & Staff Reported Satisfactions (Dv) 1980 (Pearson R^2)

	Positive Swing	Basic Home
I3s Conforming Youths*	−0.76 (0.003)	
Power-Oriented Youths		−0.82 (0.001)
NAs Conceptual Level Stage		0.72 (0.006)

Statistical Correlations Highlighted Between Resident Data (Iv) & Staff Reported Frustrations (Dv) 1980 (Pearson R^2)

Type of Resident	Personal Influence	Potential Influence	Basic Moods	Potential Moods & Anxieties	Known Frustrations Score (BNS)
I3s	−0.73 (0.006)	−0.74 (0.005)			
Conforming Youths*	−0.83 (0.001)	−0.83 (0.001)			−0.71 (0.007)
Power-Oriented Youths			0.78 (0.002)	0.81 (0.001)	
Neurotic Anxious Youths					
Conceptual Level Stage					

Source: Shawbridge Youth Centres
Note: *The higher Basic Satisfactions Score and the lower Potential Frustrations Score yielded a Pearson's Correlation Score of 0.68 or better, and significance tests of (0.011, 0.0009).
One view of the situation in the English-speaking sector of services for children in Montreal leading up to the admission of girls at Shawbridge Youth Centres can be found in Carinol (1979).

DISCUSSION

Resident Characteristics

The diagnostic characteristics of residents based on the Interpersonal Maturity Classification System: Juvenile and the Conceptual Level

Matching Model were found to interact differentially with respect to team functioning. While it was already established that these characteristics are important when making individual assignments of worker and teacher, they are also important with respect to teamworking in group care practice.

Conforming Young People

The pattern of higher satisfaction, lower frustration, and greater certainty in teams working with more of these young people is not surprising based on clinical impressions that youngsters such as these are oriented towards rules and compliance towards rules. These youths feel secure when the structure around them is clear and definite, when relationships are perceived to be safe and fair, and when the persons whom they perceive to be powerful give approval. One staff member with experience of work with conforming youngsters acknowledged that they need a firm stable parent figure with whom they feel protected, someone who can also help them learn to stand up and take care of themselves.

Power-Oriented Young People

Higher frustrations reported in teams working with power-oriented youngsters is not surprising, although the levels of frustration might have been higher. Manipulative behaviour and anger so frequently demonstrated by this group, coupled with a superficial ability to relate to in essentially power relationships, render other residents and many staff wary of these erratic and hostile behaviour patterns. Other studies show that staff who get along with these youngsters best are those who can keep "one step ahead of them" and not be easily misled by superficial acquiescence to authority (Palmer & Grenny, 1971). Practice wisdom came from one worker when declaring: "They have to know that I can and will control them, but they also need fair play."

Neurotic Sub-Types

Again the variable patterns of lower satisfaction, greater frustration, and greater uncertainty are not surprising given the clinical descriptions associated with these youngsters. Experienced workers will not be surprised to find that teams working with these youths became emotionally involved with them in such a way that their social and home life satisfactions were reduced and levels of frustration and uncertainty were increased. It is interesting to note how these symptoms are not dissimilar from those identified early on by Menzies (1970, 1977) as individual and small group transference and practitioners offer anecdotal accounts of such teamworking phenomena. Even more interesting to the authors was the apparent "contagion" with which this may occur during "off duty" (home/social life) time amongst teams working with several neurotic youths. It is as if staff teams periodically internalize, in some way, the tortured self-concepts which these youths are said to manifest and carry this emotional burden over into their relationships outside their work. One experienced worker said, *"You can't just supervise these kids, you have to develop a relationship with them and talk about the things which are important to them."*

Conceptual Level

Once again the emergent patterns came as little surprise in light of the behavioural characteristics identified by Conceptual Level. The low Conceptual Level youngster is said to be very concrete in his or her thinking, is very egocentric, and takes an anti-authority stance towards others. In addition, there is an absence of internalized, culturally accepted beliefs and values. While young persons such as these may generate high frustrations for staff at all times, noting that this would probably be greatest, according to Conceptual Level theory, when daily programming and routines are erratic or when expectations are considered ambiguous (Reitsma-Street, 1982). Higher Conceptual Level residents are thought to be more comfortable with uncertainty, for example, in a "discovery" approach to learning where they must take some initiative (Brill, 1978).

Staff Characteristics

The demographic variables and social background information collected from staff teams did not correlate significantly with any of the resident group characteristics. This was somewhat difficult to understand since variables such as sex and marital status have played so prominent a role in other studies of job satisfaction and in Fulcher's (1983) wider study of team functioning with a large international sample. It is possible that these variables were masked because of the small numbers in the sample or became less influential in mediating differences between staff and residents. At times, the sheer intensity of 24-hour involvements between neurotic youths and staff in a residential group care setting is such a powerful element in the dynamics of staff team functioning that almost everyone is affected.

The Life Events Measure

Variables derived from the Schedule of Recent and Anticipated Experiences (Holmes & Rahe, 1967) did not correlate with any of the resident group characteristics. This was not surprising in the light of findings that show how many life measures obscure or mask subjective interpretations of events by individuals, failing to assume complex associations between events, sex differences, and methodological rigour (Kale & Stenmark, 1983; Lester, Leitner, & Posner, 1983; Monroe, 1982; Zimmerman, 1983).

The Work Orientation Measures

Variables derived from the Work Orientation Schedule (Heimler & Fulcher, 1981) were highly correlated with many of the resident group characteristics under investigation. As such, this instrument would seem to provide an unobtrusive measure of quality of working life that offers distinct advantages over the more traditional job satisfaction measures. A variety of themes can be identified through the use of the Work Orientation Schedule, illuminating satisfactions, frustrations, and uncertainties in working life. These themes appear to be influential for individual workers and for group care centres as a whole, since they are instrumental in shaping patterns of team functioning and performance over time. While developmental research with this instrument has, to date, focused on groups of workers in teams, there remains considerable scope for using the Work Orientation Schedule in staff supervision, personnel management, and employment counseling in the human relations field (Fulcher, 1983).

CONCLUSIONS

Research endorsement was obtained for the practice impression of there being an important interplay between the diagnostic characteristics of residents and the patterns of staff team functioning found in any residential group care centre. Nor is this relation always considered for its impact on the quality of service outcomes and quality of working life for staff over time. These factors may be unique to individual staff members yet at any given time particular events or issues come into focus which have at least symbolic value for most members of a group care team. Such findings are consistent with what others have referred to as organizational culture (Smircich, 1983; Wilkins & Ouchi, 1983) reinforcing the notion of resource dependency (White, 1974).

Whether these influences originate from within the team, from what is happening within the resident group, from the wider organization, or from the social policy environment in which service organizations and group care centres are located, the results may at times draw team members together or they may promote destructive levels of turbulence or maladaptation in teamwork (Menzies, 1970, 1977). Based on the results of this study, an awareness about quality of working life frustrations and satisfactions in the staff team, coupled with increased understanding of the diagnostic characteristics of residents, could be used to strengthen team cohesion, promote reciprocal support of staff members, and increase the level of purposeful activity directed towards residents by staff teams.

A note of caution is still indicated. Teamwork is an ongoing process intimately related to quality of working life satisfactions and frustrations amongst staff. It is not something that happens at a single training session. Regression or fade-out, particularly after off-site team building sessions, is well known to researchers and students of organizational and management behaviour (Boss, 1983). A combination of staff development and training, involving management and supervisory structures as well as carefully identified consultative supports and follow-up, is fundamental. With such caution in mind, the following suggestions can still be made about team supervision in group care.

1. Teams working with neurotic youths are likely to require supervision of a depth-oriented and psychodynamic nature geared towards helping workers clarify what is happening with and between members in the resident group while at the same time sharing their own feelings about residents, particularly when such feelings risk interfering with "off duty" time.
2. Teams working with power-oriented young people may become stalemated at times over how best to channel their collective behaviour. Workers may be readily inclined to reinforce immediate

control measures. Such workers will often require support to reinforce longer-range goals associated with personal growth and development needs of these young people, not just their need for close supervision.

3. Teams working with lower maturity, conforming young people may need to ensure that such youths do not become overly dependent upon the staff working with them. Both workers and residents may settle into a comfortable and relaxed symbiotic collaboration in ways that resemble surrogate parenting. The relatively poor showing on recidivism measures for conforming youngsters who have been in treatment-oriented programs show that many remain highly vulnerable to conformity with delinquent and criminal peers upon leaving care.

Perhaps the most significant outcome of this study was that measures of team functioning were highly sensitive (if not yet fully understood) to differences among residents in group care practice. These findings are consistent with those identified by Eisner (1982) employing similar measures to those used in this study. The assessment typologies were robust and were reliably identified using appropriate classification methods. The assessment typologies were also validated alongside a host of differential outcome measures, including behavioural management, academic-vocational achievements, and reduced recidivism. Further refinement and uses of this team functioning assessment methodology was highly indicated in the development of human service practice and research.

NOTE

1. One view of the situation in the English-speaking sector of services for children in Montreal leading up to the admission of girls at Shawbridge Youth Centres can be found in Carinol (1979).

REFERENCES

Andre, C. R., & Mahan, J. A. (1972). *Final report on the differential education project.* Educational Research Series, No. 11 Sacramento: California Youth Authority.

Argyle, M. (1972). *The social psychology of work.* New York: Penguin Books.

Bales, R. F. (1950). *Interaction process analysis.* Cambridge, MA: Addison-Wesley.

Barkwell, L. (1976). Differential treatment of juveniles on probation. *Canadian Journal of Criminology and Correctionsm, 18*(4), 363-378.

Boss, R. W. (1983). Team building and the problem of regression: The personal management interview as an intervention. *The Journal of Applied Behavioral Science, 19*(1), 67-83.

Brill, R. W. (1978). Implications of the conceptual level matching model for treatment of delinquents. *Journal of Research in Crime and Delinquency, 12*, 229-246.

Bronfenbrenner, U. (1979a). *The ecology of human development*. Cambridge, MA: D. C. Heath.

Bronfenbrenner, U. (1979b). Contexts of child rearing: Problems and prospects. *American Psychologist, 34*(10), 844-850.

Burford, G. (1990). *Assessing teamwork: A comparative study of group home teams in Newfoundland and Labrador*. Unpublished doctoral dissertation, University of Stirling, Stirling, Scotland.

Carinol, B. (1979). Children's rights: Social action to change conditions in juvenile detention centers. In B. Wharf (Ed.), *Community work in Canada*. Toronto: McClelland & Stewart.

Davis, L. E., & Chernis, A. B. (Eds.). (1975). *The quality of working life* (Vols. I and II). New York: Free Press.

Eisner, S. (1982). *The interplay between the Heimler scale of social functioning and the interpersonal maturity level classification system*. Unpublished masters thesis, Universite de Montreal, Montreal, Quebec.

Fulcher, L. C. (1979). Keeping staff sane to accomplish treatment. *Residential and Community Child Care Administration, 1*(1), 69-85.

Fulcher, L. C. (1983). *Who cares for the caregivers? A comparative study of residential and day care teams working with children*. Unpublished doctoral dissertation, University of Stirling, Stirling, Scotland.

Fulcher, L. C. (1988). *The worker, the work group and the organisational task: Corporate re-structuring and the social services in New Zealand*. Wellington: Victoria University Press.

Fulcher, L. C. (1991). Teamwork in residential care. In J. Beker & Z. Eisikovits (Eds.), *Knowledge utilization in residential child and youth care practice* (pp. 215-235). Washington, DC: Child Welfare League of America.

Fulcher, L. C., & Ainsworth, F. (1981). Planned care and treatment: The notion of programme. In F. Ainsworth & L. C. Fulcher (Eds.), *Group care for children: Concept and issues*. London: Tavistock.

Gendreau, P., & Ross, R. (1979, October). Effective correctional treatment: Bibliotherapy for cynics. *Crime and Delinquency*, pp. 463-489.

Grant, J. D., & Grant, M. Q. (1959). A group dynamics approach to the treatment of non-conformists in the navy. *The Annals of the Academy of Political and Social Science, 3*(22), 126-135.

Hall, R. H. (1969). *Occupations and the social structure*. Englewood Cliffs, NJ: Prentice-Hall.

Harris, P. (1983). The interpersonal maturity of delinquents and non-delinquents. In W. L. Laufer & J. M. Day (Eds.), *Personality theory, moral development, and criminal behavior*. Toronto: Lexington Books.

Heimler, E. (1970). *The scale of organizational functioning*. Unpublished manuscript.

Heimler, E. (1975). *Survival in society*. New York: Halsted Press.

Heimler, E. (1979). *On the emotional significance of work: An Audio-taped Interview* (27 September). Department of Sociology, University of Stirling, Scotland.

Heimler, E., & Fulcher, L. C. (1981). The work orientation schedule. In L. C. Fulcher (Eds.), *Who cares for the caregivers? A comparative study of residential and day care teams working with children*. PhD Thesis, University of Stirling, Scotland.

Hertzberg, F. (1968). *Work and the nature of man*. London: Staples Press.

Holmes, T. H., & Masuda, M. (1974). Life change and illness susceptibility. In B. S. Dohrenwend & B. P. Dohrenwend (Eds.), *Stressful life events: Their nature and effects*. New York: John Wiley.

Holmes, T. H., & Rahe, R. H. (1967). The social readjustment rating scale. *Journal of Psychosomatic Research, 11*, 213-218.

Homans, G. C. (1950). *The human group*. New York: Harcourt-Brace.

Hunt, D. (1971). *Matching models in education: The coordination of teaching methods with student characteristics*. Toronto: Ontario Institute for Studies in Education.

Hunt, D., & Hardt, R. (1967). The role of conceptual level and program structure in summer upward-bound programs. Paper presented at Eastern Psychological Association Meeting, Boston, April. From R. Brill, (1977) Implications of the Conceptual Level Matching Model for the Treatment of Delinquents. *Journal of Research in Crime & Delinquency, 12*, 229-246.

Hunt, D., Butler, L., Noy, J., & Rosse, M. (1978). *Assessing conceptual level by the paragraph completion method*. Toronto: Ontario Institute for Studies in Education.

Jesness, C. (1965). *The Fricto ranch study: Outcomes with small vs large living groups in the rehabilitation of delinquents*. Sacramento: California Youth Authority, Research Report No. 47.

Jesness, C. (1971). The Preston typology study: An experiment with differential treatment in an institution. *Journal of Research in Crime and Delinquency, 8*, 38-52.

Jesness, C. (1980). Was the close-holton project a 'bummer'? In R. Ross & P. Gendreau (Eds.), *Effective correctional treatment*. Toronto: Butterworth.

Jesness, C., Derisi, W., McCormick, P., & Wedge, R. (1972). *The youth center research project: Final report*. Sacramento: California Youth Authority & American Justice Institute.

Johnson, V. S. (1981). Staff drift: A problem in program integrity. *Criminal Justice and Behavior, 8*(2), 223-232.

Kale, W. L., & Stenmark, D. E. (1983). A comparison of four life event scales. *American Journal of Community Psychology, II*(4), 441-458.

Knapp, R. G. (1978). *Basic statistics for nurses*. Toronto: John Wiley.

Lester, D., Leitner, L., & Posner, I. (1983). Recent life events and stress scores: An examination of the Holmes and Rahe scale. *Psychological Reports*, 53-70.

Lewin, K. (1952). *Field theory in social sciences*. London: Tavistock.

Lukin, P. (1981). Recidivism and changes made by delinquents during residential treatment. *Journal of Research in Crime & Delinquency*, January, 101-112.

Maier, H. W. (1981). Essential components in care and treatment environments for children. In F. Ainsworth & L. C. Fulcher (Eds.), *Group care for children: Concept and issues*. London: Tavistock.

Mattingly, M. A. (1977). Sources of stress and burn-out in professional child care work. *Child Care Quarterly, 6*(2), 127-137.

McLachlan, J. (1972). Benefit from group therapy as a function of patient-therapist match on conceptual level. *Psychotherapy: Theory, Research and Practice, 9*, 317-323.

McLachlan, J. (1974). Therapy strategies, personality orientation and recovery from alcoholism. *Canadian Psychiatric Association Journal, 19*, 25-30.

Megargee, E. (1977). The need for a new classification system. *Criminal Justice and Behavior, 4*, 107-114.

Menzies, I. E. P. (1970). *The functioning of social systems operating as a defense against anxiety.* London: Tavistock Institute of Human Relations.

Menzies, I. E. P. (1977). *Staff support systems: Task and anti-task in adolescent institutions.* London: Tavistock Institute of Human Relations.

Monroe, S. M. (1982). Life events assessment: Current practices, emerging trends. *Clinical Psychology Review, 2*, 435-453.

Moos, R. (1975). *Evaluating community and correctional settings.* New York: John Wiley.

Morgan, G. (1986). *Images of organisation.* London: Sage Publications.

Palmer, T. (1972). *Differential placement of delinquents in group homes, final report.* Sacramento: California Youth Authority and National Institute of Mental Health.

Palmer, T. (1974, March). The youth authority's community treatment project. *Federal Probation*, 3-14.

Palmer, T. (1976). *Final report of the community treatment project, phases 1, 2, and 3.* Sacramento: California Youth Authority and National Institute of Mental Health.

Palmer, T. (1978). *Correctional intervention and research: Current issues and future prospects.* Lexington. MA: D. C. Heath.

Palmer, T. (1992). *The Re-emergence of correctional intervention.* Thousand Oaks, CA: Sage Publications.

Palmer, T., & Grenny, C. (1971). *Stance and techniques of matched Nx, Na, MP-CFC and 12 workers.* California Youth Authority. Mimeographed paper.

Palmer, T., & McShane, M. D. (2001). *Individualized intervention with young multiple offenders: The California community treatment project, issues & perspectives.* New York: Routledge.

Quay, H. (1977). The three faces of evaluation: What can be expected to work. *Criminal Justice and Behavior, 4*, 341-534.

Reitsma-Street, M. (1982). A critical review of the conceptual level matching model and its relevance for the treatment of maladjusted youth. *The Differential View: A Publication of The International Differential Treatment Association-Sixth Annual Conference Proceedings.* Issue 12, September.

Ross. A. L. (1983). Mitigating turnover of child care staff in group care facilities. *Child Welfare, 62* (Jan.-Feb.), pp. 63-67.

Ross, R., & Gendreau, P. (1980). *Effective correctional treatment.* Toronto: Butterworth.

Scheirer, M. A., & Rezmovic, E. L. (1983, October). Measuring the degree of program implementation: A methodological review. *Evaluation Review, 7*(5), 599-633.

Smircich, L. (1983, September). Concepts of culture and organizational analysis, *Administrative Science Quarterly, 28*, 339-358.

Tomlinson, P., & Hunt, D. (1971). Differential effects of rule-example order as a function of learner conceptual level. *Canadian Journal of Behavior Science*, 235-237.

Trieschman, A. E., Whittaker, J. K., & Brendtro, L. K. (1969). *The other 23 hours*. Chicago: Aldine.

Warren, M. Q. et al. (1966). *Interpersonal maturity classification system–Juvenile: Diagnosis of low, middle, and high maturity delinquents*. Sacramento: California Youth Authority.

Warren, M. Q. (1983). Application of interpersonal maturity to offender populations. In W. L. Laufer & J. M. Day (Eds.), *Personality theory, moral development, and criminal behavior*. Toronto: Lexington Books.

White, P. E. (1974, September). Resources as determinants of organisational behavior. *Administrative Science Quarterly*, 366-379.

Whittaker, J. (1979). *Caring for troubled children*. San Francisco: Jossey-Bass.

Wilkins, A. L., & Ouchi, W. G. (1983, September). Efficient cultures: Exploring the relationship between culture and organizational performance. *Administrative Science Quarterly, 28*, 468-481.

Youth Protection Act. (1979). *Quebec Youth Protection Act twenty-five years later*. Retrieved from *http://www.acjq.qc.ca/actualites/com_024.htm*

Zimmerman, M. (1983). Methodological issues in the assessment of life events: A review of issues and research. *Clinical Psychology Review, 3*, 339-370.

SECTION 3:
ORGANISATIONAL INFLUENCES
ON PRACTICE

Chapter 9

Managing Occupational Stress
for Group Care Personnel

Martha A. Mattingly

SUMMARY. Traditional clinical professions, as well as the emerging child and youth care profession, have focused primarily on the welfare of identified clients. While the personal and professional well-being of practitioners has long been addressed in the training and supervision of human service workers, serious efforts to identify problems confronting these workers and potential consequences for both staff and residents are

Address correspondence to: Martha A. Mattingly, Applied Developmental Psychology, 5807 Posvar Hall, University of Pittsburgh, Pittsburgh, PA 15260.

[Haworth co-indexing entry note]: "Managing Occupational Stress for Group Care Personnel." Mattingly, Martha A. Co-published simultaneously in *Child & Youth Services* (The Haworth Press, Inc.) Vol. 28, No. 1/2, 2006, pp. 209-230; and: *Group Care Practice with Children and Young People Revisited* (ed: Leon C. Fulcher, and Frank Ainsworth) The Haworth Press, Inc., 2006, pp. 209-230. Single or multiple copies of this article are available for a fee from The Haworth Document Delivery Service [1-800-HAWORTH, 9:00 a.m. - 5:00 p.m. (EST). E-mail address: docdelivery@haworthpress.com].

comparatively recent. This classic contribution to the literature highlights ways in which child and youth care has provided leadership on the management of occupational stress in the human services. *[Article copies available for a fee from The Haworth Document Delivery Service: 1-800-HAWORTH. E-mail address: <docdelivery@haworthpress.com> Website: <http://www.HaworthPress.com> © 2006 by The Haworth Press, Inc. All rights reserved.]*

KEYWORDS. Group care, residential care, residential treatment, group homes, youth work, youthwork, group work, at-risk youth, burnout, post-traumatic stress

LOOKING BACK

One afternoon in 1976, a graduate student came running down the hall shouting, "They said it! Somebody finally said it!" She was holding Herbert Freudenberger's (1975) seminal article that established the term "burnout" in the psychological literature. My graduate student and I now had a name for our painful personal burnout experiences. We could see ourselves in Freudenberger's description. Shortly thereafter I organized and edited a special issue of the *Child and Youth Care Quarterly* (Mattingly, 1977) (now the *Child and Youth Care Forum*) focused on occupational stress to which both Freudenberger (1977) and Maslach (1977) contributed. This was followed by the original publication of this chapter in 1981 (Mattingly, 1981). This body of work represented a turning point from an inner psychic view of job stress towards an ecological perspective.

During the last three decades the occupational stress literature has exploded. A search of PsychInfo provides access to this expanding body of work. Central to the growing understanding of burnout is the work of Christina Maslach. Among her many contributions are the identification and exploration of the dimensions of burnout (Maslach & Schaufeli, 1993) and construction of the Maslach Burnout Inventory (Maslach, Jackson, & Leiter, 1996). She is now engaged in further elaboration of the interaction between person and workplace variables (Maslach, 2003). Also, Vic Savicki's work has focused primarily on child and youth care work and has significantly enhanced our understanding of the cultural dimension of burnout (Mann-Feder & Savicki, 2003; Savicki, 1993, 1999, 2001, 2002; Savicki & Cooley, 1987; Savicki & Riolli-Saltzman, 2001).

Child and youth care has been both a leader and a beneficiary of this chain of events. Talks and workshops took place, practitioners developed personal stress resistance and recovery plans, and agencies addressed issues of job stress. It is interesting to note that self-care obligations are now included in the ethics statements for child and youth care (International Leadership Coalition, 1995), and psychology (American Psychological Association, 2002).

As child and youth care in North America establishes credentials for the professional level of practice, consideration of occupational stress becomes even more critical (Mattingly & Thomas, 2004; Thomas, 2002). It is imperative that researchers and practitioners from child and youth care explore issues of stress in practice and apply the findings to support the quality of professional life and service to children, youth, and families. What follows still helps to inform such an imperative.

INTRODUCTION

The traditional clinical professions of medicine, nursing, education, psychology, and social work as well as the emerging child and youth care profession have focused traditionally on the welfare of the patient-client. While practitioner well-being has long been generally and implicitly addressed in the training and supervision of human service providers, it is comparatively recent that serious efforts have been made to identify problems confronting these workers and to reflect on their consequences. While child and youth care is a young emerging profession, it has been at the forefront of these efforts (Mattingly, 1977a).

In general, occupational stress refers here to workers' physiological and psychological responses to situations perceived as potentially disruptive (McLean, 1974). Disruptive situations may be either desirable or undesirable. Such positive changes as going on vacation, receiving a promotion or raise in pay, or learning a new and more effective child or youth care technique produce stress. However, the concern here is with the effects of negative stress, which arise from situations perceived as undesirable, painful, and challenging to the ability of the worker to cope effectively.

The "burnout syndrome" is an extreme response to occupational pressure. It has been described as primarily an experience of exhaustion resulting from excessive demands on the worker's energy and resources accompanied by a dehumanization of the caring process (Freudenberger, 1975, 1977; Maslach, 1976; Maslach & Pines, 1977; Mattingly,

1977b). The burnout syndrome appears to be widespread among human service workers whose work requires intense interpersonal involvement (Hall, Gardner, Peri, Stickney, & Pfefferbaum, 1979; Maslach & Jackson, 1979; Mattingly, 1979; Pines & Kafry, 1978; Pines & Maslach, 1978; Seiderman, 1978; Shubin, 1978; White, 1978; Yager & Hubert, 1979). In addition, symptoms of combat neurosis,[1] an extremely similar if not identical phenomenon, have been identified in some teachers in inner-city schools (Bloch, 1978).

The problem of job stress and burnout is of special concern in professional child and youth care work. In recent years, child and youth care workers have made enormous strides toward professionalization and improvement of the quality of care expected for children. Advances have been made in the design and availability of training. But if the field is to thrive and mature, it is essential that there be a substantial cadre of experienced, educated, and committed practitioners. Retention of workers (Pritzker, 1974) and the quality of care provided by many long-term workers are well-known problems in the field. Part of this is due to rather widespread poor selection procedures, training, salaries, and working conditions. A significant contribution, however, also comes from the physical and psychological exhaustion experienced by child and youth care workers in the caring process. The result appears to be high staff turnover, potential apathy and frustration for continuing workers, and the loss of some especially able practitioners who are concerned about their effectiveness with children. It is important to keep in mind, however, that there are effective long-term workers who do not report serious personal damage from stress.

While the child and youth care profession as well as many workers and agencies has begun to address the issues of job stress and worker burnout, some resistance to its discussion is still encountered occasionally. Such considerations arouse painful memories, a sense of vulnerability, and issues of responsibility many would like to avoid. It can bring agencies and systems face to face with the need for changes that some may find more comfortable and convenient not to confront. And, finally, it can bring the profession face to face with an enormous problem requiring attention. The profession's willingness to confront these issues raises the hope that effective ways of coping with the stress of group caring work can and will be found. The benefits will be reaped by group child and youth care professionals able to work with greater dignity and mature in the skills of their chosen profession. The ultimate beneficiaries will be the children and young people with whom they work.

A REFLECTION ON SOURCES OF STRESS
IN CHILD AND YOUTH CARING WORK

Burnout is frequently used as a catchy phrase to explain various sorts of frustration and fatigue. In order to come to grips with the problem of stress it is first necessary to identify sources of stress. Each person, of course, experiences stress in an individual manner and needs to consider his/her own situation. This reflection is drawn from the literature, the personal experience of the writer, and the generous sharing of accounts by many child and youth care workers who have willingly expressed their frustration and pain.

Agency attitudes and policies contribute to the stresses experienced by child and youth care workers. The effects of an agency as a closed system are frequently seen (White, 1978). Many agencies have enduring traditions that come from more autocratic times. Others are component parts of large and cumbersome bureaucracies that have lost the ability to be flexible and responsive. Workers can begin to assess the particular structure of their agency and its relationship to the stress they experience.

An effectively closed system is characterized by a sense of isolation and rigidity. Such an agency is isolated from professional and community resources and has a major, usually unspoken, goal to remain hidden and unchanged. There is an excessive emphasis on presenting a favourable public impression, protecting the agency from criticism, and accounting for aspects of the agency that are not central to the quality of service rendered, e.g., the linen inventory, maintenance records, and grounds-keeping staff. Such agencies tend to protect themselves through a screening procedure for new staff and consultants that assures maintenance of the preferred agency attitude. This may result in the rejection of sophisticated applicants as overqualified, unlikely to work as good team members, or not familiar with "our" problems.

Events that create conflict and disequilibrium tend to be dealt with by denial and retreat to the agency ideology. Problems are identified as arising from discrete issues and persons. The ecology of the agency is not made a focus for review. A high turnover rate for child and youth care workers may be dealt with by proclaiming that no one can do such difficult work for more than a couple of years. Crisis management issues are considered client problems without consideration of deficits in the program of care and treatment offered. Persons who begin to raise issues related to the agency are frequently identified as inept and unsuited for this type of work. Supervision is often defined as an accountability review. The result is a rigid and inflexible setting that diminishes the role of the worker and truncates the support system an agency might be expected to provide.

Morale and job satisfaction tend to decline steadily from the top to the bottom of an agency hierarchy. Morale among child and youth care workers is directly related to their perceived ability to influence the decisions affecting their work (Shamsie & Lang, 1976). Within agencies child and youth care workers are frequently perceived as among the least valued of employees. The common low level of financial compensation is the most substantial evidence for this perception. Currently a child or youth care worker may not only find him or herself a devalued and, perhaps, dispensable, easily replaced employee but is also subject to increasing awareness of the central role they play in providing quality care for children and young people. While being told of her or his importance and encouraged toward professional associations and training, she or he is deprived of the economic and psychological circumstances necessary to engage in an exciting and productive career.

Workers enter the field of child and youth care with a variety of motivations. For the most part they are dedicated, concerned persons who wish to offer themselves and their resources to assist children in their development and rehabilitation. Dedication, concern, and idealism are essential for all caring work. In fact, these qualities may be a source of the motivation and energy needed for difficult caring tasks (VanderVen, 1979). Concerned child and youth care workers support the growth of each child from their own resources and talents. However, there is an inescapable stress-producing conflict between the worker's commitment to give and the reality that frequently one cannot give enough. Each person's emotional resources are limited. The refreshment provided by family, friends, colleagues, and personal interests are often insufficient. This conflict is a particular hazard for the beginning worker but one with which all caring persons struggle throughout their careers.

The idealism and dedication characterizing the decision to engage in caring work are severely challenged by numerous physical and psychological assaults on well-being and self-esteem. Upon entering the field, workers usually perceive themselves as concerned and helpful persons whom clients and society will value. By way of contrast, workers are often confronted by assaultive youth, messy and aggressive children, and ungrateful families. The nobility of caring work turns out to be a myth. Successful workers develop a personal durability as they integrate the idealistic view of caring for children with the everyday realities. However, no matter how skilled and sophisticated the worker, a kick in the shins, broken glasses, an insult or a child's lack of progress are all assaults on self-esteem that threaten workers' perceptions of their helping ability.

Experiences that enhance workers' sense of effectiveness are quite random and inconsistent. In many instances they cannot remain involved with a child for a sufficient period to see productive growth and the resolution of major difficulties. The limitations imposed by agency structure or funding sources, special client needs, and changes in family circumstances or attitudes may result in termination of the worker-client relationship. Perhaps a seed has been planted that will bear fruit in the future, but perhaps not. The worker has been interrupted in the middle of something and is denied the rewards of experiencing a job well done.

Many child and youth care workers still lack the professional knowledge that would allow them to assess the effectiveness of their everyday practice. Supervision is frequently rendered by persons neither skilled in child and youth care nor readily available. Much supervision, if it exists at all, is almost exclusively problem- or deficit-focused. Colleagues may also be unable or unwilling to provide feedback on the quality of work. This problem is likely to be especially severe for supervisors and service administrators. Thus workers are commonly left without a realistic evaluation of the quality of their work.

Child and youth care workers must also process an enormous amount of information with great speed. In the many hours of direct client contact the worker maintains a disciplined alertness and vigilance to the children or youth as well as the setting. Masses of verbal and non-verbal behaviour, the sounds and conditions of the environment, the program of the day, and the history and treatment plan for each child are registered in awareness. Situations must also be dealt with on many levels at the same time. In fact, the very basis of child and youth care practice is the use of the everyday environment to support each child's growth while completing the tasks essential for organized living. Child and youth care workers practice in "pressure cooker" environments that are characterized by rapid decision making and sustained intensive interaction.

The conflicts between client-care and custodial managerial requirements are inescapable and include such things as food preparation, acquiring a good community image with well-dressed and comported children, and maintaining a full census so that the agency and the establishment can survive financially. The nature of clinical child and youth care rarely permits the isolation of these concerns. Rather the conflicts are embodied in everyday decisions and interactions. It can be anticipated that as professional child and youth care workers have increasing participation in agency decision-making, such inevitable conflicts may become even more acute.

Daily practices are frequently open to the scrutiny of superiors, colleagues, children and, occasionally, parents and the community. There are few places to hide errors and bad days. There is no tape recorder to turn off or office door to close. In addition, the young people are affected by how the worker expresses anger, solves problems, has fun, and deals with the disliked carrots. The worker's task is difficult. To pretend or put on attitudes and feelings is difficult and often ineffective. Rather the worker is called upon to be a fully human person, honest in interactions, and concerned with personal behaviour and attitudes.

Child and youth care workers are called upon to be empathic with a person at a different developmental level than themselves (Olden, 1953). There is a professional commitment to place one's personal experience of childhood in the service of children in need and to engage, as it were, in an empathic tension. Workers must remain fully adult, not identifying with the child or allowing the child to be an inappropriate participant in their own psychological conflicts, while being in touch with childhood perceptions and feelings. Negative emotions such as anger, guilt, and potential loss of control are almost common. Such emotions are incongruent with the image of a helper of children and often frighten many workers, particularly at the beginning of their practice careers.

The worker who lives as well as works with the children whom they serve is confronted with additional hazards. Agency requirements vary greatly but three to five days a week of live-in duty at the facility are not uncommon. This may require continuous responsibility for the children or include interspersed off-duty periods in which the worker may or may not be expected to remain on site. The live-in worker's "amorphous omnipresence" (Grossbard, 1960) provides limited opportunities for withdrawal, psychological repair, or personal recovery. Interpersonal interactions are also very intense. Living quarters may allow for the constant intrusion of children's noises. Personal phone calls and visits, as well as the security of personal possessions may be severely limited. Off-duty time is open to interruption by both children and staff, often for insubstantial reasons such as finding a lost shoe or confirming the time of a parental visit. The live-in worker's perpetual exposure to the stressful environment tends to intensify all the stress producing influences (Reed, 1977).

The child and youth care worker must also sustain a professional identity with limited reinforcement from social and community sources. The common characteristics of babysitter, disciplinarian, and self-sacrificing martyr reflect the impoverished and inaccurate understanding of professional child-care work. Thus the child and youth care worker is denied realistic psychological support from these sources and must continue to reestablish basic career identity questions like "Who am I?" and "What do I do?"

BURNOUT: EXPERIENCES AND SIGNALS

Exposure to potentially harmful levels of stress is an inevitable part of child and youth caring work. A debilitating and painful response to these pressures is the burnout syndrome which is a phenomenon of physical and psychological exhaustion. Some basic components of burnout that occur with regularity have been identified and measured (Maslach, 1976; Maslach & Pines, 1977) include emotional exhaustion, depersonalization, and lack of personal accomplishment. In addition, each person's stress response has a unique individual pattern of symptoms, behaviours, and attitudes. Since most child and youth care workers are young adults, some of the traditional symptoms of stress may be masked (Hewitt, 1979). Thus any particular "burning-out" worker may experience only part of what is described here.

Burnout frequently begins as a vague subtle experience of discontent. The worker begins to have doubts about his or her caring work and may feel inadequate to and overwhelmed by the tasks, including a growing, uncomfortable rigidity of thinking and behaviour. He or she may be irritable, labile in moods, less empathetic, and behave, on occasion, in ways not congruent with personal self-image as a helper of children. Such experience is frequently confronted alone, and the worker often comes to the conclusion that she or he is unfit for the work. A severe fracture of professional identity is a common result.

As the pain and confusion increases, the worker may try to discuss these feelings with supervisors, colleagues, and friends who may respond with denial. Some talented workers report that their clinical work, though somewhat less flexible and creative, remains a good quality during a burning-out process. These persons seem to have the ability to isolate the effects of the stress they experience from their clinical work. Their pain is not apparent and their feelings are likely to be ignored.

In response to these workers, supervisors and colleagues may adopt a traditional inner psychic view and insist that the worker must deal with the personal problems that are deemed to be the source of their difficulties. The necessity for a critical self-reflective attitude has been emphasized in the training of the child and youth care worker. Thus one may be predisposed to engage in an energy-consuming self-review and perhaps seek professional assistance. Such effort even further depletes the worker's already meager energy (Freudenberger, 1975). Workers report that even skilled psychotherapists often do not recognize the stress arising from the caring commitment.

A note of caution is required here. Some workers have personal problems that do interfere with caring work. These need to be identified and dealt with. However, the customary and uncritical assumption of the inner psychodynamic view of the worker's distress effectively excludes consideration of the full circumstances of engaging in a caring commitment. Thus many, if not most, workers are denied the support and assistance to which they are entitled from agency and colleagues.

The worker may reject the suggestion to work on personal problems and choose to confront the frightening experience. Many workers have expressed a serious concern about "going crazy." This arises from the major discrepancy between the painful personal experience and the lack of interpersonal validation for such experiences.

A waning distinction between the time and place for personal life as well as a fading distinction between the psychological needs of the worker and child or young person may signal the arrival of burnout. This merger between the worker and the agency is a particular hazard for young workers. The structure of formal training that frequently demands an almost total commitment and the enthusiasm of beginning workers contribute to such hazards. The staff member may find it difficult to stop working. Careful consideration may reveal that over a period of time the worker has stopped taking lunch or rest breaks. If relief personnel are available for these periods the person may continue to hang around, including at the end of the shift and on days off, working or not.

She or he may be enthusiastic when called upon for overtime and emergency duty and volunteer to provide extra services during time off. Such behaviours and attitudes may signal that the worker lacks the energy and motivation to develop and sustain a rewarding personal life and relies on the agency to meet personal needs. Again, a note of caution is required. These comments are not intended as guidelines for worker behaviour. The caring commitment and personal interest may lead workers to appropriately offer personal time, skills, home, and family to assist a child or young person. Excessive agency regulation of these matters is usually not helpful to stress management.

Rather, workers' overinvolvement in their work may be a manifestation of the generally high level of stress in the agency and a lack of trust in supervisors' and workers' competence and judgment (Reed, 1977). These comments are intended to identify a hazard and encourage reflection about the personal meaning of such behaviours and attitudes.

Rigid and inflexible attitudes with a stubborn resistance to change are also part of the burnout phenomenon. As the worker's interaction with the setting becomes more stressful, personal resources are diminished and exhaustion approaches. Workers may find themselves without the flexibility needed to be confident and effective. The worker may retreat to a position of "knowing it won't work" or that "it has already been tried before" when innovations are suggested. Attempts at change are resisted. The burning-out worker literally cannot depart from the usual work pattern and experiences innovations as personally unmanageable (Freudenberger, 1975).

Rigidity is frequently also reflected in the worker's vocabulary. Language may become more evaluative and distancing with the use of stereotyped phrases and words. This is particularly, but not exclusively, evident in regard to perceptions of the client (Maslach, 1976; Maslach & Pines, 1977). Stereotyping statements can be simple such as "a quiet child" and "disruptive child" or they can be very sophisticated such as in repeated referrals to unresolved Oedipal conflicts or separation issues. The worker is exhausted and does not possess the energy necessary to process the complex data of the situation. Partial perceptions are channeled into preconceived categories. This allows the exhausted worker to garner psychological energies for the purpose of and continuing to serve clients.

Burning-out workers are also vulnerable to a substantial misevaluation of their abilities and prerogatives. Some workers grow increasingly unsure of themselves. They become overly concerned about personal deficiencies and may imagine errors in practice. They may become unduly apologetic to colleagues, supervisors, and children, requesting additional supervision designed to elicit approval and reassurance. Such workers start underestimating themselves.

Alternatively, overestimation was graphically described by one burning-out worker. A serious ice storm struck the area on an evening when her group was scheduled for an off-campus activity particularly valued by children and staff. In spite of warnings in the news media, she loaded the van and started down a long treacherous hill. At one point when the van had slid off the road, she sent a very disturbed child out to evaluate the situation. Finally, after surmounting numerous hazards the group arrived safely at its destination. It was not until months later that this exceptionally well-trained and experienced worker was able to analyze that situation. She had felt almost completely directed by the schedule that called for this particular activity on that particular evening. This well-trained and experienced worker dangerously overestimated her ability to surmount real hazards and seriously misjudged the evaluative capacity and ability of her child-helper. One need only reflect for a moment on such considerations as safety for the young, disturbed children, suicide supervision, and confronting violent youth to be struck by the dangers for both child and worker that can result from misjudgment.

Trust in one's colleagues and reliance on their skills, goodwill, and ability to help evaluate one's work are perceived by child and youth care workers as a major source of support, and the loss of trust in other members of the working team and the assumption of a self-sufficient attitude often result from overestimation. "If I want it done right I'll have to do it myself," or "If only Johnny had been assigned to me, all that trouble wouldn't have happened." Such thinking further isolates the burning-out person from the support of colleagues requiring the exhausted worker to expend even more energy.

It is not unusual for several members of a work group to burn out simultaneously. The staff support system begins to deteriorate, and group collusion becomes a predominant feature of staff relationships. Staff meetings may become brief or are cancelled frequently for superficial reasons. Meetings that are held may be stereotypical and repetitive. Participants frequently express the feeling of having attended the same meeting before, perhaps even many times. On occasion staff and committee meetings may become preoccupied with numerous details and become very long yet unproductive. Worker interactions, both professional and social, are marked by urgent, compulsive, repetitive displays of feeling. Stories comparing hazards, noble feats in the face of danger, and bizarre or amusing client behaviour are told incessantly.

Short-term tension reduction and a personal sense of relief may result. All of these interchanges are characterized by an inattentive attitude in which participants do not focus on client concerns or listen effectively to one another. Collusive relationships become dangerous when they substitute for genuine concern for colleagues.

Excessive stress is also likely to be manifested in physical symptoms. With almost startling regularity health problems begin or intensify during the burning-out process. No particular health problems have been identified as closely associated with the burnout process in child and youth care workers, probably because of their young average age. Workers are most often just aware of an increase in illness and medical contacts. Sometimes the problems are difficult to diagnose and seldom is there opportunity for discussion about the relationship between job stress and health difficulties. An increase in accidents and injuries has also been speculated as well as an increase in the use of escape routes such as food, tobacco, alcohol, and other mood altering or tranquilizing drugs (Freudenberger, 1977; Maslach, 1976).

STRESS RESISTANCE AND RECOVERY

The caring commitment makes many demands upon the energy and resources of group care workers. It is generally thought that many effective workers feel driven from the field in a state of exhaustion and confusion. Others become the exhausted, cynical, and apathetic walking wounded. An increase in workers' capacities for stress resistance and recovery can preserve their freedom to sustain a caring commitment and/or to follow the directions of their personal development. Each person can imagine a special setting and wish to be magically transported. The proverbial South Sea island with its white sand, gentle winds, and waving palms presents an idyllic relaxed image. But effective stress management depends rather on a thoughtful and disciplined process. With careful attention, individual workers, professional groups, and agencies can develop practical and helpful plans.

An articulated level of personal awareness is essential for all interpersonal helping work (Freudenberger, 1977). Reflection can begin with a consideration of personal motives and needs in relation to caring work. Why am I doing this? What do I need from the work? What are my rewards? Vague notions and traditional clichés such as "I like children" or "I just enjoy helping" do not constitute the results of a serious reflection. It is sometimes useful to think about particular clients and situations that have been especially rewarding or unpleasant. A meticulous detailed description will highlight important dimensions which affect the worker's practice.

It is also helpful to identify and perhaps even to describe in writing areas of particular competence. It may be that there is only limited external help available for this process in that supervisors and co-workers might not be sufficiently skilled in group care work to highlight competence. Even the professional literature is limited and often not widely known. Lack of clarity or misunderstanding about areas of personal competence serve to deprive workers of substantial and realistic experiences wherein self-esteem and professional effectiveness can be rewarded.

The structure and quality of personal life is a major factor in the ability to manage stress effectively. Patterns once useful may become detrimental as personal circumstances change. Some unproductive habits were probably established by accident. Group care workers are frequently tempted into junk food meals and irregular eating. The ever-present coffee pot, cups of tea, or availability of soft drinks are invitations to excessive caffeine consumption. Appropriate amounts of sleep and general health care are also important but often neglected. Nutrition and sleep habits may require additional attention when live-in schedules, rotating shifts, and split shifts result in disrupted patterns of daily living.

Rewarding personal activities need to be identified and planned. The determination of group care workers to participate in professional training often intensifies this problem. During any serious professional training period the demands are such that personal interests are frequently set aside in order to fulfill training requirements. Also the excitement engendered in a beginning period of work can preoccupy young practitioners. Thus during an intense period of training, professional activity, and enthusiastic work involvement, a worker's participation in rewarding personal activities may become severely limited. In seeking to restore a balance between personal and professional activity, previous interests should be considered as well as explorations of new directions resulting from personal growth and maturation. Traditional hobbies are, of course, possibilities but developing new career interests or writing a book might also be refreshing. The possibilities are limited only by the scope of imagination.

It is a common experience for workers to be preoccupied with work-related thinking and feelings and to feel continuing tension long after leaving the work site. Effective transition allows the worker to put aside job concerns and to engage more fully in personal life (Maslach, 1976). The process of worker transition receives little attention and, perhaps, is assumed mistakenly to occur automatically. Each person can identify a desired style of transition but must recognize that the same procedure may not always be effective. Child and youth care workers have shared the following transitional measures: settling the concerns of the day by talking about them, a rigorous closure on work which avoids any discussion of it, changing clothes, physical exercise, shopping, listening to music, playing a musical instrument, blocking work-related thinking by engaging in cognitive activities not related to work or having a social drink.

The transition process is especially difficult for persons who end the work period at odd times such as early morning or late at night and those with rotating shift schedules (Kroes, 1977). Only by developing and maintaining effective patterns of transition can the benefits of personal life make a full contribution to stress management in the child and youth care field. And the importance of such transitions cannot be emphasized enough.

Group care workers frequently feel exhausted by the end of their work period. It is difficult to muster the necessary energy and enthusiasm for exercise. Thirty minutes of vigorous exercise three times a week is commonly suggested. Resistance to regular physical activity can sometimes be seen in unrealistic planning and the expectation that it will be enjoyable. Particularly at the beginning there will be no perfect day and it will not feel right. Many workers find that after the exercise habit is instituted, it becomes positively enjoyable and a highly valued period in the personal schedule. In addition it is helpful to develop personally compatible and practical relaxation techniques that can be used when needed, including formal meditation techniques, prayer, and other religious exercises, solitude, listening to music, and soaking in the tub.

Vacation or holiday time, now almost universally available to child and youth care workers, is an important asset to be used in behalf of personal restoration and growth. Much has been written about the difficulties many persons have in using holiday time effectively. Again personal reflection and understanding are important. Some persons prefer short vacations to longer ones. Some prefer high levels of planned recreational activity while others prefer a restful, more spontaneous pace. Effort should be directed towards understanding personal style and needs and then to coordinate these with family and friends.

As discussed earlier, rigid and inflexible attitudes, stereotypical thinking, perceptual rigidity, and diminished creativity are part of the stressful experience. Exercises and activities that employ imaginative thought will aid cognitive and perceptual flexibility. In this regard benefits offered by the arts–drama, music, and painting–are well known. Small personal exercises can also be developed. For example, imagine that you can fly. What would it feel like? Cold? Hot? Windy? Would you fly on a carpet, in a personal carrier, or like Superman? Where would you go? Or imagine you have just become a millionaire. Each person can, no doubt, create various exercises of personal interest. It has also been suggested that participation in a pre-constructed fantasy in which the participant is successful may be useful at stressful points during the work day. Standke (1979) presented the example of thinking about climbing a difficult hill during which obstacles must be overcome. Perhaps future workers will take fantasy breaks by withdrawing briefly to a quiet, comfortable area to develop a scene in imagination. This technique, while requiring further investigation, has the advantage of being usable in close proximity to the daily realities of occupational stress.

In addition, imaginative exercises can be used by personal or professional groups and agencies to facilitate the creative exploration of problems and solutions. One such exercise suggests that participants have unlimited resources and can redesign their current agency or plan a new one. Participants are encouraged to share ideas as they occur without evaluating their practicality. Some notions are refreshingly fantastic: close the agency and buy everybody a family, fund research in self-esteem transplants, buy a politician, send the difficult kids to the moon, buy an airplane and have seasonal programs in different parts of the world. This exercise (Kroes, 1977) helps to free participants from their everyday concerns. Embedded among the absurd suggestions are usually some creative ideas that can be used as a basis for a second stage of discussion that addresses the issues in a more realistic fashion.

Support from family, friends, colleagues, the profession, agency, and community are important contributions to workers' caring commitment. Since there are such widespread misconceptions of group care work, extra effort is required to give family and friends a more accurate understanding. Perhaps a visit to the agency or a planned discussion will allow them to respond more effectively. A spirit of trust and generosity can develop in collegial relations. Group care workers should be available to associates with an attitude of willingness, confidentiality, and concern. Even though professional workers are clinically trained listeners, professional work practices are not always used with colleagues. Each worker has the right–as well as the need–to turn to colleagues and expect to be respectfully heard.

Co-workers should be assisted in taking earned compensatory time, sick time, vacations, and other benefits without being made to feel guilty for abandoning clients and fellow workers. To be sure, inappropriate and unreliable workers appear in agencies from time to time.

Such persons require supervisory attention but should not be permitted to create a distrustful atmosphere. Off-duty time should be fiercely guarded. All workers are responsible for the protection of off-duty colleagues and should expect the same consideration in return. Participation in a professional association can also provide the opportunity to develop support between colleagues, keep up with new ideas, and create and sustain a professional identity while also influencing agency and community perceptions of group care workers.

A well-managed agency contributes to stress reduction (Ayres, 1977). Job descriptions should exist for all positions. Personnel policies, including such items as benefits, grievance procedures, and general agency procedures, should be available. In the past many agencies were quite lax about these. Pressure from funding agencies and a general concern with accountability have resulted in most agencies having such documents available. However, availability is only the first step. These documents need to be reviewed for their reality and implementation. Do job descriptions provide accurate guidelines so that agency and workers share a common and appropriate view of workers' duties? Can compensation time really be taken by the worker who has earned it? Can sick time be used when needed? Can vacations be planned in advance with a consideration of the needs of both clients and workers? Or are the specifications of these items mere papers written to satisfy regulating bodies but with little relationship to the realities of work?

Appropriate task-related policies and procedures also facilitate stress-management by freeing the worker from unimportant or inefficient decision-making and coordinating complex agency enterprises. Creative energy is then available for matters which require it. Policies and procedures should be reviewed in this light and revised or eliminated if they are not facilitating. Workers frequently feel that direct care of clients as well as their information and insights are not valued by the agency. Participation in those aspects of agency and client planning that are relevant to direct care work can provide for an appreciation of the complex caring system, a sense that caring work is taken seriously, and give the agency the benefit of the workers' knowledge and creativity.

Scheduling is another issue that is critical for agencies while also having a major impact on the personal life of workers. Group care, particularly for residential clients, presents the difficult problem of planning for continuous attention to client needs. Work patterns seem, all too often, to be determined by administrative convenience and a wish not to be accused of unfairness. Resulting patterns are frequently unrelated to the needs of the clients or the care workers. For example, excessively long periods of on-duty time, such as ten days on and five days off, may be scheduled. In such cases, the worker may spend most of the off-duty period simply recovering from exhaustion and restoring personal relationships. Another destructive pattern, particularly when the duty extends over twenty-four hours, is four days on-duty and four days of off-duty. This does not allow for any consistency of specific days of the week off-duty. Thus the worker is effectively excluded from almost all organized activities such as classes, choirs, and sports groups that meet on regular days of the week. The rotating shift may also create additional problems of disrupted personal schedules and physiology.

Scheduling needs to provide for a brief withdrawal from especially stressful situations. Time involved in direct client contact is related to the worker's level of stress (Maslach, 1976). Variation in work diminishes the impact of client contact and, if well planned, such variation can add novelty and challenge for the worker. For example, direct care work might be combined with planning in-service training, ordering supplies, or participating in other administrative or case management duties. Discussions of scheduling in group care work to date have been simplistic and little has been done with flexitime, compressed time, and job sharing which have been successfully enacted in other areas of employment, including those responsible for continuous client care (Cohen & Gadon, 1978). Creative experimentation is badly needed.

Appropriate supervision provides an assessment of work including recognition of strengths, identification of weaknesses with assistance for their correction, and a supportive forum for expressing and dealing with the intense feelings that arise in group care work. It requires a supervisor who is clinically skilled in group care work and who has a balanced sensitivity for the client, the worker, and the agency. Regular effective supervision, encompassing all these factors, is rarely available on a regular basis. The supervisory process must often be initiated by the worker (Mattingly, 1977b; Nelson, 1978). The availability of supervision is also influenced by budget constraints. Workers, professional groups, and agencies all have potential influence in assuring that effective supervision is readily available to increasing numbers of group care workers.

Professional group care workers should also be engaged in a continuing effort to identify both new directions and unsatisfactory aspects of their practice. The inadequate preparation of some workers, changes in client population, or alterations in services delivered will also result in the discovery of areas requiring training. For example, the reception of increasing numbers of aggressive clients may require the acquisition of appropriate management skills. Provision of services to adolescent parents may motivate the traditional youth worker to acquire information about parenting and early childhood. Unfortunately, much reflection and supervision may only serve to identify vague problematic areas yet fail to clearly specify learning needs so that appropriate information and training can be sought.

It is important to recognize that philosophical, ethical, legal, and theoretical information are also essential to effective group care practice. Such information should be kept in mind when formulating study plans. Workers and agencies can then develop specific study plans. Individual workers frequently have professional study plans that are independent from the agency. This allows the plan to be tailored to personal style and interest as well as to focus on skills and knowledge relevant to future career plans.

An effective study plan must be realistic in terms of the time and energy available. It needs to be concrete, embody the principles of effective educational design (VanderVen & Mattingly, 1979), and have a timetable including a termination point. This allows participants to experience the pleasure of completion and accomplishment. Some suggested formats include readings, asking a skilled or knowledgeable worker to teach others, a small study group, an agency in-service program, as well as programs offered by professional associations and educational institutions.

Group care worker associations can encourage training programs to include a range of clinical and indirect skills that will allow for reasonable flexibility in choosing the type of client and setting for work. In addition, professional associations can provide a forum for the discussion of occupational stress and encourage its inclusion in induction and in-service training. This will provide workers with an understanding of the stressful conditions they are likely to encounter and increase their ability to cope effectively (McLean, 1974).

CONCLUSION

Group child and youth care workers, along with many other human service personnel, have made substantial progress in exploring the stressful nature of their work. The topic appears with increasing regularity in in-service training and the programs of professional associations. Agencies are sometimes willing to engage in self-review and to promote appropriate discussion. Individual workers can engage in effective personal planning. Thus both workers and agencies can move beyond the isolation, confusion, pain, and helplessness that have all too frequently characterized the process of burning out.

The somewhat dramatic images called forth by the term "burnout" can, however, contribute to its use as a vague term for dissatisfaction or frustration. The systematic study of occupational stress for caregivers has only just begun. The experience has not yet been fully described. The situations that care givers find distressing have not been adequately identified. Only a little is known about the conditions which aggravate or assuage the process. Coping strategies amongst effective long-term workers, supervisors, and administrators have yet to be studied. Further specification of the stress and burnout process will allow workers and agencies to plan more precisely. The result, hopefully, will be an increase in workers' effectiveness and satisfaction with substantial benefits accruing for children, young people and their families.

NOTE

1. Combat neurosis was a term that emerged following World War II referring to the pattern of physiological and psychological symptoms that were identified in military casualties as resulting from exposure to the severe environmental pressures of combat. The earlier term, "shell-shock," was used following World War I (Babington, 1997). "Post-traumatic shock disorder" is now the commonly used term for such conditions but the condition is not limited to military experiences (Schiraldi, 2000). Instead, PTSD may be diagnosed with respect to a variety of traumatic shock experiences and the longer term impact these might have on personal well-being and behaviour.

REFERENCES

American Psychological Association. (2002). Ethical principles of psychologists and code of conduct. *American Psychologist, 57,* 1060-1073.

Ayres, P. R. (1977). *Staff stress in day care: The director's role.* Unpublished Master's thesis, University of Pittsburgh.

Babington, A. (1997). *Shell-shock: A history of the changing attitudes towards war neurosis.* Barnsley, South Yorkshire, England: Pen & Sword.

Bloch, A. (1978). Combat neurosis in inner-city schools. *American Journal of Psychiatry, 135*(10), 1189-1192.

Cohen, A. R., & Gadon, H. (1978). *Alternative work schedules: Integrating individual and organizational needs.* Reading, MA: Addison-Wesley.

Freudenberger, H. J. (1975). The staff burnout syndrome in alternative institutions. *Psychotherapy: Theory, Research and Practice, 12*(I), 73-82.

Freudenberger, H. J. (1977). Burnout: Occupational hazard of the child care worker. *Child Care Quarterly, 6*(2), 90-99.

Grossbard, H. (1960). *Cottage parents: What they have to be, know, and do.* New York: Child Welfare League of America.

Hall, R. C. W., Gardner, E. R., Peri, M., Stickney, S. K., & Pfefferbaum, B. (1979). The professional burnout syndrome. *Psychiatric Opinion, 16*(4), 12-17.

Hewitt, L. H. (1979). *Work characteristics, quality of supervision and job stress in child care.* Unpublished Master's thesis. University of Pittsburgh.

International Leadership Coalition (1995). Code of ethics: Standards for practice of North American child and youth care professionals. *Child and Youth Care Forum, 24*(6), 371-378. Retrieved January 17, 2005, from www.acycp.org.

Kroes, W. H. (1977). *Society's victim–the policeman.* Springfield, IL: Charles C. Thomas.

Mann-Feder, V., & Savicki, V. (2003). Burnout in Anglophone and Francophone child and youth workers in Canada: A cross-cultural comparison. *Child & Youth Care Forum, 32*(6), 337-354.

Maslach, C. (1976, September). Burned-out. *Human Behavior, 5,* 16-22.

Maslach, C. (2003). *Burnout: The cost of caring.* Los Altos, CA: Institute for the Study of Human Knowledge.

Maslach, C., & Jackson, S. (1979). Burned-out cops and their families. *Psychology Today, 12*(12), 58-62.

Maslach, C., & Pines, A. (1977) The burnout syndrome in the day care setting. *Child Care Quarterly, 6*(2), 100-113.

Maslach, C., Jackson, S. E., & Leiter, M. P. (1996). *The Maslach burnout inventory (3rd ed.).* Palo Alto, CA: Consulting Psychologists Press.

Maslach, C., & Schaufeli, W. B. (1993). Historical and conceptual development of burnout. In W. B. Schaufeli, C. Maslach, & T. Marek, (Eds.), *Professional burnout: Recent developments in theory and research* (pp. 1-16). Washington, DC: Taylor & Francis.

Mattingly, M. A. (Ed.). (1977a). Symposium: Stress and burnout: [Special issue]. *Child Care Quarterly, 6*(2), 88-137.

Mattingly, M. A. (1977b). Sources of stress and burnout in professional child care work. *Child Care Quarterly, 6*(2), 127-137.

Mattingly, M. A. (1979). Stress in work with children. *Children in Contemporary Society, 12*(2), 21-24.

Mattingly, M. (1981). Occupational stress for group care personnel. In F. Ainsworth & L. C. Fulcher (Eds.), *Group care for children* (pp. 151-169). London: Tavistock.

Mattingly, M. A., & Thomas, D. (2003). The promise of professionalism arrives in practice: Progress on the North American certification project. *Journal of Child & Youth Care, 19,* 209-215.

Mattingly, M. A., & VanderVen, K. D. (1979). Meeting the treatment needs of children through educational preparation of child care practitioners. *Proceedings of the Fifth Annual Inter-Association Child Care Conference.* Valley Forge, PA.

McLean, A. (1974). Concepts of occupational stress. In A. McLean (Ed.), *Occupational stress.* Springfield, IL: Charles C. Thomas.

Nelson, J. E. (1978). Child care crises and the role of the supervisor. *Child Care Quarterly, 7*(4), 318-326.

Olden, C. (1953). On adult empathy with children. *Psychoanalytic Study of the Child, 8,* 111-126.

Pines, A., & Kafry, D. (1978). Occupational tedium in social services. *Social Work, 23*(6), 499-508.

Pines, A., & Maslach, C. (1978). Characteristics of staff burnout in mental health settings. *Hospital and Community Psychiatry, 29*(4), 233-237.

Pritzker, NJ Children's Hospital and Center. (1974). *The new child care worker: An agent in delivery of human services: The future professional.* Presentation at the 1974 American Orthopsychiatric Association Annual Meeting, Chicago: Author.

Reed, M. J. (1977). Stress in live-in child care. *Child Care Quarterly, 6*(2), 114-120.

Savicki, V. (1993). Clarification of child and youth care identity through an analysis of work environment and burnout. *Child and Youth Care Forum, 22,* 441-457.

Savicki, V. (1999). Cultural work values for supervisors and managers: A cross-cultural look at child and youth care agencies. *Child and Youth Care Forum, 28,* 239-255.

Savicki, V. (2001). A configurational analysis of burnout in child and youth care workers in thirteen countries. *Journal of Child &Youth Care Work, 15/16,* 185-206.

Savicki, V. (2002). *Burnout across thirteen cultures: Work, stress, and coping in child and youth care workers.* Westport, CT: Praeger.

Savicki, V., & Cooley, E. J. (1987). The relationship of work environment and client contact to burnout in mental health professionals. *Journal of Counseling & Development, 1,* 249-252.

Savicki, V., & Riolli-Saltzman, L. (2001). *Optimism and coping: Moderation of situational factors in burnout.* Poster Presented at Western Psychological Association Conference, Lahaina, Maui, HI, May 2001.

Schiraldi, G. R. (2000). *The post-traumatic stress disorder sourcebook: A guide to healing, recovery, and growth.* Lincolnwood, IL: Lowell House.

Seiderman, S. (1978). Combating staff burnout: Day care and early education, *Summer,* 6-9.

Shamsie, J., & Lang, G. (1976). Staff attitudes and management styles in psychiatric hospitals. *Canadian Psychiatric Association Journal, 21,* 325-328.

Shubin, S. (1978) Burnout: The professional hazard you face in nursing. *Nursing, 8*(7), 22-27.

Standke, L. (1979, February). The advantages of training people to handle stress. *Training/HRD,* 23-26.

Thomas, D. (2002). The North American certification project in historical perspective. *Journal of Child & Youth Care Work, 17,* 7-15.

VanderVen, K. D. (1979). Developmental characteristics of child care workers and design of training programs. *Child Care Quarterly, 8*(2), 100-112.

White, W. L. (1978). *Incest in the organizational family: The unspoken issue in staff and program burnout.* Unpublished paper presented at the 1978 National Drug Abuse Conference, Seattle, WA.

Yager, J., & Hubert, D. (1979). Stress and coping in psychiatric residents. *Psychiatric Opinion, 16*(4), 21-24.

Chapter 10

Patterns of Career Development in Child and Youth Care

Karen D. VanderVen

SUMMARY. Patterns of career development in the field of child and youth care are reexamined in relation to roles that involve working directly with children in specific settings as well as in relation to roles that involve working indirectly in support of children through working with other adults, be these parents, other caregivers or professionals. Other career roles involve working in support of human service systems that impact on the care of children and young people and influence family welfare. Finally, some career roles involve working at the macro level to formulate policies that shape the culture of caring communities to support the health and well-being of children. Each career role presents important challenges and offers valuable opportunities for influencing the lives of children, young people and their families. *[Article copies available for a fee from The Haworth Document Delivery Service: 1-800-HAWORTH. E-mail address: <docdelivery@haworthpress.com> Website: <http://www. HaworthPress.com> © 2006 by The Haworth Press, Inc. All rights reserved.]*

KEYWORDS. Group care, residential care, residential treatment, group homes, youth work, youthwork, group work, at-risk youth, career development, practitioner, professionalization

Address correspondence to: Karen D. VanderVen, Psychology in Education, WWPH 5940, University of Pittsburgh, Pittsburgh, PA 15260.

[Haworth co-indexing entry note]: "Patterns of Career Development in Child and Youth Care." Vander-Ven, Karen D. Co-published simultaneously in *Child & Youth Services* (The Haworth Press, Inc.) Vol. 28. No. 1/2, 2006, pp. 231-257; and: *Group Care Practice with Children and Young People Revisited* (ed: Leon C. Fulcher, and Frank Ainsworth) The Haworth Press, Inc., 2006, pp. 231-257. Single or multiple copies of this article are available for a fee from The Haworth Document Delivery Service [1-800-HAWORTH, 9:00 a.m. - 5:00 p.m. (EST). E-mail address: docdelivery@haworthpress.com].

doi:10.1300/J024v28n01_04

REFLECTIONS ON CAREER DEVELOPMENT
AFTER TWO DECADES

On re-reading "Patterns of Career Development in Group Care," much if not most of this material still rings true. It offers a framework for viewing what functions are needed in the field and how worker's experience and personal growth enable them to grow into particular work roles and to "cover" them, so to speak, for what those work roles require. Yet the world is different than it was then, and so it's a good idea to look at what changes have taken place and implications these pose for career development in the future. Three new themes are worth highlighting: shifts in the nature of the work, complexity of the work tasks and career longevity.

Changes in the Nature of the Work

The earlier chapter (VanderVen, 1981) begins with the phrase, "group care of children," implying that this is an established occupation. The article states that group care is a "mainstay of children's services," although it will be "subject to change under the impact of altering societal influences" (p. 201). Indeed, much has changed in how the work is conceptualized. First of all, there has been a loosening of the boundaries in what people think constitutes group care. No longer are residential programs considered the primary employers of group care workers. They may work in a variety of venues including streetwork, home care, day care, and treatment settings. Nor are children and young people necessarily the primary clients. Clients may be young pre-school age children, young adults, adults and, increasingly, older adults. The increased flexibility in practice sites and populations gives a great deal more career mobility to practitioners.

Not only can they move vertically through the different indirect roles such as supervision, administration, consultation, and training, but they can also move horizontally to work with different age or client groups and settings. It is still important to focus on the unique nature of the work we do and its identified competencies rather than where and specifically with whom the work is done.

Complexity

Subsequent to the publication of this chapter there has been a major paradigm shift in the worldview of those who study human development, social sciences, and human services. From following the rational-empiricist tradition of using scientific methods to look for predictability, sequential cause and effect, and knowledge without a specific context, it is now recognized that the reality of the world is far more chaotic and complex, filled with unpredictability and a non-sequential relationship between cause and effect. What are the implications for career development of such a new worldview?

For those involved in professional preparation, this means that there are new perspectives as to what constitutes a profession and new opportunities for us to pioneer a transformed concept of profession that is more contextual, individual, and flexible than the traditional sociological model. It also means that career patterns within the field are now and will be less linear and prescribed than in previous years. Rather than perform one job function and, possibly, progress on or up to another, one might follow a "blended" career path in which several functions might be performed simultaneously. However, the group care field still needs a career pathway that allows practitioners to grow into performing functions of greater complexity and responsibility while still remaining in *direct* contact with children and young people. In the Bronfenbrenner schema, these practitioners might still be working with children in the micro-system but would hold advanced and highly responsible roles requiring both experience and advanced professional preparation. They would handle the most difficult and complex children and young people, serve as practice consultants and resources to others, and perhaps have specialties such as in-depth skill at understanding and working with a particular problem or issue.

Longevity

There is increased longevity in domains that affect career patterns. First of all, many people are living longer, and it follows that retirement patterns, along with career patterns, are changing. What does that imply? First of all, practitioners in child and youth care work require new guidelines for shaping and planning a lifetime career. Retirement no longer means moving to the tropics. It can mean leaving one job to recreate a new, possibly related occupation. Because it appears that many people are choosing to remain employed longer, then one needs to consider career options that can utilize their wisdom and their particular assets. Perhaps in the future we will see people retired from administrative or full-time practice positions into private practices, consulting practices, entrepreneurial activities, or developing new kinds of volunteer programs.

The other aspect of longevity relevant to career development in this field is the increased need for child and youth care work to define itself by the unique services it can provide rather than by age group and to work towards serving the growing cadre of people who are working and living longer but still eventually find their way into group care facilities such as nursing homes, intermediate care programs, assisted living, and the like.

I have often said that the core of "child and youth care work" models the most needed human service of the future because of its focus on the life space, use of relationships and activity, and its fluid boundaries that can resonate with a rapidly changing world. Time will tell how those who create and develop their careers might further advance the significance of this work in the future.

INTRODUCTION TO THE ORIGINAL 1981 PUBLICATION

The significance of group care of children as a mode of service provision is highlighted by Bronfenbrenner (1979) who stated, "Besides home, the only setting that serves as a comprehensive context for human development is the children's institution" (p. 172). On the premise that group care is not only a mainstay of children's services, particularly in its newer community context, but also that it will be subject to change under the impact of altering societal influences, it is then crucial to consider the preparation and maintenance of group care practitioners capable of responding to the demand for group care services in years to come. This chapter describes a conceptual formulation for defining skills and attributes required at various levels of group care work based on a review of human services trends.

CHILD ECOLOGY AND OTHER TRENDS IN THE DELIVERY OF GROUP CARE SERVICES

Perhaps one of the most important theoretical advances in the field of child development has been the recognition that to have a significant impact on children's development requires a comprehensive ecological approach that influences all of the environmental systems that impinge on children. The ecology of group care and its relevance to practice is illustrated by several examples. In the area of residential treatment, historical precedents were set by the early child guidance movement in which individual therapy with identified children was considered the primary mode of treatment. Applied to the residential setting this meant providing a custodial or at best hygienic environment for children while they awaited their treatment sessions.

In the last several decades, this orientation has changed as is well documented by Davids (1975). Today, multiple influences such as increased professionalism in the child care field (Beker, 1979) and developments in the concept of the therapeutic milieu, have contributed to the emergence of group care workers as the key personnel with potential to affect the total milieu of children in care. This meant that "the other 23 hours" (Trieschman, Whittaker, & Brendtro, 1969) and not simply the clinical hour became the core of a child's treatment.

Another example was provided by group care programs for young children such as Head Start. These were designed as early intervention services that promoted ongoing and positive development of cognitive, social, and other abilities children need for later school success. Evidence demonstrated that the effectiveness of these programs was related to the degree to which the services targeted not only the children themselves but also their living situations, health status, and economic factors. Such examples all demonstrated that successful promotion of children's development and positive mental health must be aimed at both the child as well as the child's total environment.

The ecological formulation highlighted ways in which the environments where children grow and interact are composed of a *hierarchy of settings ranging from immediate influences to the broadest context of society.* This view articulated by Bronfenbrenner (1977, 1979) argued "that the person's development is profoundly affected by events occurring in settings in which the person is not even present" (1979, p. 3), and Brim (1975) described "macro-influences" or broad reaching societal factors that affect the course of children's development.

Whittaker (1979) was among the increasing number who recognized implications arising from the concept of ecology for designing and implementing children's services. This requires that group care practitioners embrace a concept of group care that transcends its direct delivery in an immediate setting and also that they be educated with the prerequisite skills and attributes necessary to function at different hierarchical levels in the ecological system. Because these qualifications are so varied, it is not possible to inculcate them solely in an initial training effort. Thus, education must be concerned not only with initial preparation but with promoting ongoing personal and professional development that will help ensure that practitioners have the abilities to address the career demands at each level.

A full consideration of the needs for preparing group care practitioners also requires consideration of other trends in human services design and delivery. These include developments in at least five areas. First, work in the areas of children's mental health and positive development increasingly focus on the prevention of disorders as well as on the cure of identified and well-established conditions. Thus, the well-known mental and public health model of primary, secondary, and tertiary prevention has had particular relevance for education of group care practitioners.

Historically, training for group care personnel was directed toward skills primarily oriented towards tertiary prevention. Such skills were aimed at the rehabilitation of disorders that were already present, the aim being to reduce their severity and degree of disability. This function was analogous to that of the direct care worker in a residential context involved with children who have already evidenced the need for therapeutic or rehabilitative approaches. Activity in secondary prevention–attempting to reduce the duration of impairment in cases already identified–and primary prevention–reducing the actual incidence of disabilities–did not traditionally come under direct purview of those directly involved in group care service delivery.

This was, and still is, particularly true of those who have entered this field as direct care workers in specific settings for relatively brief periods but who left it early due to lack of education, stress, limited career opportunities, and other factors that have contributed to a short working life of group care workers. The result has been a weakening of their representation in more responsible and influential roles beyond the direct care level. If the provision of group care services for children is to develop an orientation to primary prevention, then at least *some* practitioners must be qualified to work with the broader social system. This development is important since the broader social system has a strong indirect influence on patterns of service response. Even those who have criticized the concept of primary prevention have noted how certain children's programs with a group focus have served an effective primary prevention function, such as carefully designed settings for homeless infants (Lamb & Zusman, 1979).

Closely allied with the concept of primary prevention was a second trend in service design and delivery: encouraging positive development, even in children with identified disabilities. This involves providing a constructive and educative environment, not just directing efforts at rehabilitation of a psychiatrically diagnosed syndrome. It has also formed the basis for effective tertiary prevention (remediation) as applied to group care of children. Hobbs' concept of Re-Ed (1974) that Whittaker (1979) described as "having the most direct and immediate bearing on the development of community-based group care settings for troubled children" (p. 72), was an educative approach emphasizing "competence across the total spectrum of the child's development" (Whittaker, 1979, p. 71).

Hobbs named particular biases as characteristic of this approach, including biases towards learning, towards growth and social systems intervention, and away from dynamic psychology and formal psychiatric diagnosis. The philosophic underpinnings of the Re-Ed approach and similar approaches posed great implications for group care delivery. They suggested a crucial teaching and development function for group care practitioners to fulfil. This is not to say that workers would not require understanding of children's psychodynamics but that professional skills aimed at social competencies and re-education for children in social and cognitive abilities are particularly important for the new roles in which practitioners will be expected to work.

A third trend that influenced service design and delivery was the growing recognition that perspectives on children and their needs espoused by particular disciplines or associated with diagnostic labels have prevented effective service design and delivery (Arthur & Birnbaum, 1968; Hobbs, 1974; Schopler & Reichler, 1976; Vinter, 1973). This trend led to the development of generic perspectives. Hobbs documented the deleterious effects on children of specific diagnostic labels that do not actually "fit" a child's characteristics and capabilities, that may stigmatize them, and that may result in an extremely poor balance between a child's needs and the services they actually receive. Similarly, working with children through the sole perspective of one discipline may omit significant variables and influences in their lives. Because some factors may not fall within the scope of a particular discipline, insufficient account is taken of these in designing interventions and inadequate service responses.

Thus, effective work with children must rely on educational preparation of practitioners that develops and maintains a broad knowledge base and a systems perspective so that the restrictions imposed by narrow visions can be ameliorated. Because such a mature mode of functioning is rarely characteristic of beginning workers, it is necessary for career mobility in the field to offer opportunities that retain practitioners in the mainstream of group care work while they develop professional maturity through continuing education and experience. If the group care worker increasingly functions as the coordinator and integrator for a child's total life experience in the milieu (Barnes & Kelman, 1974) then such workers are the ideal professionals in whom to encourage the development of a broad, encompassing perspective.

The social upheavals of the 1960s helped to shape a fourth trend that influenced the balance of decision making in the human services. Previously policy and treatment decisions were made solely by professionals, with clients as passive recipients. In line with the wider consumer movement, clients became increasingly involved as participants in decisions and actions that affected their lives. This shift in service delivery posed several important implications for group care.

The first concerned the role of parents. Prior to the advance of participatory models, parents were considered to be the primary cause of their children's problems. As a result, there was little professional empathy with the parents of a child needing special help. Therefore, parents were not involved as collaborators in the treatment process. However, parent involvement, a cornerstone of programs such as Head Start, has become a much more central part of group care programs for older and/or exceptional populations (VanderVen & Griff, 1978).

Such parent activities include participation in administrative planning and decision making, sharing in the design and delivery of specific services, and in the securing of resources for programs. Parents have become actual partners in the implementation of treatment plans and direct service activity. Professional work with parents has included training them in specific skills (Conte, 1978) beyond those used by helping professionals, relying less on the amelioration of pathology.

Children, too, in keeping with the child advocacy movement, now participate more directly in decisions concerning the services they receive and the quality of such services. Advances in this area were described by Goldsmith (1976) including, for example, children joining in treatment planning conferences, commenting on behaviour records, and participating in other activities previously considered sacrosanct to professionals, particularly with child clients. The growing significance of this concept of client participation was articulated by Fischer and Brodsky (1978) as the Prometheus Principle. This referred to informed participation that allies human service consumers alongside their course of treatment in reviewing and responding to information collected about them and the decisions and actions that are predicated on such information.

The movement toward increased client involvement posed important implications for professional development of group care practitioners. Test scores, diagnoses, and traits were reduced in their importance as daily life events became the central focus of activity and collaboration with clients (Fischer & Brodsky, 1978). The education and development of group care workers has had to prepare them to function in such collaborative roles, and the skills that group care workers already had in milieu work made them particularly suited to such developments.

No discussion of significant trends in group care would be complete without consideration of the growing pressures for demonstrating accountability or the degree to which programs have been expected to achieve the outcomes for which they have been funded (Whittaker, 1979). Accountability required new attitudes and skills amongst group care practitioners, even at the direct care level. Cost-effectiveness and evaluation were not concerns that were readily congruent with the general orientation of human services workers. Initiatives aimed at demonstrating accountability in group care services involved the application of managerial concepts such as goal and objective setting, care and treatment planning, team organization, budgeting, and resource allocation to the conduct of the program. Goal-oriented activity focused on helping children meet specific objectives became increasingly the norm of practice regardless of whether direct care workers participated in setting the objectives that now guided their activities.

The attitudes and skills involved in goal and objective setting had not been traditionally taught or inculcated in group care workers. This was also true in other human service professions such as social work (Patti & Austin, 1977) and psychiatry (Klerman & Levinson, 1969). One reason for the lack of attention to such material in human service training was the clash that many clinically oriented or humanistically inclined professionals felt towards anything that smacked of business management or even financial matters. Thus, the ability to respond to requirements for accountability required a tremendous shift in orientations to professional practice and modes of functioning.

ATTRIBUTES AND SKILLS REQUIRED OF GROUP CARE PRACTITIONERS

The preceding discussion of trends in human service provision since the 1970s, with its prime focus on an ecological framework, has identified areas in which group care practitioners require appropriate attributes and skills in order to have a far reaching and lasting impact on the lives of children with whom they work. The following section builds on Bronfenbrenner's description of hierarchical levels in a total ecological system, highlighting the need for group care practitioners at *each* level if truly effective care is to be assured. The requirement is for persons with prerequisite skills and attributes who can operate within the various ecological levels, recognizing that differences do exist from level to level.

Level 1: The Microsystem–Direct Work with Children

The microsystem refers to the immediate environment containing a child "and the complex of relations between the developing person" (Bronfenbrenner, 1977, p. 517). Elements of the microsystem include physical features of the setting, role relationships among persons immediately involved in the setting, and activities conducted in that setting. The microsystem would include home and school classrooms (Bronfenbrenner, 1977, 1979) while in an extended group care context they would include settings such as the day care centre, the residential treatment centre, or the hospital. To be effective, practitioners at this level need to be highly prepared in direct caregiving skills that are designed to make children feel special and nurtured (Maier, 1977, 1978).

Some components of this primary care for children in their immediate settings have been described by Maier (1979) as including the provision of bodily comfort, responding to each child's unique individuality, ensuring predictability and dependability, and giving personalized behaviour training. In addition, such practitioners require skills associated with *environmental design* and *activity programming* so that they can use equipment, playthings, developmental media, and other elements in their settings to help children develop a sense of competence and social skills. Such workers also require an awareness of their own *professional identity* as group care workers as well as knowledge about the roles and functions of other adults with whom they work collaboratively in the children's settings. Knowledge of the structure and dynamics of *teamwork* is also important for microsystem workers in view of the significance that all relationships have within the microsystem.

These areas of skill are related to current trends in human service delivery. Workers employed in settings such as infant and pre-school day care are performing a *primary prevention* function for these children through the positive nurturing they offer in a facilitating physical environment. Workers in settings dealing with children with special needs in residential treatment centres may employ a primarily *rehabilitative* (tertiary prevention) role. In all modes of microsystem practice, group care workers are closely involved in encouraging *positive development*, as the ideal persons whose skills and resources can facilitate children's developing social competence.

Because these workers may be unfamiliar with practices that encourage client participation, *client participation* skills have become essential for microsystem level group care workers. This may include working conjointly with parents and allowing children to participate actively in making decisions that influence their lives in such settings. Planning skills associated with setting and working towards specific goals and objectives with children are also needed, consistent with trends towards strengthening the roles of group care workers in the microsystem as *coordinators and integrators* of children's total life experiences in care. Practitioners at this level should be encouraged to develop a *generic perspective* to their work so as to gather and synthesize information from various others in the child's life space, and to use this responsively in the group care environment.

Level 2:
The Mesosystem–Indirect Work with Children and Work with Adults

The mesosystem "is comprised of *interrelations* among major settings which contain the developing person at a particular point in his or her life . . . (or) a system of microsystems" (Bronfenbrenner, 1977, p. 515). Such interrelations or linkages exist for children between their homes, schools, recreational facilities, service agencies, and similar institutions. The mesosystem still contains the developing child within its linkage system, even though the interrelations *within* a setting with a hierarchy of role functions were not included in the microsystem. The interrelations and patterns of interaction between the serving adults in the settings are characteristic of the mesosystem.

Skills required for practice in various relationships within the mesosystem are thus radically different from those of the microsystem. Workers are required to move from providing *direct* care to providing *indirect* care or, as Dockar-Drysdale (1973) suggested, working through intermediaries. The practices are *indirect* since the mesosystem worker is primarily involved with facilitating the quality of care delivered by others. The worker may serve as the supervisor or teacher or may have administrative responsibility for services. Care and attention is directed towards the organizational structure and climate she or he creates, knowing how this indirect care exerts an influence on the effectiveness of primary care givers and their work in that setting. The worker's responsibilities for staff development and supervision as well as attention to program design and coordination relate closely to the requirements for accountability. In many respects the modes of working are very similar to those characteristic of workers in the microsystem, the major difference being that work activity is directed towards other adults and, thus, indirectly with children.

The mesosystem worker requires organizational skills that include the ability to gather and synthesize information in the activity of coordination of links within and between specific settings. Communication skills are also required so that the mesosystem worker employs the greatest number of ways of making contact with others, conveying information to the best advantages for children being served. Knowledge of organizational structure is required as is knowledge of the relationships between specific organizational features and the quality of care being delivered. Skills in team building are vital, since group care delivery at the indirect level involves collaboration of members from various disciplines and backgrounds (VanderVen, 1979a).

Team building with other adults is an extension of work in the microsystem where group care workers serve as an integrator of services offered to children by various disciplines. To the extent that teams involve all appropriate workers in the setting, this may be considered an extension of the client participation principle. Similarly, an understanding of work group dynamics is necessary for mesosystem practitioners. Knowledge and skill in education of adults is also essential for the mesosystem worker, paralleling those required of the microsystem worker engaging with children. This includes the ability to assess learner characteristics and design, effectively deliver, and evaluate instruction. The mesosystem worker, too, is concerned with the building up of competence and mastery among those personnel with whom they serve as immediate supervisors or teachers.

The mesosystem worker requires skills in working with parents who are essential collaborators for group care settings that provide services to children. This extends the principle of primary work with other adults. All of these functions require that group care practitioners working in mesosystem roles have the ability to identify and empathize with adults and their concerns, just as the microsystem worker must do with children. As group care workers affect relationships and linkages in the mesosystem through working with other adults, they move more directly towards primary prevention functions. Through encouraging others in their ability to provide quality services, their sphere of influence is extended, thereby influencing wider systems that affect children.

Level 3: The Exosystem–Work with the Human Service System

The exosystem is

an extension of the mesosystem embracing other specific social structures, both formal and informal that do not themselves contain the developing person but impinge upon or encompass the immediate settings in which that person is found, and thereby influence, delimit, or even determine what goes on there. (Bronfenbrenner, 1977, p. 515)

The skills required for practice in the exosystem are logical extensions of those used in the mesosystem. Because the area of concern is a system, the transition process for practitioners moving from one level of practice to another is not as dramatic, although the complexity of the systems may vary. Exosystem workers require skills in *organizational* matters, although now at a managerial level, in terms of carrying out major planning and problem solving functions. Here involvement of the practitioner is in activities that influence the design of entire caring systems such as a network of day care centres or group homes.

Work at this level contrasts with mesosystem roles where a worker normally functions within the organizational structure of one setting or a specific program. Skills required include those of coordination and communication but are applied across a wider service network. Additional skills in financial planning, budgeting, and administration and, perhaps, fundraising are required at the exosystem level.

Political activity is another potential sphere of engagement that comes into the scope of the exosystem worker. For practitioners to influence the exosystem, political skills in negotiation, policy design, lobbying, and debate are crucial. While group care has always been subject to political activities, it has become increasingly politicized over the past quarter century with the formation of social policy and enactment of legislation exerting important influences on child and family life. Defining the exosystem for group care practitioners includes the naming of government agencies as exosystem structures.

Thus, workers in this sphere exert an influence over the pattern of group care services at earlier levels through assuming instrumental roles in agencies that control and shape the nature of child and family life in the country. Such an orientation has not been a traditional one for group care practitioners. Examples of exosystem roles include local and regional politicians, governmental officers concerned with health, education, and welfare planning and, perhaps, researchers or writers on group care practices whose work is widely disseminated. Communication and organizational skills acquired in earlier work are therefore re-applied in wider contexts. The relationships between client participation skills and political action are obvious, as successful workers in a political context involve constituents in a variety of ways. Accountability for practitioners in the exosystem involves the ability to evaluate the successes of broad-reaching programs, information which can then be used as a basis for policy-making and legislative design. The need for generic perspectives in such complex activity is obvious. Those who work within the exosystem have opportunities to influence primary prevention. It is at this level that far-reaching decisions on social and economic policy are made and these reach incisively into the very quality of child and family life.

Level 4: The Macrosystem–Work Within the Culture

The macrosystem

> refers to the overarching institutional patterns of the culture or sub-culture, such as the economic, social, educational, legal and political systems, of which micro- meso- and exo-systems are the concrete manifestations. Macrosystems are conceived and examined not only in structural terms, but as carriers of information and ideology that, both explicitly and implicitly, endow meaning and motivation to particular agencies, social networks, roles, activities, and their interrelations. (Bronfenbrenner 1977, p. 515)

The capacity to influence global attitudes and viewpoints about a culture or subculture is, of course, an achievement that is made by very few individuals. Those in society who do ultimately have such an influence are· usually not those who have followed a career in group care with children. Rather, such people may be entertainers, political figures, writers, industrial leaders, and others who have achieved a national prominence. Dr. Benjamin Spock, author of *Baby and Child Care*, which sold millions of copies over the years, has been cited as a major influence on child care practices and attitudes towards child rearing. As such, Spock might be considered as someone in the field of child care who has had an impact on the macrosystem.

It is not beyond the realm of possibility that others might emerge within the broad field of group care practice whose work will ultimately have similar impact. It is through the emergence of such persons, albeit few at this level, that impact can be made on "the place or priority (which) children and those responsible for their care (receive) in such macrosystems" influencing "how a child and his or her caretakers are treated and interact with each other in different kinds of settings" (Bronfenbrenner, 1977, p. 515).

ENCOURAGING PERSONAL
AND PROFESSIONAL DEVELOPMENT

It is obviously impossible to inculcate in one group care practitioner all of the skills and attributes necessary for practice at the various ecological levels in an initial educational effort. Furthermore, many of the requirements for practice in the wider spheres of influence require a certain perspective and maturity which can be achieved only by special preparation and experiences gained over an extended period of time. Implications are apparent, therefore, for any concerned with extending the professional impact of group care practitioners to be able to ensure longevity in the field for a substantial cadre of its initial (microsystem) practitioners. This may be achieved through providing activities that facilitate an extended process of personal and professional development into new modes and levels of practice.

Advances in developmental theory can be applied to the tasks of promoting personal and professional development of group care practitioners. One of these is the increasing recognition that children, with their particular temperamental and behavioural characteristics, can have an impact on their caregivers (Thomas, Chess, & Birch, 1968; Bell & Harper, 1977) in the same way that the caregivers and their practices have an impact on children. "Actual behavior is a function of a continuous process of multidirectional interaction or feedback between the individual and situations he or she encounters" (Magnussen & Endler, 1977, p. 4). Such an interactive process suggests that any *ongoing* professional development of workers with children should take account of how involvement with child care work is likely to have a transforming impact on their own development as persons and as practitioners.

Another advance in developmental theory that is relevant to group care practitioners concerns the extension of child development concepts into adult development. In this way, the adult, like the child, is involved in an ongoing process of growth and change throughout the life cycle. The life cycle itself can be conceptualized in stages, as proposed in Erikson's (1950) well-known formulations about adult development as well as in the formulations by Levinson et al. (1978). In the field of adult development, the relationship between personal growth and change is integrally linked with professional development. A change in one area impacts on another and the educational process itself is considered to be an influence on personal development. Specific changes related to the ability to practice take place in students during their initial period of professional preparation. Such changes have been documented by studies in professions such as medicine (Zabarenko & Zabarenko, 1978), occupational therapy (Butler, 1972), and nursing (Olesen & Whittaker, 1968).

Entry into professional practice itself constitutes a stage of development as described by Babcock (1964). Ongoing professional activity is marked by transitional periods when practitioners move from one mode of practice to another, as indicated in such articles as "Becoming the Director: Promotion as a Phase in Personal-Professional Development" (Klerman & Levinson, 1969) where changes from a primarily clinical to administrative approach in psychiatrists' careers were considered.

In the field of child care, Bayduss and Toscano (1979) and Vander-Ven (1979a) articulated the developmental characteristics of child care practitioners in relation to educational preparation and modes of practice. Similarly, Katz (1977) described developmental stages among preschool teachers. That adult workers can be influenced in their own personal and professional development by the very fact of having contact with children represents a core issue for the group care field, as do the ways in which workers proceed through stages of personal and professional development as the result of educational preparation and experience. It is thus possible to formulate a set of developmental characteristics for group care practitioners at various stages in their personal and professional development. These relate to acquiring and utilizing attributes and skills required for practice at the various levels set out earlier. Implications for supportive education and professional development can also be highlighted.

Major Life Issues for Workers at Level 1

A large proportion of group care practitioners involved in either preparation for microsystem work or who have entered the field as direct care workers without initial preparation are young people. In line with Erikson's (1950) formulations concerning life stage development, they may still be in the process of consolidating their own sense of personal identity and may also be involved in resolving issues of authority and individuality away from their own parents. These dynamics of personal development are often characteristic of the microsystem group care worker, particularly in the beginning while actually participating in the setting.

At Stage 1, workers usually have limited aspirations for professional development and expanded role functions. Attention is more singularly focused on the practical demands of specific children with whom she or he is working. This strong identification with *childhood as a life stage* (VanderVen, 1978) is a normal characteristic of such practitioners. They see and approach situations from children's perspectives. At times they may overidentify with children, acting as a peer rather than an adult counterpart, possibly colluding with children against other adults instead of differentiating their role.

Related to this characteristic is a counter-identification with adults and the system, perhaps reflecting still unresolved ties with parents and authority figures. It may be reflected in the general tendency to view other adults as rigid and possibly even bad for the children. Parents are seen as being at fault for causing their children's problems, and supervisors and administrators may be seen as agents of a repressive bureaucracy. Interestingly, such disdain seems to give these new workers the special energy which inspires dedication and vitality in their direct care work, seemingly giving them strength to withstand numerous realistic frustrations in the work. Such workers may form collusive relationships with peers that challenge agency policies and mores, especially when such workers are treated as low-status employees. In more democratically run programs, front-line workers more often find peers to be a strong source of support.

Avoidance of adult functions frequently means that the level of aspiration of workers at this level does not extend beyond direct care work. The traditional reward system in group care practice does not always include opportunities for career mobility. These factors, combined with others, contribute to direct care work being highly stressful (Mattingly, 1977), and many young workers have left the field before their development might have encouraged assumption of role functions at a wider level. This has contributed to contemporary situations where practitioners assigned to indirect roles, with potential to influence the broad group care system, have limited experience of group care work. Thus, the educational and employment system has a responsibility for encouraging microsystem workers to make a continuing contribution to the field.

Beginning microsystem workers may hold a strong rescue fantasy: their conviction that they, with their tremendous warmth and dedication, can make up to the children what their deprived pasts have failed to give. Such workers may feel that agencies and others are depriving children of life entitlements. Policies equalizing treatment for all children or guidelines for professional relationships are considered unreasonable, since they fly in the face of their wish to give. Once again, a moderate rescue fantasy should not be seen as negative. It might even be conceived as an essential ingredient for successful performance of a worker's major nurturing role, in line with the characteristics of primary care outlined by Maier (1979).

In a similar way "unproductive humility" (VanderVen, 1978) is also characteristic of many direct group care practitioners. In their dedication to a specific group of children, direct care workers may hold the conviction that advancement, pursuit of additional resources, or participation in political activity is self-seeking. Such workers often fail to take advantage of real opportunities for professional advancement that might be available. They are saying, in effect, "What, little me? I can't do that!" An example might be the practitioner who is invited to participate in a workshop in an area of her or his experience but refuses for no justifiable reason, thereby limiting their potential for advancement.

Microsystem practitioners generally have an *affective* orientation to the work (VanderVen, 1978, 1979b) that involves responsiveness to feelings, interpersonal relationships, and group processes. Educationally, clinical material and experiential teaching strategies appeal to the Level 1 worker's *affective* stance. Cognitive activity–theory, research, writing–may be seen by such workers as irrelevant to genuine practice in the field and thus be rejected. Similarly, the microsystem practitioner is more likely to reflect an *expressive,* as contrasted to an instrumental, approach to activities. A beginning worker in the microsystem more commonly espouses a singular approach to group care practice, seeing others' ways of viewing and caring for children as negative.

For example, she or he might strongly embrace a particular approach because of limited exposure to other approaches. Such ardent acceptance is often related to a particular developmental stage and may also contribute to a sense of identity that aligns with others who share similar views against those who do not. Related to this is the characteristic of being non-synergistic, based on King's (1975) formulation of synergy or the ability to see things from a variety of perspectives. The initial practitioner therefore tends to see things in a one-or-the-other perspective, such as "parents are bad," "organizations stifle," or "commitment is good" rather than adopting a comprehensive stance and seeing both the strengths and weaknesses of different approaches.

Advances in the fields of adult development and education have highlighted considerations about learning styles characteristic of adults at various stages in their own development. An attempt can be made to relate these to group care practitioners. At the microsystem level, workers' learning styles probably relate most closely to Kolb's (1976) concept of *accommodator*. Here the greatest interest lies in doing things and being involved in new experiences which can then be adapted to new circumstances. The accommodator solves problems utilizing intuitive rather than analytic abilities. Perceptions of field-dependent learners (Witkin, Moore, Goodenough, & Cox, 1977) are shaped by what is around the worker or by the organization of the surrounding field.

Because field dependent learners are sensitive to social cues and interested in others, one can hypothesize that many group care practitioners are field-dependent learners. This is not inconsistent with Witkin et al. (1977) who described field-dependent learners as having a "with people" orientation (p. 12). The learning styles of group care practitioners pose implications for the design of their educational experiences. These learning styles may also change through growth and experience, suggesting that different instructional modes may be more effective with different workers of varied experience.

Major Life Issues for Workers at Level 2

In general, workers in the mesosystem may be dealing with different life issues than those working in microsystems. It might be hypothesized that these workers may have mastered the developmental tasks of Level 1 in passing on to Level 2. Their major life issues may concern establishment and maintenance of a completely adult mode of living: finding a home which is at least semi-permanent, getting married or forming a steady relationship and, perhaps, becoming a parent, consistent with Erikson's Stage of *Intimacy*. Sometime during this period the practitioner is capable of broadening their perspectives beyond the initial level. Professional requirements for Level 2 work, with its emphasis on working with other adults who are providing direct care of children, means that the practitioner needs to assume a different viewpoint towards both parents and those with administrative and supervisory responsibilities.

Effective mesosystem workers need to develop a more expanded concept of their own professional development and role function. There is concern with the care required for various groups of children, but this concern is focused through a specific investment and encouragement towards the effectiveness of other adults who have primary care giving responsibilities. Thus, developing mesosystem workers shift from identification with childhood as a life stage to *identification with adulthood as a life stage*. Here, workers see and approach situations from both children's as well as adults' perspectives, able to empathize with other adults *vis-à-vis* children, as well as that of children *vis-à-vis* adults.

In contrast with the microsystem worker, mesosystem workers are less likely to collude with children against other adults. This may reflect partial resolution of earlier developmental issues around authority and separation from their own parents. Such practitioners are more likely to empathize with parents and the many stresses and difficulties of the parental role, especially around parenting a difficult child or one with special needs. Similarly, mesosystem workers are more capable of practising and identifying with the role of the supervisor, administrator, or teacher in involvements with other adults. Effective mesosystem workers develop a more extended level of aspiration. If they have remained in the field of practice, they are more likely to have integrated factors previously described which contribute to the "short career life" of direct care workers. Prospects for a longer term career commitment in this field have been realised.

Mesosystem workers, like microsystem workers, may continue to hold a rescue fantasy, albeit now with a different form and content. There may be a realization or feeling that both children and their parents are victims–possibly of society–and workers wish to alter the system that is not treating their clients properly. This provides emotional fuel for their investment in assisting the development of other adults working with children. They want to influence many elements working effectively to enact change. The "non-productive humility" of Level 1 workers is rapidly disappearing in the mesosystem practitioner.

The necessity for initiative-seeking and authoritative, instrumental behaviour is recognized and utilized in order to have a wider influence. Effective mesosystem workers may be able to function this way because at this stage they are cognitively ready to assume a broader generic perspective. The benefits of more than one approach may be appreciated and integrated into a personal philosophy of care.

This may occur because the primarily affective orientation of Level 1 shifts towards a more cognitive one. Without abandoning concerns about feelings, relationships, and processes, practitioners at this point become more receptive to theory, research results, and the value of presenting ideas in writing. Such cognitive development contributes to an ability to think synergistically or from a variety of perspectives. Both the viewpoints of children and adults can be seen and appreciated, as can the strengths and weaknesses in particular developmental or therapeutic approaches. Kolb's work on adult learning suggests that learning styles can actually change through the transformation of ongoing experiences.

Thus, it is possible to hypothesize that some mesosystem practitioners begin to manifest divergent learning styles (Kolb, 1976) where one is interested in people and can view concrete situations from many perspectives. Such learners may still be field-dependent, however, since it is suggested that this general orientation is fairly stable (Witkin et al., 1977). In that education for group care practitioners is assumed to be continuous no matter what levels of operation, characteristic learning styles at this stage continue to have important implications.

Major Life Issues for Workers at Level 3

By the time practitioners assume work roles in the exosystem, effectiveness is quite likely to reflect differences in personal development and professional orientation when compared with microsystem and even mesosystem workers. Considerable growth and transformation have likely taken place by the time a person comfortably and adequately performs in exosystem activities. Exosystem workers may reflect characteristics of Erikson's (1950) stage of *generativity* in which a genuine concern for the well-being of the next generation is held to be important. A stable life style and ongoing professional advancement have contributed towards an even broader perspective than is commonly characteristic of mesosystem workers. There is not only investment in the development and direct support of those with primary responsibilities for group care service delivery but also concern about the adequacy of systems which influence the extent to which these adults can be effective.

Effective exosystem workers are likely to have consolidated a distinctive professional identity as group care practitioners through sustained involvement in practise at this level. Identifications have continued to shift from identification with children to identification with adults and now *identifying with systems*. This does *not* mean that there is failure to see flaws in the system that contain and impact on children and families. Rather, these very systems become the area in which work is directed. Having developed greater ability to recognize relationships between caring systems and the quality of direct care provided, effective workers seek to exert an influence in the exosystem to encourage positive change requiring many new personal skills and attributes.

Exosystem workers, like colleagues working in narrower spheres of activity, continue to hold a rescue fantasy that provides the emotional energy to work in a frustrating and challenging context. Concerns are with children, families, and those who work within the system to provide positive care. It is reflected in a wish to work within an organizational context where no direct or clinical contacts are the objects of work efforts.

Effective exosystem workers are likely to reflect a strong instrumental orientation, recognizing that only through exerting initiative, direction, and authority can they operate within organizational contexts that are characteristic of the exosystem. It is acceptable to move away from direct client interaction and also to function in discordant relationships with others. Exosystem practice requires the exercise of power and control and this does not always lead to popularity. Thus, the practitioner evolves considerably in the progression from Level 1 to Level 3.

In the initial level, concerns were with warm peer relationships even when used as a vehicle for expressing disdain for those at higher levels. At Level 3, a practitioner may have to perform without such a support system and function in ways that require considerable maturity and vision. Cognitively, the exosystem worker is deliberately concerned with a wide variety of theoretical and empirical information. This is needed as a background for complex planning and decision making. Cognitive modes of working are likely to be well integrated into the practitioner's professional orientation. Like Level 2 workers, those in the exosystem continue to manifest synergistic thinking although it is likely to be even more encompassing for complexities in organizational structure and interrelationships between clients must be perceived.

Relationships between specific organizations serving a clientele and networks which link various organizations together must also be perceived. Such synergistic thinking is essential for complex financial planning and effective work in the political sphere as well as in giving direction to a central organisation that coordinates service delivery across a large number of subordinate agencies. It can be hypothesized that the learning styles of effective exosystem practitioners take on characteristics of the *assimilator* (Kolb, 1976) where there is both capacity and, frequently, the requirement to create conceptual models that assimilate disparate observations, experiences, and empirical data into an integrated perspective that can be communicated effectively to a diverse and complex constituency.

Major Life Issues for Workers at Level 4

Because few group care practitioners are likely to be found working in the macrosystem and actually influencing this sphere, it is difficult to articulate specific developmental characteristics in detail, although some general projections might be in order. In terms of personal development, it can be proposed that the individual will have mastered tasks in Erikson's stage of *generativity* and may still be in that stage while others may have embraced the life stage of *integrity* and completion. Professional activity for successful macrosystem workers is likely to extend to a variety of indirect activities with children, families, and with other adults serving in various capacities in professional associations, leadership or support roles across different organizations and actively participating in broader social networks or child advocacy roles.

There is likely to have been experience across a range of professional practice activities, including both direct and indirect practices, thereby contributing to a real sense of professional consolidation. Interestingly, a worker at this level is probably not subject to some of the isolation and hostility experienced by exosystem workers since they are likely to be eminent in professional circles and thereby shown respect.

Traces of orientation to initial microsystem work have long since been transformed in the macrosystem practitioner. Unproductive humility has given way to a *sense of entitlement*. Such persons may recognize that they have made important contributions and there is an expectation of respect by others. The orientation of macrosystem practitioners is likely to have moved from the initial identification with childhood to *identification with the human condition*. They are able to stand back and reflect, with empathy, on a wide variety of experiences. An instrumental mode continues through wishing to communicate ideas generated through a wealth of experiences. For some, this might be manifested through publications whilst others may maintain extensive contacts across a wide audience of practitioners and the general public, through lectures, public appearances, and the like.

CONCLUSION

To significantly influence the quality of human services delivered to children requires a comprehensive ecological approach that can influence each of the environmental systems that impinge on children and affect their lives. Such efforts will be even more effective if they accommodate important trends in developmental theory and human service delivery. Because group care is an established feature of service delivery for children, it is essential that group care practitioners demonstrate skills and attributes necessary for effective work not only with children directly but also with the environment, which exerts an indirect but highly potent influence. This requires engagement in an ongoing process of personal and professional development since the need for ecological interventions at successively complex environmental levels cannot be met by those prepared for, or engaging at beginning levels of practice.

Because the group care field has still not developed ongoing educational and staff development efforts to the same extent as other more established human service disciplines, it is important that those concerned with advancing the field mount efforts to develop such initiatives. Special attention needs to be given to career development activities, such as the development of appropriate levels and content of education, job structuring and enrichment, and facilitation of relevant personal skills and interpersonal relationships. While some progress has been made in increasing educational opportunities and developing professional associations, much more is still required to strengthen responsive services across the group care field and achieve increased professionalism in the delivery of services for children. At the very least, group care practice with children has become a "semi-profession" (Etzioni, 1969) where, in terms of responsibility, status and impact, advancement in the field requires moving successively away from clients to engage in the various levels of the ecological hierarchy highlighted in this chapter. There is still a need to strengthen and expand involvement in areas of indirect practice and to encourage the development of indirect practice skills and competencies. It is still hoped that effective practitioners will soon be found operating at all levels, thereby enhancing the quality of care available and further extending career opportunities for highly regarded professionals in the group care field.

REFERENCES

Arthur, B., & Birnbaum, J. (1968). Professional identity as a determinant of the response to emotionally disturbed children. *Psychiatry, 31*, 138-149.

Babcock, C. G. (1964). *Having chosen to work with children: The common problems that face the professional person.* Unpublished paper presented for the Extension Division of the Child Therapy Program. Chicago: The Institute of Psychoanalysis.

Barnes, F. H., & Kelman, S. M. (1974). From slogans to concepts: A basis for change in child care work. *Child Care Quarterly 3*(I), 7-24.

Bayduss, G., & Toscano, J. A. (1979). The development of child care workers: Correlates between occupational and social-emotional growth. *Child Care Quarterly, 8*, 85-93.

Beker, J. (1979). Training and professional development in child care. In J. K. Whittaker (Ed.), *Caring for troubled children.* San Francisco: Jossey-Bass.

Bell, R., & Hurper, L. (1977). *Child effects on adults.* Hillsdale, NJ: Lawrence Eribaum.

Brim, O. (1975). Macro-structural influences on development: The need for childhood social indicators. *American Journal of Orthopsychiatry, 45*, 516-524.

Bronfenbrenner, U. (1977). Toward an experimental ecology of human development. *American Psychologist, 32*, 513-530.

Bronfenbrenner, U. (1979). *The ecology of human development: Experiments by nature and design.* Cambridge, MA: Harvard University Press.

Butler, H. F. (1972). Student role stress. *American Journal of Occupational Therapy, 26*, 399-405.

Conte, J. R. (1978). Helping groups of parents change their children's behavior. *Child & Youth Services, 2*, 1-9.

Davids, A. (1975). Therapeutic approaches to children in residential treatment. *American Psychologist, 32*, 809-814.

Dockar-Drysdale B. (1973). Staff consultation in an evolving care system. In J. Hunter & F. Ainsworth (Eds.), *Residential establishments. The evolving of caring systems* (pp. 39-56). Dundee, Scotland: University of Dundee, Department of Social Administration.

Erikson, E. H. (1950). *Childhood and society.* New York: Norton.

Etzioni, A. (Ed.). (1969). *The semi-professions and their organization.* New York: Free Press.

Fischer, C., & Brodsky, S. (Eds.). (1978). *Client participation in human services: The Prometheus principle.* New Brunswick: Transaction Books.

Goldsmith, J. (1976). Residential treatment today: The paradox of new premises. *American Journal of Orthopsychiatry, 46*, 425-433.

Hobbs, N. (1974). Helping disturbed children: Psychological and ecological strategies. In M. Wolins (Ed.), *Successful group care.* Chicago: Aldine.

Katz, L. (1977). *Talks with teachers.* Washington, DC: National Association for the Education of Young Children.

King, M. (1975). *For we are: Towards understanding your personal potential.* Reading, MA: Addison-Wesley.

King, M., & VanderVen, K. (1980). Creative behavior is involved in personal growth, development, and values of child care practitioners. *The Creative Child and Adult Quarterly, 5*(2), 86-93.

Klerman, G., & Levinson, D. (1969). Becoming the director: Promotion as a phase in personal-professional development. *Psychiatry, 32,* 411-27.

Kolb, D. (1976). *Learning style inventory.* Boston, MA: McBerard.

Lamb, H. R., & Zusman, J. (1979). Primary prevention in perspective. *American Journal of Psychiatry, 136,* 12-17.

Levinson, D. J., Darrow, C. N., Klein, E. B., Levinson, M. H., & McKee, B. (1978). *The seasons of a man's life.* New York: Alfred Knopf.

Magnussen, D., & Endler, N. (1977). Interactional psychology: Present status and future prospects. In D. Magnussen & N. Endler (Eds.), *Personality at the crossroads: Current issues in interactional psychology.* Hillsdale, NY: Lawrence Erlbaum.

Maier, H. W. (1977). The child care worker. In J. Turner (Ed.), *Encyclopedia of social work.* New York: National Association of Social Workers.

Maier, H. W. (1978). Piagetian principles applied to the beginning phase in professional helping. In J. F. Magary, M. K. Poulsen, P. J. Levinson, & P. A. Taylor (Eds.), *Piagetian theory and the helping professions.* Los Angeles: University of Southern California Press.

Maier, H. W. (1979). The core of care: Essential ingredients for the development of children at home and away from home. *Child Care Quarterly, 8,* 161-173.

Mattingly, M. (1977). Sources of stress and burn-out in professional child care work. *Child Care Quarterly, 6,* 127-137.

Olesen, V., & Whittaker, E. (1968). *The silent dialogue.* San Francisco: Jossey-Bass.

Patti, R., & Austin, M. (1977). Socializing the direct service practitioner in the ways of supervisory management. *Administration in Social Work, 1,* 267-280.

Schopler, E., & Reichler, R. (Eds.). (1976). *Psychopathology and child development: Research and treatment.* New York: Plenum Press.

Thomas, A., Chess, S., & Birch, H. (1968). *Temperament and behavior disorders in children.* New York: New York University Press.

Trieschman, A. E., Whittaker, J. K., & Brendtro, L. K. (1969). *The other 23 hours.* Chicago: Aldine.

VanderVen, K. (1978). *A paradigm describing stages of personal and professional development of child care practitioners with characteristics associated with each stage.* Paper delivered at Ninth International Congress of the International Association of Workers with Maladjusted Children, Montreal.

VanderVen, K. (1979a). Towards maximum effectiveness of the unit team approach in residential care: An agenda for team development. *Residential and Community Child Care Administration, 1,* 287-298.

VanderVen, K. (1979b). Developmental characteristics of child care workers and design of training programs. *Child Care Quarterly, 8*(2).

VanderVen, K., & Griff, M. (1978). *Expanded roles for child care workers: Work with families.* Unpublished paper.

Vinter, R. (1973). Analysis of treatment organizations. *Social Work,* 3-15.

Whittaker, J. K. (1979). *Caring for troubled children.* San Francisco: Jossey-Bass.

Witkin, H. A., Moore, C. A., Goodenough, D. R., & Cox, P. W. (1977). Field-dependent and field-independent cognitive styles and their educational implications. *Review of Educational Research, 47,* 1-64.

Wolins, M. (1974). *Successful group care: Explorations in the powerful environment.* Chicago: Aldine.

Zabarenko, R., & Zabarenko, L. (1978). *The doctor tree: Developmental stages in the growth of physicians.* Pittsburgh, PA: University of Pittsburgh Press.

Chapter 11

The Economics of Group Care Practice:
A Reappraisal

Martin Knapp

SUMMARY. For the past two decades, economic influences have significantly impacted the provision of health and welfare services for children, young people and their families in communities around the world. The dynamic of cost has reshaped both the nature and provision of group care services, promoting de-institutionalization and transforming the nature of caring services offered in local communities. In a reappraisal of themes identified in his seminal contribution more than two decades ago, this leading authority looks back at key themes impacting on the economics of social care that shape group care services for the new millennium. *[Article copies available for a fee from The Haworth Document Delivery Service: 1-800-HAWORTH. E-mail address: <docdelivery@haworthpress.com> Website: <http://www.HaworthPress.com> © 2006 by The Haworth Press, Inc. All rights reserved.]*

KEYWORDS. Group care, residential care, residential treatment, group homes, youth work, youthwork, group work, at-risk youth, accounting, cost of care, management and human services

Address correspondence to: Martin Knapp, Professor of Social Policy, London School of Economics, Houghton Street, London WC2A 2AE, UK.

[Haworth co-indexing entry note]: "The Economics of Group Care Practice: A Reappraisal." Knapp, Martin. Co-published simultaneously in *Child & Youth Services* (The Haworth Press, Inc.) Vol. 28, No. 1/2, 2006, pp. 259-284; and: *Group Care Practice with Children and Young People Revisited* (ed: Leon C. Fulcher, and Frank Ainsworth) The Haworth Press, Inc., 2006, pp. 259-284. Single or multiple copies of this article are available for a fee from The Haworth Document Delivery Service [1-800-HAWORTH. 9:00 a.m. - 5:00 p.m. (EST). E-mail address: docdelivery@haworthpress.com].

REFLECTIONS AFTER TWENTY-FIVE YEARS

When my original chapter was published in 1981 the number of economic studies in the child care area could be counted on the fingers of one hand. Today one would still need only three or four hands for a similar count such has been the disappointing response by economists to the pressing needs for more focused analysis in this field. Until quite recently, there has also been only lukewarm interest from non-economics researchers to include an economics component in their studies. This stands in very marked contrast, for example, to the thousands of health economists across the world. Indeed, a look at how the subject of health economics has developed over a 25-year period reveals enormous methodological and empirical breakthroughs. My first reflection, therefore, is one of disappointment that research in this area remains quite scarce (Knapp & Lowin, 1998; Romeo, Byford, & Knapp, 2004).

Meanwhile, cost pressures remain, cost analysis among micro and macro planners has developed, cost awareness among decision makers has grown, although largely–as just noted–in an evidence-free environment. Indeed, whereas in the early 1980s many decision makers in the child and family welfare sector would have reacted with horror to the suggestion that financial considerations should have a part to play in the prioritization and allocation of services, the reaction today would be healthier and more positive. There is often a more mature recognition that deploying resources cost-effectively makes it possible to reach more families given fixed funds, fixed amounts of skilled staff time, and so on. In other words, improving the efficiency with which funds, staff time, and other resources are used actually extends the reach of budget-constrained agencies.

Another change over the past 25 years has been movement away from simply focusing on costs to inquiring about cost-effectiveness. Decision makers, and those researchers who feed evidence to them, are less likely to be interested in simply measuring the costs and understanding how they vary, which was the main focus of my original chapter, and much more interested in understanding how costs are linked to child and family outcomes. It is never sufficient to make decisions solely on the basis of cost information, and I would argue that it is also never sufficient to build policies or implement practice changes solely on the basis of outcomes. What is needed is to blend the resource side with the outcomes side; that is, to look at the cost-effectiveness of different ways of using available resources.

This focus on cost-effectiveness must not be misunderstood. The first consideration in deciding which services, care settings, therapies, or medications to use in addressing the needs of the individual or family should be the expected outcomes. Which intervention or arrangement is most likely to maximize the improvement in individual and family quality of life, for example? Second, if improvements in quality of life can be achieved, what is the most cost-effective way to achieve them? Put more bluntly, what are the costs of achieving particular improvements in quality of life, and is it worth spending that amount of money? It is precisely this kind of question (Is it worth it?) that decision makers face every day.

Cost (or cost-effectiveness) has always been an issue in group care and in the human services more generally. However, the first edition of *Group Care for Children: Concept and Issues* was one of the very earliest to give the topic attention. What we now need is a more concerted response from the research community.

INTRODUCTION

In recent years it has been rare indeed to find a change or development of child or youth care policy or practice that has not had to run the gauntlet of a long line of "But what does it cost?" questions. The economic problems that beset Western economies in the mid-1970s–precipitated by the so-called oil crisis–forced upon public, private, and voluntary providers of care a degree of cost consciousness hitherto unknown in the post-war period. It is true that for years each new policy initiative and each new extension of existing policies had to be evaluated within cost constraint, but such constraint was never as tight as the constraints faced by the start of the 1980s.

Many an eminently reasonable policy change has been postponed, rejected, and at times even abused because it was felt to be too expensive. As a consequence, cost constraint became the subject of considerable criticism, and the penny-pinching politician, the short-sighted accountant, and the hard-headed economist came to be viewed as the chief villains of the piece. Social care services had long been felt to be the preserve of the social worker or the student of social policy. These services, it was argued, should not be the testing ground for economic theories or cannon fodder for central government fiscal policies. Costs, in short, are anathema to social care.

The move towards cost-consciousness has, at least to the economist, three saddening features: unwarranted denigration, unfortunate belatedness, and unselective over-reaction. The denigration, rather than applause, which greets each new attempt to impose a degree of cost effectiveness or economic rationality upon child and youth care policies is the most immediately recognizable feature of recent trends.

Criticism about the introduction of economic arguments into policymaking stemmed in part from a feeling that services as indubitably and inherently desirable as child and youth care should be above the vicissitudes of national economic welfare, such that public expenditure cuts should fall elsewhere. Similarly, private and voluntary caring agencies should be compensated for their unavoidable difficulties.

Such arguments unfortunately confused ideology and rationality. Nobody would deny the need for child and youth care or other personal social services, but it is dangerous and foolish to argue that certain activities are beyond economic analysis. Very few activities in modern society are costless. Resources, including child and youth care services, are scarce and therefore have a positive value or cost to society. Allocating resources in one way immediately implies the rejection of alternative allocations. The late 20th century recession heightened our awareness of scarcity, and it is scarcity which commonly signals the arrival of the economist. If there is a wish to make the best use of scarce resources, if there is a wish to deploy available group care services in such a way as to maximize their effectiveness or their success, then efforts must be made to ensure that value for money is being achieved; in other words, it is necessary to take a long and careful look at the cost implications of each policy decision.

The second and related saddening feature of late 20th century experience has been the fact that child and youth care administrators, just like the administrators of other welfare services, only turned to a careful examination of the costs of their services at a time of economic adversity. Most children and young people in care in the United Kingdom are the responsibility of local authorities, and these authorities sailed through the halcyon days of growth of expenditure and expansion of services with barely a fleeting backward glace at the cost trail left behind. When recession bit, and bit deep, it was these public providers of care who were shown to be least prepared for the challenge. Recession revealed an embarrassing ignorance of the basic principles of economic management and a distinct lack of both the necessary data and information required for sensible policy making and the requisite expertise for gathering and applying such knowledge.

Little can be done about the second of these features, and one can only hope that the gradual acquisition of information and expertise and the gradual realization of the need for careful cost planning will help to remove the first feature. It is the third feature that is the subject of this chapter. Faced with a shrinking budget and a growing potential clientele, politicians, administrators, and lower-level managers have grasped unselectively the nettles of cost information readily available or collected. Unfortunately there has been very little discrimination among available information sets and even less apparent understanding of the problems associated with applying such information in practice. Residential care has been given the "Too Expensive" label, higher staffing ratios have been criticized for wasting valuable skilled resources, maintenance expenditure has been halved in the name of efficiency, and new capital projects–of which there have been precious few–have been pruned and delayed in the name of cost reduction.

The sad fact about all this generally well-intended, frenetic activity is that it has been largely misplaced and misdirected. Not only have administrators made either improper or inadequate use of the cost information currently available to them, but also this information is really not the kind of cost information that they should be using in the first place. If the intention is *really* to get value for money, if one *really* wants to ensure that available care resources are used in the best possible way, then it is necessary to make specific collections of information which allow for proper and reliable computation and comparison of group care and child welfare costs.

In what follows, the intention is to set out an ideal cost measure for use in child and youth care planning. It will be seen that the collection of information necessary to obtain such a measure is itself costly, and for that reason administrators may, initially at least, prefer to make use of information already available in the annual accounts drawn up by his or her treasurer. The analysis moves on to a consideration of the uses of cost data that is routinely available, with brief commentary about the types of routine information of *most* use for rational planning purposes. Our major concern here, however, will be to explain how to use available information *sensibly* and highlighting three key issues: variability, comparability and predictability. This leads an examination of three popular techniques of cost analysis, techniques that have long been employed in more conventional areas of economists' concern but which have just as much validity when studying the "production of care services" or the "production of wellbeing" (Knapp, 1979a, 1984).

THE ECONOMIST'S DEFINITION OF COST

"What does it cost to provide residential care for a mentally handicapped child?" This apparently straightforward and unambiguous question might be answered with an apparently straightforward and unambiguous answer, like "one hundred Pounds Sterling, Dollars, or Euros per week." But this and other similar questions deceive by their simplicity, for they really hide a multitude of other questions. One hundred Pounds Sterling, Dollars, or Euros per week is similarly a screen–a smoke screen of little intrinsic value in itself–that hides the answer: the *real cost* of care.

To illustrate what is meant by the real cost of care, let us take up an example familiar to students of economics and of English literature: the tale of Robinson Crusoe. Suppose that Crusoe, on that eventful Friday when he first saw the footprints in the sand, had found not a fit, athletic man but instead a severely mentally handicapped child. Would Crusoe have thanked us for giving him one hundred Pounds Sterling, Dollars, or Euros per week in order for him to care for that unfortunate child? Not at all, for money was useless to him on his desert island. Much more useful would have been a gourd of goat's milk or a net of fish, for in caring for the mentally handicapped child, Crusoe would have to give up the time he would otherwise have spent milking or fishing. The *cost* to Crusoe of caring for the mentally handicapped child could not be reckoned in Pounds Sterling, Dollars, or Euros but only in terms of what he had lost (the milk and fish) by not using his time and energy in an alternative pursuit (milking and fishing).

Of course, Daniel Defoe's hero did not find a mentally handicapped child, but this distortion of a familiar story well illustrates the economist's meaning of cost. The cost of an article, a resource, or a service cannot, in general, be reckoned merely by reference to its price but must be gauged in terms of what is given up in order to have the article, resource, or service. Sometimes the price paid will be a good approximation to the value of what has been given up, but this is by no means always the case. Many resources and services are not bought and sold on the open market, and those that are have prices that are frequently and largely influenced by market distortions. This definition of cost– what the economist sometimes calls the *opportunity cost*–will be seen to be intuitively appealing, to have considerable validity in the context of social care, and to possess a certain indispensability when one tries to assess "efficiency," or at least in attempts to get value for money.

When faced with a mentally handicapped child, Crusoe had given up his milking and fishing in order to provide care: The giving of care had cost Crusoe the milk and fish he had not been able to collect. A little nearer to home one can imagine a child welfare agency having to decide whether to build a new secure unit for disruptive young people or to use the available financial resources to open three new day care units. In this sense, the cost of the secure unit is equal to the three day units foregone, and the cost of a day unit is equal to one-third of a secure unit.

Alternatively, consider the case of the qualified social worker waiting in court to attend a five-minute hearing for a juvenile client charged with shoplifting. The time spent in court might alternatively have been spent visiting the mother of another young person on his or her caseload or, perhaps, attending an afternoon seminar on intermediate treatment work with juvenile delinquents. The cost of the court attendance is thus to be reckoned in terms of the opportunities missed by not visiting the other client or not attending the seminar. In each of these cases, one is expressing the cost of supplying a service or employing a resource in terms of the value of opportunities that have been missed. For this reason the economist's conceptualization of cost is called the *opportunity cost*:

> The cost of using a resource in a particular service or mode of care is not (in general) the money cost or price of the resource, but is the benefit foregone, or opportunity lost, by not using the resource in its best alternative use.

The value of this cost definition is that it emphasizes the fact that our need for cost information stems from our need to choose between alternative claims, wants, or needs. Scarcity implies choice, and the act of choice gives us our definition of cost. From this chain of logical statements one can identify a number of implications and characteristics of our opportunity cost definition. Opportunity costs are context specific, they are inherently subjective, they require knowledge of the alternatives open to us, and they are rejected benefits and thus measurable in terms of benefits.

In practice, these are not problematic, for the context specificity of opportunities makes the computations relatively easy. Generally one uses the going currency to measure opportunities–Pounds Sterling, Dollars or Euros–either because market prices are reasonably accurate enough to allow such measures to be used or because money is a convenient common *numeraire* in which to express these various costs. One

characteristic of opportunity cost is very important–they are subjective–
and it is this characteristic which leads one irrevocably to a consideration of the differences between private and social costs.

The distinction between private cost and social cost can be viewed
from two perspectives, depending on whether one is talking about bare
expenditures, that is, accounting costs, or about opportunity costs. For
example, one might ask the head of a children's home to tell us the annual cost of running the home. Consulting the financial accounts, she
would be able to list expenditures on staff, provisions, laundering, elec-
tricity and gas, and so on. The same question posed to the director of social services or the director of the child welfare agency might elicit a
slightly different answer, for the director would probably add expenditure on peripatetic teachers and social workers and the cost of central
administration to the head's list.

These two services are financed by the social services department or
care agency but do not appear in the financial accounts of the children's
home. One might then ask the Secretary of State or Governor the same
question and further costs might be added, including the cost of doctors'
visits to the home. It is clear that in Britain the Secretary of State's list of
expenditures covers all, or at least most, of the services received by residents living in a children's home. This list of expenditures is thus much
closer to the *social* cost of care than either of the other two lists. Clearly,
when reckoning the cost of a service it is necessary to include *all* costs
or items of expenditure.

Of course, as argued elsewhere in this chapter, it is necessary to look
beyond the monetary "veil" of expenditure figures and instead try to
calculate opportunity costs. The distinction between private and social
costs then becomes rather more marked. The *private opportunity cost* of
employing a resource in a given use is the value of that resource in the
next best alternative use available to the employer. For example, the private opportunity cost to a social services department of using a minibus
to ferry handicapped children to and from day centres might be the
value of using the minibus to deliver meals to elderly people in their
own homes. In contrast, the *social opportunity cost* of employing a resource in a given use is the value of that resource in the next best alternative use available to the *whole society*. It may be, for example, that if the
minibus were not used to transport day centre clients then it would be
employed to take school children to and from a local swimming pool.

Which costs should one be looking at in an analysis of child and
youth care services? First, as argued above, one should be concerned
with *opportunity* costs and not accounting costs or expenditures if one is

to use costs as a true reflection of the value of the resources. Secondly, one should be looking at *social* opportunity costs–the value of alternative uses of resources available to the whole society. By their very nature, most child and youth care services are *social* services and so to concentrate only on opportunity costs to the child welfare agency or the group care centre would be illogical indeed. One should look at *all* the resources used in providing a given service, whether or not they are financed out of the agency's budget, and consider their alternative uses to society as a *whole*.

A word of warning would not go amiss at this point. It is quite likely that the efforts expended in calculating opportunity rather than accounting costs will not be appreciated by holders of the purse strings. Much of the research conducted by child and youth care agencies, whether public, voluntary or private, is interested only in expenditure or accounting costs, and any challenges to such a perspective may not be greeted with open arms. Research emphasis of this kind is usually explained or excused by reference to constrained budgets, but it should be recognized as somewhat myopic and socially inefficient and actually lead to the misallocation of scarce resources.

EXPENDITURES AND ACCOUNTING COSTS

Opportunity costs are not, unfortunately, readily observable or measurable. For some resources or services there may be a market price which is sufficiently free of distortions to be a useful and reliable indicator of opportunity cost, but many resources used in the provision of child and youth care services simply are not bought and sold on the open market, and even those that are may have prices so distorted by market imperfections that they are far from reflecting the social opportunity cost of employment. However, because opportunity cost collection actually imposes an opportunity cost on the administrator, one might feel that annually collected and published expenditure figures will suffice. These expenditure figures, typically appearing in the annual accounts of each child or youth care agency and, probably, each separate group care unit, might be referred to as *accounting costs*. It is these accounting costs that are being quoted when an answer of one hundred Pound Sterling, Dollars, or Euros per week is given to the question about residential care costs.

Accounting costs clearly have a number of potential uses for the child or youth care administrator and planner, but it is rare to find them quoted sensibly or employed properly to their full advantage. Capital costs are often omitted or misquoted, current costs are frequently incomplete, and most cost figures tend not to be qualified by reference to the myriad of factors that influence them and which, therefore, make bare comparisons a hazardous practice. Capital figures quoted in annual accounts are generally listed as debt charges and revenue contributions to capital outlay. These items of expenditure, notional or otherwise, are principally determined by the age or vintage of the capital resources and the discounting procedures adopted by the accountant.

A common form of depreciation accounting is straight-line charging, capital resources being assumed to depreciate steadily and linearly over time. This method therefore assumes that all depreciation is physical deterioration that accompanies the mere passage of time and the value losses occasioned by technological progress (obsolescence). Use-depreciation, the deterioration attributable to actually operating or using the capital, is not separately recorded. If one is to make sensible and valuable use of costs data, it is necessary to be sure that any capital cost information one uses is accurate and valid. As well as these problems of interpretation of published capital figures, the conventional form of accounts will ignore various current overhead and incidental costs.

The costs of group care should ideally include administrative costs and the costs incurred in the employment of peripatetic skilled social workers, teachers, child psychiatrists, pediatricians, and so on. Excluding these cost elements will partially invalidate comparisons between, for example, residential and day care services, where the incidence of these peripatetic and overhead services will probably be very different. The major problem on this count is to decide where to stop the process of counting. Does one, for example, need to include the costs of collecting taxes when assessing the overall cost of a publicly provided child or youth care service? The answer, of course, is "yes" and "no," for one *should* be including these costs if they were making a comparison *between* private and public services, and one can clearly omit them for the reason that they do not vary if one is comparing between public care services.

A third difficulty encountered in the use of accounting costs arises because there are a myriad of factors that exert an influence upon the costs and expenditures of a child welfare agency or group care centre and it would be folly indeed to make a comparison between service types without taking these into account. It is to these variations and the factors that account for them that attention now turns.

FACTORS INFLUENCING THE COSTS OF GROUP CARE

It is a source of considerable dismay to note the number of times bare comparisons are drawn between current expenditures on different child and youth care services without qualification for the many influential factors liable to render any such comparisons irrelevant. It does not take a great deal of research to find evidence of great variations in cost for any one service, various both between and within administrative boundaries. Consider, for example, the figures presented in Table 1, taken from an annual publication of personal social services expenditure in England and Wales.

Table 1 shows the net cost per child week for six different group care services provided by English and Welsh local authorities. Average, minimum, and maximum expenditures are tabulated. The extent of the variation between local authorities is very marked indeed. Part of this variation is almost certainly due to differences in the classification of services between authorities. For example, an "ordinary" community home may provide extensive observation and assessment services but

TABLE 1. Variations in Expenditure per Child Week Between English and Welsh Local Authorities

| Service[b] | Expenditure per child week[a] | | |
	Mean	Minimum	Maximum
Hostels and Community Homes	72.54	39.96	167.14
Observation and Assessment Centres	120.58	57.08	267.73
Residential Nurseries	109.41	54.88	230.63
Community Schools	107.26	40.49	277.70
Homes for Mentally Handicapped	101.28	55.01	237.86
Day Nurseries[c]	30.70	11.35	52.35

[a]Net cost per child week excluding capital charges, in pounds sterling, 1977-1978, averaged over all relevant care units in a local authority.
[b]Services provided by local authority only.
[c]Net cost per child day multiplied by 5.
Note: For more information, see Chartered Institute of Public Finance and Accountancy, 1979.

not be classified as such. This would push up the expenditure of what is apparently a non-specialist residential home and thus distort the figures. This problem of classification highlights the real and major problem of making cost comparisons: One can only draw meaningful conclusions from comparisons if one is comparing like with like!

There are clearly a large number of factors which must be taken into account before one can claim to be comparing like with like, and in an attempt to impose some order on these factors, a simple theoretical framework is adopted as described by the author elsewhere (Davies & Knapp, 1980; Knapp, 1979a, 1984). The theoretical framework assumes that child and youth care services are directed at a number of objectives. These objectives might include improvements in physical, psychological, emotional and social well-being, in educational progress, in behaviour and maturity, and so on. The success of a child and youth care service can thus be couched in terms of the extent to which such objectives are attained.

Of course, the degree of success attained by the child or youth care agency will be dependent upon a number of factors, which one can arrange in three broad groups: the personal characteristics of the children (age, sex, reasons for being in care, background experiences, personality traits, and so on), the various dimensions of social environment or caring milieu (regime, social control and independence, privacy, stimulation and participation, interaction and communication, flexibility, homogeneity) and, thirdly, the characteristics of the physical or resource environment (including staff characteristics, attitudes, and experiences not covered by social environmental features). The boon of such a theoretical framework is its isomorphic correspondence with the economist's theory of production.

Where the economist would talk of inputs combining together in various proportions to produce outputs, one can conceive of the various personal, social, and resource characteristics combining and interacting with each other in order to determine the degree of success achieved by the child welfare agency or group care centre. By reference to the economist's discussion of cost variations, of which there are many, this correspondence between our simple theoretical model of child and youth care and the economic theory of production allows us to disentangle the many cost-influencing factors in order to draw meaningful comparisons of relevance for policy making in this difficult area.[1]

Attention now turns to a brief discussion of the major influences upon the costs of child and youth care taking advantage of the insights afforded by the correspondence between explaining child and youth care success and explaining variations in output in more conventional production processes. In this discussion, attention is directed towards the average cost per child week in a "short-run" model of cost determination. In other words, it is assumed that there are certain capital resources necessary for the provision of child and youth care services which cannot be increased in the immediate future. It takes time to design, construct, and open a new children's home or day service unit, and the assumption here is that the child welfare administrator must accept the currently available stock of homes or units as fixed. This assumption allows us to ignore the capital cost implications of alternative designs of building while including the *current* resource implications of capital outlay. The former are more appropriately the concern of the architect than the economist. In this short-run world one can distinguish seven groups of cost-influencing factors: some of them are causally influential and most of closely inter-related.

Resource Prices

In Table 1 the range of variation in average cost per child week was set out for six publicly provided services in England and Wales. What was not recorded is the fact that for four of the five residential services tabulated the maximum expenditures per child week were incurred by London Boroughs and the minimum expenditures by local authorities in the very north of England.[2] It is well known that employers of care staff in all the personal social services must pay much higher rates in the southeast of England than elsewhere. Thus, much of the nationwide cost variation is attributable to differences in area wage rates. The first thing one should do when comparing service costs, therefore, is to standardize all cost figures for geographical (and other exogenous) resource price differences. Of course, the child or youth care agency may itself be partly responsible for pushing wage rates higher in its own area than in other areas of the country or region. Labour markets for even the most skilled care staff tend to be localized and a heavy demand for skilled staff may well force wages up.[3]

Geographical variations in cost attributable to differences in price levels were identified and modeled in a national study of observation and assessment centres (Knapp, Curtis, & Giziakis, 1979). When drawing comparisons between the costs of services within a local authority area, price variations may be much less important although the non-pecuniary ramifications of a standard pay structure, for example, should be examined.

Charges

Again referring to Table 1 one will notice that the statistics published annually for English and Welsh local authority child and youth care services do not distinguish between gross and net expenditures per child week. Ideally, one should be concerned with *gross* costs, for these give a better indication than net costs of the resources employed in the care process. If one is also interested in the respective shares of total expenditure incurred by the care agency and the child or young person's family then at a *second* stage once could examine costs net of charges. It is important, however, to keep these two stages independent and to examine them separately.

Charging policies tend to vary quite markedly between different public providers, between public, voluntary, and private agencies, and over time. Different charging structures may be a consequence of a whole host of factors, including the ability of the young person's family to contribute to the costs of care and the provider's ability to attract gifts and charitable funds, and there is no reason for these to be systematically or consistently related to gross costs or the effectiveness of the child or youth care agency. If therefore one wishes to use cost figures as indicators of the resources employed in the care process, and this is really the only major justification for using them, then it is gross and not net costs that one should be examining. Criticisms of the rising costs of care in recent years lose much of their substance if one takes notice of the fact that revenue from charges has risen less rapidly than gross cost. The oft-quoted rate of inflation of net costs thus exaggerates the changing true resource consequences of care over a period of time.

Thus far, our discussion of cost-influencing factors has been concerned with the *definition* of cost and not its determination through the processes, characteristics, and effectiveness of care. The two factors distinguished above serve to illustrate the need to start off with a definition of cost that is consistent between care agencies, areas, and time periods. Unfortunately, even this most basic of requirements is violated in many commentaries on social service costs and the usefulness of such figures as those presented in Table 1 is thus called into question. Assuming that one is now in a position to draw up consistently defined costs, what other factors are liable to cause costs to vary?

Outputs

The word "output" is used as a convenient shorthand term for the degree of success achieved by a care unit in reaching its explicit or implicit policy objectives. Two types of output may be distinguished. *Final outputs* measure the changes in individual well-being, adjustment, behaviour, and so on, as compared with the levels of well-being (etc.) in the absence of a caring intervention. Final outputs thus relate success to the ultimate and individual-level goals of care. The second type of output is the *intermediate output* which is an indicator of the care services themselves, or workload, rather than the effects of these services on the children. Intermediate outputs are thus concerned with lower-level, service delivery objectives.

Obviously, if one's aim is to furnish the policy maker with information and recommendations for improving the delivery of child and youth care services, then one should be trying to measure final–and not just intermediate–outputs. One can, for example, picture two identical children's homes facing identical prices and receiving identical children into care. One home, however, may have an annual expenditure figure vastly in excess of the other simply because the head of the home feels that staff should have more time to spend with the children and therefore the home needs more staff. A bare comparison of intermediate outputs–the number of children in care, weighted perhaps by their ages, sex, and dependency–will not shed any light on the reasons for the differences in cost.

On the other hand, if the subsequent development of the young people is taken into account, if their abilities to behave and interact in some "normal" manner is reckoned, then the home with more staff and thus higher expenditure will probably also be the home with the higher final outputs or outcomes: that is, greater success in achieving ultimate child and youth care objectives. There are of course a number of fundamental problems that have been ridden roughshod over in this preliminary discussion of the output concepts: the identification and agreement, if that is possible, of service objectives and the measurement of success being principal among them, but the general thrust of the argument should be clear and, hopefully, widely accepted.

How then does the cost of care vary with the level of output? Firstly the two will generally be positively related, higher costs being associated with higher final and intermediate outputs. Secondly, one can expect the cost of each marginal or additional unit of output to differ from the cost of the previous unit. Consider for simplicity a very simple intermediate output indicator: the number of children in a home. One would reasonably expect to observe economies of scale in child and youth care, cost per child falling gradually as more children are accommodated in the home. These economies result from the more extensive use of fixed capital resources (with a fixed cost), from the fact that variable resource inputs increase less than proportionately with outputs, from the specialization of staff and other resources in areas of greatest competence made possible by larger scale,[4] and the bulk buying of some consumables.[5]

Remaining in this intermediate output world it is also possible to identify one or two reasons why the average cost per child may tend to rise beyond a certain scale of home: The burden of management and administration may increase to such an extent that inefficiencies creep in, the supply prices of scarce resources will be forced up by excess demand, and general inefficiencies will arise with resource implications. These are the conventional arguments used by economists to explain the observed curvilinear relationship between average cost and scale (Silbertson, 1972) and these would seem to be the factors accounting for similar observations in previous work on public child care costs (Knapp, 1977; Knapp, Curtis, & Giziakis, 1979).

If one moves from intermediate to final outputs, the arguments about scale economies become more complicated and more interesting. If output is conceptualized in terms of child development then one must concern themselves with the organizational and personal ramifications of large scale. In their classic study of residential care for the mentally handicapped, King, Raynes, and Tizard (1971) found no association between home size or living unit size and a child management practices scale, and Sinclair and Heal (1976) reached a similar conclusion from research on community homes. However, Grygier (1975) found that size was associated with low participation rates in activities, low cooperation with educators, and disciplinarian attitudes in his work on Canadian Training Schools. Furthermore, the Curtis Committee Report (1946), which provided the blueprint for the Children Act of 1948 and, thus, the first major statement of the British government's philosophy of child care, proposed that large institutions be abandoned in favour of small family group homes with no more than twelve children under the charge of a married couple. A government study of British observation and assessment centres argued that:

> An assessment centre should not be so large that it is in danger of becoming institutionalized nor so small that it would be uneconomic to provide the staff and specialist facilities necessary for thorough observation, diagnosis and assessment. For these reasons, we suggest that for an assessment centre an upper limit of about sixty

places is appropriate. We realize that the size of any one centre will be determined to some extent by its geographical situation and by the area it serves, but we think that some children will need a range of facilities and expertise greater than that which could be provided in a small assessment centre. Within any centre there is likely to be some breakdown into smaller groups for various purposes. (Department of Health and Social Security, 1971, p. 69)

The introduction of final output considerations–or service outcomes–thus complicates the picture greatly, but it is this complication which holds the key to the successful marriage of the economic, sociological, and psychological approaches to the organization and planning of child and youth care services.

Activity

As well as the level of output, whether intermediate or final, it has been suggested that the costs of providing a service are also related to the *rate* of production of output. In a group care context, one should thus examine the influence of the rates of admission, turnover, or occupancy and the average length of stay. There are costs associated with receiving a child or young person into care, particularly because more staff resources are required to help the young person adjust to his or her new environment and because of administrative duties, and for this reason one might expect higher admission or turnover rates to push up average costs. The argument for examining the occupancy rate is that there are many costly resources, principally staff resources, which are geared to a particular level of operation and which cannot easily be adjusted to short term changes in occupancy rates. If a home is temporarily under-occupied, in so far as it has more spare places than usual, then other things being equal one would expect to see the average cost per child being slightly higher than usual. Finally, one should also be looking at the association between cost and average length of stay, more especially in group care centres with a specialist function. Thus, for example, the common problem of the "silting up" of observation and assessment centres because of difficulties with delays in assessing young people and placing them in suitable caring environments has the effect of "wasting" the skilled resources available in these centres and pushing costs about the expected level (Brown, 1976; Harris, 1978; Knapp, Curtis, & Giziakis, 1979).

Aspects of Care

Probably the most important of all the influences upon the cost of child and youth care, and certainly the influence of most importance to policy makers, is the level of final output or service outcomes discussed in *Outputs* above. However, final outputs are also the most difficult to conceptualize and measure. Without the facilities afforded by a fairly expensive, longitudinal study of a large number of group care centres, it will probably be impossible to include valid and reliable indicators of final output in, say, a costs study. However, the alternatives open to policy or practice researchers are capable of providing a number of valuable insights into the cost-output relationship. From previous research on child development, on the effects of interactions and attitudes in group care, of regime and independence, stimulation, and privacy, it should be possible to draw up a list of factors and practices which have been found to be ameliorative in the developmental and caring processes.

Drawing on longitudinal research of the type conducted by Skeels (1942; Skeels & Dye, 1939) and Tizard (1970, 1974; Tizard, Cooperman, & Tizard, 1972) provides insights of this kind (see also Rutter & Madge, 1976; Whittaker, 1978). The aim would be to identify care practices and other incidental factors associated with successful child or youth care and development, collect information on these practices and factors in the course of a relatively inexpensive cross-sectional research study, and examine their influence upon the costs incurred by the group care centre. This clearly takes us back to our discussion of the analogy between the economist's theory of production and the child and youth care process for, basically, one would be aiming to collect information on the non-resource correlates of successful care.[6] It should be emphasized that the availability of a reasonably comprehensive set of reliable final output indicators would obviate the need for such input and intermediate indicators.

Child or Youth Characteristics

One important set of factors that influence the success or failure of child and youth care are the characteristics of the children and young people themselves. Basic characteristics like age, sex, and handicapping conditions have obvious staffing implications, but aspects of personality and attitudes may also be important. Because of their impact on final output it would probably be unnecessary to include these factors as well as final output indicators, but this is partly an empirical matter. In previous research on observation and assessment centres the sex ratio of children was significantly related to average cost, and work on old people's homes found resident dependency to be a very important influence (Davies & Knapp, 1981; Knapp, Curtis, & Giziakis, 1979).

Much of the observed variation in child or youth characteristics between centres and areas can be attributed to differences in policy. In England and Wales, local authorities often adopt quite different strategies for child care, some preferring to maintain a relatively large residential care sector, others favouring foster care or supervision at home. The relative size of assessment and other specialist facilities also varies between areas. These policy differences will be translated into differences in the characteristics of children and young people found in any one type of care facility because of the different roles that these facilities must therefore play (Davies, Barton, & McMillan, 1972). In addition, differences in demand or, more correctly, need between areas pose important ramifications for child and youth care policies and thereby costs (Bebbington, 1976; Bebbington & Giziakis, 1979; Curtis, 1979).

Capital Stock

Some aspects of the capital stock, particularly the design of the building and the durable resources used for care, will have implications for staffing, for energy resources, and thus for costs. Furthermore, these influences will probably not be picked up by the other cost-influencing factors mentioned above. Homes with oil-fired central heating will now appear to be rather more expensive relative to other homes than they were. Of rather more importance in view of the labour-intensiveness of child and youth care are the staffing implications of building design. The implications for child and youth care costs are probably not dissimilar to those for the costs of care for old people, where the combination of a poorly designed building and dependent clientele push up staffing requirements (Knapp, 1979b).

USING COST INFORMATION FOR POLICY MAKING

These seven groups of cost-influencing factors vary in a number of ways. Of immediate interest is the variation in the availability of information to the policy maker. As argued before, the most important group of factors is the set of final output indicators, but these are notoriously hard to obtain and even those child welfare agencies with comprehensive record systems may be hard pressed to accurately assess the development of the children or young people in care and, thus, the success of the agency in pursuing its ultimate objectives. In contrast, most care agencies will have in hand reliable information on certain basic child or youth characteristics (age, sex, reasons for care, background), on operating characteristics and activity indicators (admission and discharge rates, occupancy levels, lengths of stay), on charges and input prices, and on certain other aspects of care.

Armed with this information it would then be possible so to standardize the available expenditure figures as to make comparison between care units, agencies, and time periods very much more valuable for policy purposes. Until these basic factors are taken into account, many of them being outside the domain of control of the unit or agency itself, it is simply absurd to make recommendations on the basis of bare expenditure figures. Unfortunately, it is all too common to observe this method of policy making in practice.

For the purposes of policy making there are three major cost analytic techniques used by the economist: cost-benefit analysis, cost-effectiveness analysis, and cost-function analysis. The basic principles and uses of these three methodologies have been set out and discussed in the context of child and youth care on a previous occasion (Knapp, 1979a) and the arguments are not repeated here. It is sufficient to note here that cost-benefit and cost-effectiveness analyses are designed to answer questions about a small number of alternative projects or care services, such as "Is care service A worthwhile?," "How much of A is worthwhile?" and, "Is A more worthwhile than B?" In each case the criterion "worthwhile" is defined in terms of cost-benefit differences or cost-effectiveness ratios. Cost-effectiveness analysis differs from cost-benefit analysis in so far as the benefits or outputs of the project or care service are not valued in monetary terms.

Cost-effectiveness analysis cannot, therefore, answer questions of the first variety, for costs are not immediately comparable with outputs. The relative analytical and computational ease of the cost-effectiveness method must thus be balanced against the greater power of the cost-benefit method, and for this reason economists have sought far and wide for methods of valuing outputs and service outcomes in monetary terms. Pearce (1978) and Williams and Anderson (1975) give good accounts of the progress that has been made in this difficult area of benefit valuation.

The third method of analysis, cost-function analysis, is rather more basic than the other two and provides a useful methodology both for standardizing bare cost figures for the variety of influential factors discussed above and for examining the cost-output relationship. The statistical technique used is multiple regression analysis. To describe the technique one may adapt Dean's (1976) argument by working through the eight stages of cost function analysis, illustrating each stage with a brief account of a study of English and Welsh community home costs undertaken by the author (Knapp, Curtis, & Giziakis, 1979).

1. *Select a care unit suitable for analysis:* Ideally one should be looking at largely autonomous care units such as separate residential homes or day units. Homes adopting "family group" designs probably do not keep separate accounts for each group, so that cost information would not be available for a more disaggregated research design. In the community homes study, the individual home was chosen as the relevant unit of analysis. At this stage one should ensure that one has observations on enough care units to undertake multiple regression analyses.

2. *Decide on the measurement of output:* The researcher must decide whether to seek information on final outputs or indicators of aspects of care that have previously been shown to be associated with final outputs. Only measures of intermediate output (child days), activity (occupancy rates), child characteristics (at a local authority level), and policies (again at a local authority level) were used in our community homes work.

3. *Determine the time unit of observation:* Child and youth care practices and policies vary almost daily within agencies and within units, but expenditure figures are rarely available for periods of less than one year. Only annual expenditure date was available for the community homes study. Much of the true variation in cost and, thus, the true cost-output relationship will be missed if the true unit of observation is too long.

4. *Choose the period of analysis:* In this case our concern was with the choice between a cross-sectional or longitudinal design. While expenditure figures may be available for a number of years, it is rare indeed to find sufficient information on the major causal factors for each of a number of time periods to undertake a longitudinal study. The community homes research was conducted on a sample of 1099 homes with data for 1977-78. The two alternative

designs allowed for slightly different policy questions to be answered.

5. *Decide on the measure of cost:* Ideally one would use social opportunity cost figures, but the cost of collecting these figures can be considerable and one must generally rely on expenditure figures. Our earlier discussion of expenditures and accounting costs described the major elements of cost to be included. In our community homes study all current expenditures were included, with the exception of debt charges and revenue contributions to capital outlay. Overhead administrative costs and capital costs were not included, although ideally these would not be omitted. The cost concept of interest should also be selected at this point, the choice being between average cost and total cost.

6. *Deflate the cost data:* At this stage the first two of the influential factors described above are introduced, correcting the expenditure figures for charges (to give us gross costs) and for resource prices. Deflation may be achieved directly by weighing the cost figures or indirectly by including price data in the regression equation, the method used in the community homes study since resource price information was available at a local authority level.

7. *Match costs with outputs and other factors:* Provided that there are no problems of associating an output observation with a cost observation (such as time lags in payments for resources) one may proceed with the multiple regression analysis. The output variables and data for the other cost-influencing factors are now used as regressors to "explain" variations in the standardized cost factors.

8. *Select the form of the function:* The researcher must now exercise considerable ingenuity and expertise in order to obtain that form of the multiple regression equation which best fits the available data and which accords most closely with reality. It is at this stage that the vast "science" of econometrics comes into play, and this final stage can take a long time to complete, particularly if, as in the community homes study, the number of influential factors is large and their influences various and highly inter-correlated.

Having completed these eight stages, the researcher will have a single equation linking the average or total expenditure by a child or youth care agency or centre in a given time period to a number of influential factors. This *cost function* relationship can then be used to cast light on a number of policy issues.

Firstly, cost functions ensure that costs are viewed and compared within a proper theoretical context: Extraneous and exogenous influences upon the cost of care are taken into account before policy implications are examined. If the "production of welfare" analogy is accepted as a valid representation of the child and youth care process, then the cost function follows logically and immediately. The cost-function approach coordinates and synthesizes the myriad of potential influences upon cost. An immediate corollary is that the estimated function allows us to assess and quantify the impact of the various causal factors upon cost. If the balance of care between residential, day, and foster care is to be altered, the cost function will tell us the cost or resource implications of the policy change. Similarly one is able to assess the cost implications of policies to use small rather than large group care centres or homes, to locate regional assessment centres or secure units in rural rather than urban areas, to convert existing premises into day units rather than erect new purpose-built units, and so on. An important implication of this property is the fact that the cost function allows one to allocate joint costs.

Within a residential home or a day unit, the children or young people exhibit a great variety of needs and characteristics. The estimated cost function allows the researcher and policy maker to assess the resource implications of care for each child or each need characteristic. This property is especially valuable for comparing costs between modes of care where the varieties and balances of needs and characteristics probably differ to a considerable degree. In this way child and youth care policies can be examined from an economic perspective at an *individual* level.

There may be a number of alternative modes of care for a child or young person with a given set of personal characteristics and needs. The policy maker should be concerned to allocate services to clients in order to achieve the best possible use of the available resources. This requires that the pattern of care services be as near as possible to achieving the ultimate objectives of the system whilst making efficient use of the scarce, and therefore costly, resources that are available. Only by taking account of the cost-influencing factors described earlier can one hope to achieve an efficient allocation of society's resources and also desirable repercussions for the caring process. Child and youth care agencies that impose charges can make use of an estimated cost function to set differential charging rates tailored to the particular characteristics of clients and services. This may be particularly useful for public authorities sharing regional assessment or other specialist facilities.

Until fairly recently the economic element in the planning of welfare service policies was relatively minor. Public expenditure cutbacks and the general economic recession have forced upon policy makers the need to examine economic and cost factors rather more carefully. In this chapter some of the principles of cost analysis have been set out and illustrated with respect to child and youth care services. The principal aim of economic analysis is the efficient allocation of scarce resources. Of course, efficiency is a very difficult concept to define and operationalise in a care context, but the economic approach—and thus the cost function approach—to planning child and youth care services represents nothing more than an attempt to explain and formalize a decision making process that has in the past been almost entirely implicit and informal and hence wasteful of available resources.

Wasting resources in one location—using more resources than needed to achieve a given set of objectives—leaves fewer resources for use in other locations. In other words, fewer services can be provided and the needs of fewer children or young people met whether through public, voluntary, or private care. By taking a closer and more careful look at child and youth care costs, it may be possible to waste fewer resources and meet more needs.

NOTES

1. The analogy drawn in particular is between the economist's production function and the child or youth care researcher's attempt to "explain" success in terms of care styles and milieux. In our discussion of cost variations one thus draws on the vast and various cost function literature to indicate the main influences on cost and their position in a logical framework of explanation and comparison. It should be emphasized that one should always be looking at the cost *function* and not the cost *equation* (cf. Hall, 1978), the latter being no more than an accounting identity that provides little or no information of value for policy making. A recent and very comprehensive account of cost function methodologies is provided by Dean (1976).

2. The exception was residential care for mentally handicapped children.

3. Even with nationally or regionally agreed wage scales, competition among employers will tend to push up the 'real' price of staff. This may come about by employers taking on slightly inferior staff, by regarding posts, or by offering non-pecuniary advantages such as accommodation, less disruptive hours, and so on. Non-pecuniary competition of this kind in the market for qualified social workers characterized the London authorities a few years ago.

4. A small home may not keep a child psychiatrist fully occupied on tasks for which she is especially qualified and she may thus perform "ordinary" care tasks more suit-

able undertaken by other care staff. In a larger home the child psychiatrist would be more fully and usefully employed (Harris, 1978).

5. This is a contentious issue, as witnessed by the cornflakes served for breakfast in children's homes in Northern Ireland. Economies were sought through the bulk-buying of provisions and supplies for homes but resulted in cornflakes which arrive in plain boxes marked "not for resale," catering managers imposing portion control on units, and government-issued soap and other toiletries. These supplies were felt to "work against . . . increasing some semblance of normal home life for the children in the home" (*Social Work Today*, 9 (30), 4 April 1978: p. 5).

6. The resource correlates of successful care are already included in the study for, by very definition, they are included in the cost figures. One should not therefore make the mistake of double-counting by including them as causal determinants of cost (cf. Hall, 1978).

REFERENCES

Bebbington, A. C. (1976). *Policy recommendation and the needs indicator for social service provision for children.* Discussion paper 34. University of Kent at Canterbury, Personal Social Services Research Unit.

Bebbington, A. C., & Giziakis, F. (1979). *Social services expenditure in England and Wales: The years 1974-75 and 1977-78.* Discussion Paper 119. University of Kent at Canterbury, Personal Social Services Research Unit.

Brown, P. (1976). *Finding children in need.* London: Tavistock Institute of Human Relations.

Chartered Institute of Public Finance and Accountancy. (1979). *Personal social service statistics: 1977-78 actuals.* London: CIPFA.

Curtis, S. E. (1979). *The needs indicator approach to the study of social services for children.* Discussion paper 140. University of Kent at Canterbury, Personal Social Services Research Unit.

Curtis Committee Report. (1946). *Report of the care of children committee.* London: Her Majesty's Stationery Office.

Davies, B. P., Barton, A., & McMillan, I. (1972). *Variations in children's services among British urban authorities.* London: Bell.

Davies, B. P., & Knapp, M. R. J. (1980). Hotel and dependency costs of residents in old peoples' homes. *Journal of Social Policy, 7*(1), 1-22.

Davies, B. P., & Knapp, M. R. J. (1981). *Old peoples' homes and the production of welfare.* London: Routledge & Kegan Paul.

Dean, J. (1976). *Statistical cost estimation.* Bloomington: Indiana University Press.

Department of Health and Social Security. (1971). *Care and treatment in a planned environment.* London: Her Majesty's Stationery Office.

Grygier, T. (1975). Measurement of treatment potential: Its rationale, method, and some results in Canada. In J. Tizard, I. Sinclair, & R. V. G. Clarke (Eds.), *Varieties of residential experience.* London: Routledge & Kegan Paul.

Hall, A. (1978). Estimating cost equations for day care. In P. K. Robins & S. Weiner (Eds.), *Child care and public policy.* Lexington, CT: Heath.

Harris, J. M. (1978). Child observation and assessment centres: Psychiatrists' and social workers' difficulties. *British Journal of Psychiatry, 132*(1), 195-199.

King, R. D., Raynes, N. V., & Tizard, J. (1971). *Patterns of residential care*. London: Routledge & Kegan Paul.

Knapp, M. R. J. (1977). A cost function for children's homes. Discussion paper 81. University of Kent at Canterbury, Personal Social Services Research Unit.

Knapp, M. R. J. (1979a). Planning child care services from an economic perspective. *Residential and Community Child Care Administration, 1*(3), 229-248.

Knapp, M. R. J. (1979b). On the determination of the manpower requirements of old people's homes. *Social Policy and Administration, 13*(3), 219-236.

Knapp, M. R. J. (1984). *The economics of social care*. London: Macmillan.

Knapp, M. R. J., Curtis, S. E., & Giziakis, E. (1979). Observation and assessment centres for children: A national study of costs of care. *International Journal of Social Economics, 6*(3), 128-150.

Knapp, M. R. J., & Lowin, A. (1998). Child care outcomes: Economic perspectives and issues. *Children and Society, 12*, 169-179.

Pearce, D. (1978). *The valuation of social cost*. London: Allen & Unwin.

Romeo, R., Byford, S., & Knapp, M. R. J. (2005). Economic evaluations of child and adolescent mental health interventions: A systematic review. *Journal of Child Psychology & Psychiatry, 46*(9), 919-930.

Rutter, M., & Madge N. (1976). *Cycles of disadvantage*. London: Heinemann.

Silbertson, A. (1972). Economies of scale in theory and practice. *Economic Journal, 82*(1), 369-391.

Sinclair, I., & Heal, K. (1976). Diversity with the total institution: Some evidence from boys' perceptions of community homes. *Policy and Politics, 4*(1), 5-13.

Skeels, H. M. (1942). A study of the effects of differential stimulation on mentally retarded children: Follow-up report. *American Journal of Mental Deficiency, 46*, 340-350.

Skeels, H. M., & Dye, H. B. (1939). A study of the effects of differential stimulation on mentally retarded children. *Proceedings and Addresses of the American Association on Mental Deficiency, 44*, 114-136.

Tizard, J. (1970). The role of social institutions in the causation, prevention and alleviation of mental retardation. In H. C. Haywood (Ed.), *Social-cultural aspects of mental retardation*. New York: Appleton-Century-Crofts.

Tizard, J. (1974). Longitudinal studies: Problems and findings. In A. M. Clarke & A. D. B. Clarke (Eds.), *Mental deficiency: The changing outlook* (third edition). London: Methuen.

Tizard, B., Cooperman, O., Joseph, A., & Tizard, J. (1972). Environmental effects on language development: A study of young children in long-stay residential nurseries. *Child Development, 43*, 337-358.

Whittaker, J. K. (1978). The changing character of child care: An ecological perspective. *Social Service Review, 52*(1), 21-36.

Williams, A., & Anderson, R. (1975). *Efficiency in the social services*. Oxford: Basil Blackwell: London: Martin Robertson.

Chapter 12

Conclusion–Looking Ahead

Leon C. Fulcher
Frank Ainsworth

SUMMARY. Attention is drawn to important themes thought likely to influence the continuing development of group care services for children and young people in the decade ahead. These include a poorly educated workforce, autonomous training, multi-disciplinary approaches, centres of excellence, diversified programs, new trends and issues shaping the future, and group care practice and the law. *[Article copies available for a fee from The Haworth Document Delivery Service: 1-800-HAWORTH. E-mail address: <docdelivery@haworthpress.com> Website: <http://www.HaworthPress. com> © 2006 by The Haworth Press, Inc. All rights reserved.]*

KEYWORDS. Group care, residential care, residential treatment, group homes, youth work, youthwork, group work, at-risk youth

At the end of our 1985 volume, *Group Care Practice with Children*, six themes were identified as thought to impact on the group care field as a whole. Here we update those themes to assess changes that have oc-

Address correspondence to: Leon C. Fulcher, 64 Cameron Street, Dunfermline, Scotland KY12 8DP, UK.

[Haworth co-indexing entry note]: "Conclusion–Looking Ahead." Fulcher, Leon C., and Frank Ainsworth. Co-published simultaneously in *Child & Youth Services* (The Haworth Press, Inc.) Vol. 28, No. 1/2, 2006, pp. 285-294; and: *Group Care Practice with Children and Young People Revisited* (ed: Leon C. Fulcher, and Frank Ainsworth) The Haworth Press, Inc., 2006, pp. 285-294. Single or multiple copies of this article are available for a fee from The Haworth Document Delivery Service [1-800-HAWORTH, 9:00 a.m. - 5:00 p.m. (EST). E-mail address: docdelivery@haworthpress.com].

doi:10.1300/J024v28n01_06

curred during the past twenty years, as well as highlighting other, newer themes that require attention. These themes are (a) a poorly educated workforce, (b) independent child and youth care training, (c) an absence of multi-disciplinary approaches, (d) centers of excellence, (e) a diversified range of programs, (f) new trends and issues shaping the future, and (g) group care practice and the law.

A POORLY EDUCATED WORKFORCE

With few exceptions worldwide, child and youth care practitioners working in group care settings remain a significantly undertrained occupational group, a position which continues to amaze and appall given the complexity of educational and therapeutic tasks such workers are expected to perform. Some exceptions can be found amongst child and youth care training programs in Canada, Ireland, and in Western Europe and also in some measure in the United Kingdom. Even in these places a large proportion of direct care personnel still enter practice in group care programs without formal qualifications. The situation in the U.S., New Zealand, and South Africa is even more unsatisfactory while in Australia there is no accredited training for group care practitioners. The few university-based youth work programs that do exist in Australia give scant attention to the theory and practice of group care even though some qualified youth workers find employment in such programs for children and youth. This situation is very disappointing more than 20 years after the publication of *Group Care for Children* and *Group Care Practice with Children.* Even the richest and most highly developed Western countries are, alas, still failing to address the education and training needs of the group care workforce for children and youth in any coherent fashion.

The development of the occupation and profession of group care as well as child and youth care continue to be thwarted by two sets of factors. The first factor, as we argued in 1985, involves the way in which the field had been conceptualized around one primary setting, residential programs, and with particular client groups such as maladjusted adolescents rather than from general principles that apply across group settings and client populations. A second difficulty at that time was the absence of any clear model of practice that identified the knowledge and skills required of practitioners in group care. Our hope was that a practice curriculum published in the early 1980s (Central Council for Education and Training in Training in Social Work, 1983) might go some way towards responding to this deficiency. Such a hope was clearly overly optimistic and little appears to have changed. Illustrating this point is the way that the Scottish Institute for Residential Child Care at Strathclyde University is subsumed within faculties of education and social work, with the result that group care practice is assigned minority status instead of being accorded independent professional standing. Education and training for residential child care is developed with social work.

AUTONOMOUS CHILD AND YOUTH CARE EDUCATION

In some countries such as the Scandinavian countries, France, Germany and, more recently, Canada and Ireland, professional training programs for child and youth care workers are well established, some for nearly half a century. Unfortunately, many of these are not free-standing educational programs. Therefore research and educational traditions specifically tailored to the needs of the group care field have been thwarted. Without such developing professional recognition and independent accreditation for child and youth care workers practicing in the group care field, as commonly found in Sweden and Norway, then enhanced professional recognition for the field remains an illusive prospect.

THE ABSENCE OF MULTI-DISCIPLINARY APPROACHES

The group care field requires independent educational programs that combine an emphasis on child and adolescent development alongside knowledge and technical skills needed to provide educational and therapeutic services for children, young people, and their families. It follows that such programs need to be broader than education or social work, since child and youth care practice in group care is neither exclusively office-based (counseling) nor classroom-based (teaching) activities. Indeed, daily living becomes the stage for this work where skilled interventions require an integration of knowledge from a broader range of perspectives. Some of these perspectives are drawn from education, psychology, and social work, but these are by no means their exclusive preserve. Child and youth care practice needs to be firmly rooted in the physical environment of practice. The aim is to promote living and learning opportunities through the course of daily activities, promote behaviors that reinforce personal development, and steer children and youth toward healthy adult lives.

Unfortunately, programs embedded in schools of education, psychology, or social work often lack such a multi-disciplinary approach. Instead, their foundation discipline tends to dominate and prescribe learning requirements, thereby relegating the interdisciplinary perspectives needed by child and youth care to positions of less importance. Until independent child and youth care programs are established that maintain a commitment to multi-disciplinary education and training then aspirations for professional recognition of group care or child and youth care practice will remain a distant dream.

CENTRES OF EXCELLENCE

Twenty years ago, it was claimed that specific centers were needed for the study of group care practice where personnel with proven track records of scholarly and professional achievement could offer inservice training, qualifying studies, and consultancy services to allied programs. The analogy that was used by Beker (1981) was the teaching hospital in the medical system. We think this analogy is still correct. Centers that may claim this status do exist, but they are few. The Walker Home and School in Massachusetts, Boys' Town in Nebraska, the Casey Foundation with operations in various parts of the U.S., Kibble Education and Care Centre near Glasgow, and the National Children's Home, Cotswold Community in England in our view fit this category and there are no doubt more. While these centers represent important examples, they remain rare when compared with the number of children and young people in care in their respective countries. Noticeably, a feature of each of these centers is that each is funded by voluntary organizations, although they do provide services on a fee for service basis to public agencies. We know of no state or government managed centers of excellence.

A DIVERSIFIED RANGE OF PROGRAMMES

Many have argued that the service systems which sponsor child and youth care would need to offer a diversified range of programs for children and young people in receipt of residential education or treatment. While some diversification has occurred, most notably in the non-institutional sector, policy options have more commonly moved towards developing community-based alternatives to group care, and such developments have occurred mostly for ideological reasons. Countries like Australia have seen an abandonment of residential programs and have moved to an almost total reliance on foster care with arguably catastrophic results (Ainsworth & Hansen, 2005). In New Zealand the trend has been towards contracting out of residential group care to the voluntary and private sectors, with social policy advocates favoring kinship care and non-residential group care placements.

In North America the shift has been toward mental health and health-related programs that qualify for health insurance funding. In fact, in most U.S. states, community funding for residential group care placements remains contentious. Thus most states support fewer large group care programs than twenty years ago with length of treatment and cost factors regrettably now the dominant issue in decision making rather than effectiveness. This means that while there are fewer placements there may actually be more programmes, but these are smaller programmes than before.

NEW TRENDS AND ISSUES SHAPING THE FUTURE

Current trends include:

- In Western countries there is a continuing move from large to small service units and towards more individualized and personally tailored services.
- The shift from rural to urban and community-based services has, if anything, intensified.
- The tradition of monocultural services has given way to demands for more culturally sensitive and responsive practices.
- Where services were once driven by professionals informed by largely expert models of practice, there have been important shifts towards the rights of service users and for enhanced consumer participation in service planning and decision-making.
- Instead of removing children and young people from the parental home and developmentally unhelpful family influences, there is some recognition that family members need to be included as essential partners in education and treatment services designed to address these issues.[1]

- Twenty years ago there were also large numbers of services funded long-term via ongoing annual government grants including services sponsored by well established nonprofit voluntary organizations. Now growing numbers of local community-based initiatives operate under individual contract for service arrangements that are reviewed annually against government determined performance criteria that focus on service outcomes and effectiveness.
- There is also a growing number, especially in the U.S., of private, fee-for-service and for-profit agencies dependent on health insurance income sources.
- Once there were also services shaped primarily by religious conviction, professional values, and codes of practice. Now these services must respond to new demands for performance accountability and complex regulatory requirements that are not always compatible with such values.

A NEW FRONTIER: GROUP CARE PRACTICE AND THE LAW

In the busy world of front-line services for children and young people it is easy to become preoccupied with immediate educational and therapeutic tasks and ignore important contextual issues about professional negligence and duty of care responsibilities. Such responsibilities are assigned to child and youth care organisations and their practitioner workforce whenever a court or parents place a child in an education or treatment program. These are responsibilities in our view that are too readily relinquished to managers and policy makers with little thought being given to them by direct service practitioners. Yet, a cursory examination of duty of care responsibilities and the legal accountability it implies shows that they are having an increasing impact on every moment of direct service. In fact, issues of negligence and duty of care are now more than ever at the centre of practice (Fulcher, 2002).

This was not always such a prominent issue as indicated by its absence in our two earlier volumes (Ainsworth & Fulcher, 1981; Fulcher & Ainsworth, 1985). Indeed, even in this volume there is little mention of how the law has had an impact on the child and youth care field over the last two decades. Yet legal practitioners with an interest in children's rights who draw much of their inspiration from the United Nations Convention on the Rights of the Child now have a significant voice in every area of human service practice including group care practice. For example, it is now quite common for children and young people entering a group care program to be given a written statement of their rights (entitlements) and to be told of a complaints procedure should they feel that they are being mistreated by program staff.

Such practice is one small indicator of the way organizations have responded to legal advances. However, what these rights statements seek to do is not only to protect the rights of children but also to manage risk for the employing organization. In such instances, the risk involves legal action against the organization by a child, parent, or children's advocate group for negligent practice or a failure in the duty of care. Unfortunately while protecting an organization such risk management actions add to the vulnerability of direct care practitioners. This is because it opens the possibility for an organization to defend itself against legal action by citing such statements of rights as evidence of the organization's good intentions. It then follows that any failure to follow the organization's rights statement was solely the result of errors committed by individual practitioners.

Of course, claims that a worker's actions were not endorsed by the employing agency are unlikely to lead to a completely successful defense in such situations. In addition, even when governments contract out services they may not be able to avoid liability for the work of the actual service provider. But this is a complex matter that will only be decided on a case by case basis and the outcome may vary across jurisdictions.

None of this augers well for direct practice or for the careers of individual practitioners who may get caught up in a legal action. Faced with possible legal action, workers are more than likely to respond with self-protective and ultra-cautious behaviours that are not necessarily the most helpful responses for children and young people in a group care program. Alas, at its worst, practitioners are told that they must never touch a child or young person, offer physical comfort during times of distress, or enter a child's room alone in order to safeguard against allegations of abuse. All such responses may add up to an uncaring program environment and to practices that while legally safe are sterile and unresponsive.

Just as inhibiting to the building of professional child and youth care practice in Western countries have been the incessant inquiries by government into cases of abuse in large institutions run historically by state and religious orders. Such inquiries have highlighted experiences that remain ever present in the minds of a generation of children and young people who in an earlier era suffered negligence and horrendous breaches of the duty of care. These inquiry reports have frequently resulted in multi-million dollar payouts to those who suffered in this way or recommendations to government for schemes to compensate those severally affected by such experiences (Senate Affairs Reference Committee, 2004). And virtually all such reports are emblazoned with the rhetoric of the United Nations Convention on the Rights of the Child by children's rights lawyers and other advocates. Virtually all of these initiatives have been driven by members of the legal profession who have pressed for much needed reforms of the group care sector. Unless group care personnel, as well as child and youth care workers take their duty of care seriously within the law, their futures will continue to be challenged.

While in our view very few child and youth care workers would deliberately contemplate breaching their duty of care to children and youth, the sad fact remains that some may already unwittingly have done so, and on too many occasions. Moreover, past actions are increasingly the subject of legal complaint and these actions can no longer be defended by claiming that they were good enough at the time. The standard of care remains constantly open to ongoing scrutiny by the courts. As a consequence, the actions of child and youth care workers and employing organisations require daily vigilance if practice is to achieve a defensible professional standard. Children and young people deserve nothing less.

A NEW AGENDA FOR THE FUTURE

More than ever before, the field of group care warrants close consideration for the positive contribution it makes to the continuum of services much needed by children, young people, and their families in the education, health care, social welfare, or justice system. Ideologies that have driven service reforms over the past quarter century have commonly assumed that group care is a negative choice in the continuum of service alternatives, only to be used as a last resort after all other options have failed. Such simplistic reasoning ignores the many positive examples of proactive group care programs available, as well as the many instances of close working partnerships between group care programs and family members.

In the Preface to our first volume, we acknowledged that the materials contained there were as much "a product of travel as it was of academic contemplation and practice" (Ainsworth & Fulcher, 1981, p. xii). Travel began with each editor taking up residence in the other's country and extended through many transatlantic journeys. Our claim was that such travels promoted an overview of group care work with children and young people in Great Britain, Ireland, Canada, and the U.S. and gave incentive to the development of our ideas in the first place. There was also a desire to try and achieve some deeper under-standing and synthesis of different approaches found in our respective countries.

A quarter century later we have extended our travels and practice experiences and acquired dual nationalities. For the past twenty years, one of us lived in different states in Australia and the other in New Zealand while carrying out practice research in Malaysia, China, and the United Arab Emirates. As noted in 1981, "an interest-ing feature of cross-cultural work is that in learning about group care for children in another context, what one acquires is a new way of viewing that with which one is already familiar–familiarity that all too often results in an unseeing eye" (Ainsworth & Fulcher, p. xii). Such a commitment to comparative methods of analysis remain, such that instead of evaluating certain aspects of practice as better or worse, the major question remains: What accounts for such differ-ences and their resulting outcomes?

In a world increasingly shaped by globalization and world travel it is easy to perpetuate the myth that one country's solutions (com-monly "my" country or the services with which I am familiar) fit all. Developing countries frequently look to the West for modernization pathways and, while growing numbers of Western consultants readily act on such requests, a good number do so with little thought given to cross-cultural differences. If three decades of international travel and professional practice has taught us anything it is that the more we know, the more we know what we do not know. In that sense instead of seeking to confirm what is known about responsive group care services for children, young people, and their families, it is paradoxical that many professionals from across the human service spectrum continue to make a concerted effort to explore virtually ev-ery service option other than group care including, unbelievably, iso-lating troubled youth in rented houses and even motel rooms with twenty-four hour supervisory staff. Our hope is that the papers in this volume will be viewed as a renewal and a continuation of our attempt to articulate the positive contribution that child and youth care prac-titioners and group care programs can make to the lives of troubled children, young people, and their families.

294 *Group Care Practice with Children and Young People Revisited*

NOTE

1. This particular movement still has a long way to go. Unfortunately parent blaming continues unabated in child and family services, many of which are by now largely forensic and investigative child protection services. The ethos of child care and practical support for families suspected of child abuse or neglect have given way to these newer, but not necessarily more successful, service models.

REFERENCES

Ainsworth, F., & Fulcher, L. C. (Eds.). (1981). *Group care for children: Concept and issues*. London: Tavistock.
Ainsworth, F., & Hansen, P. (2005). A dream come true–no more residential care: A corrective note. *International Journal of Social Welfare, 14*(3), 195-199.
Beker, J. (1981). New roles for group care centres. In F. Ainsworth & L. C. Fulcher (Eds.), *Group care for children: Concept and issues* (pp. 128-145). London: Tavistock.
Central Council for Education and Training in Training in Social Work. (1983). *A practice curriculum for group care, paper 14.2: Staff development in the social services*. London.
Fulcher, L. C. (2002). The duty of care in child & youth care practice. *Journal of Child & Youth Care Work, 17*, pp. 73-84.
Fulcher, L. C., & Ainsworth, F. (Eds.). (1985). *Group care practice with children*. London: Tavistock.
Senate Affairs Reference Committee. (2004). *Forgotten Australians: A report on Australians who experienced institutional or out-of-home care as children*. Canberra: Commonwealth of Australia.

Index

T - #0482 - 101024 - C0 - 212/152/18 - PB - 9780789032805 - Gloss Lamination